Making a Difference
for America's Children

Speech-Language Pathologists
in Public Schools

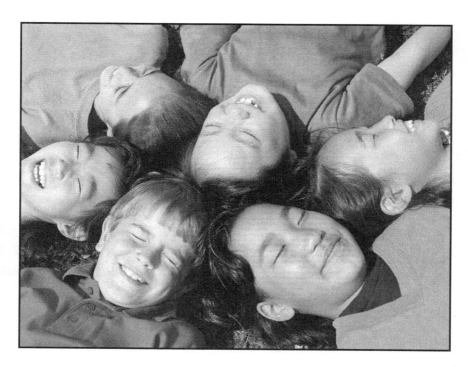

Barbara J. Moore-Brown, Ed.D., CCC-SLP
Judy K. Montgomery, Ph.D., CCC-SLP

Thinking Publications • Eau Claire, Wisconsin

With a foreword by Thomas Hehir, Ed.D., Harvard University

10   09   08   07   06   05   04   03   02   01   10   9   8   7   6   5   4   3   2   1

Library of Congress Cataloging-in-Publication Data

Moore-Brown, Barbara J., date.

    Making a difference for America's children : speech language pathologists in public schools / Barbara J. Moore-Brown, Judy K. Montgomery.

        p. cm.

    ISBN 1-888222-52-2 (pbk.)

    1. Speech therapy for children—United States. 2. Communicative disorders in children—United States. 3. Handicapped children—Education—United States. I. Montgomery, Judy K., date. II. Title.

LB3454 .M66 2001

371.91'42—dc21

                       00-051214

Printed in the United States of America

Cover Design by Debbie Olson

Technical Editing by Sarah Thurs

Photos by Sharon Donnelly (pp. 1 [bottom], 4, 9, 21 [middle], 25, 38, 46, 49 [top and middle], 56, 77, 79 [top and middle], 89, 116, 121, 140, 148, 149, 162, 182, 196, 205, 208, 226, 239, 242, 244, 259, 269 [middle], 283, 291, 294, 319 [middle and bottom], 322, 334)

THINKING PUBLICATIONS®

A Division of McKinley Companies, Inc.

424 Galloway Street • Eau Claire, WI 54703
(715) 832-2488 • FAX (715) 832-9082
Email: custserv@ThinkingPublications.com

COMMUNICATION SOLUTIONS THAT CHANGE LIVES®

To those speech-language pathologists throughout
the country with whom we have been honored to work.
Your work has been the inspiration of this book.

And to the next generation of speech-language pathologists.
May these words create the inspiration within you to blaze new trails for children
with communication disorders in your work in schools.

Finally, to our husbands, Roy and Ken,
for your love, support, and understanding when we conspire.

Contents

List of Figures and Tables

Tables

Foreword

I recall a meeting I had with the district's speech-language pathologists back in 1990 when I was the associate superintendent of the Chicago Public Schools. This was my introductory meeting with the group, and I was concerned over the reception I would receive. I was keenly aware of their very heavy caseloads as we were trying hard to bring the district into compliance with IDEA and we did not have a sufficient number of speech-language pathologists. We had worked out a plan with the state speech consultant to hire bachelor's level speech assistants to help meet our needs, but even that would not be enough. In a very real sense, every person in the room was gold to the district. We could not afford to loose one of them, and frankly I wanted each of them to recruit their friends. Therefore, I knew my remarks to the group would be crucial. I wanted them to understand how deeply we appreciated their services to Chicago kids. Prior to the meeting, one of the district's speech administrators, Suellen Hurt, had assured me that my anxiety was misplaced, "Tom, these are highly dedicated, professional people who are committed to our kids and families."

I began my remarks talking about our plans to hire speech assistants and went on to detail our plans for improving special education within the district. I specifically spoke about the need to move to more inclusive service delivery. I related inclusive education to the need for kids to have typical speech models. Applause filled the room. These folks of course knew the importance of that and were looking forward to these opportunities for the kids they served. I also talked about the advances in technology, particularly augmentative communication devices and the critical role they would be serving in bringing these liberating devices to children. Again, applause. I ended my talk looking forward to the opportunity to talk to them individually at the reception that was to follow. Clearly Suellen had been right.

As I was meeting these folks individually, I was intrigued by the question of why these people were working for us, dealing with all the challenges of working in urban schools, when they could potentially make more money working in hospitals or for HMOs. So I decided to ask one of the speech-language pathologists directly. She responded quickly and in an animated manner. She said the answer was simple, "Working in schools is simply better!" She went on to say how she had worked with some children and families for years and had had the great joy of witnessing their language development and subsequent success in school. She went on to say that she had worked in a hospital setting before and was not afforded such an opportunity. "I know I make a difference here."

This anecdote came to mind immediately when I read Barbara Moore-Brown and Judy Montgomery's book. This book captures the spirit exemplified by this speech-language pathologist in Chicago. Speech-language pathologists make a huge difference in the lives of children throughout

America's schools. Further, school-based speech-language pathologists are fundamental to the preschool and early intervention programs so crucial to the ultimate success of students with disabilities.

An important feature of this book is the clear vision of the role speech-language pathologists in schools: central to the education of many students with disabilities, not an appendage to programs. This distinction is crucial; too often some schools view related services as "add-on" programs. This is a huge mistake. Language is the foundation upon which much of educational progress rests. And, for many students with disabilities, language and speech are deeply connected to their disability. Therefore, the speech-language pathologist in an educational setting can be the critical element in ensuring their success in school and ultimately in life. Thus the speech-language pathologist is faced with both an awesome responsibility and a great opportunity to truly make a difference in the educational lives of children.

This book not only provides a compelling vision of an exciting profession, but is also full of common-sense, practical information. I am particularly impressed with the way in which the authors have summarized the legal context of special education. Special education law and the legal decisions that surround it are complex. Professionals working in this field obviously have to understand this important aspect of the job. However, some descriptions of the law get bogged down in legalese and minutia. Here, that is not the case. The treatment of the law in this book is comprehensive and intelligible, providing the "big picture" view. A central point made in this discussion is that the law is dynamic; interpretations change and the law can be amended. It is important that speech-language pathologists recognize this as they embark on their career. They must keep up with developments in this area; these developments will effect their job.

Consistent with the central message that runs throughout this text, speech-language pathologists are indeed essential to the success of children with disabilities. This book does a terrific job of grounding the profession within the context of standards-based reform in general education. Children with disabilities need to benefit from all school reform efforts. It is no longer acceptable to put these children off to the side. Simply put, programs for children with disabilities should not only address the needs that arise out of their disabilities, but also should be based on the curriculum being taught to nondisabled students. And, schools need to be held accountable for that learning. Again, Barbara and Judy have provided a wonderful overview of school reform environment at the beginning of the new century.

In conclusion, this is a terrific introduction to an exciting and important profession. Those of you who choose to become school speech-language pathologists are entering a profession with a proud past and a great future. Along with other special educators, speech-language pathologists have helped open the doors of education to millions of children with disabilities. You are entering a profession that truly makes a difference.

—Thomas Hehir, Ed.D.
Lecturer on education, Harvard University
Former director of the U.S. Department of Education,
Office of Special Education Programs

Preface

From the very beginning, we shared a common passion—school-based speech-language pathology. We had worked for many years as speech-language pathologists in 10 different school districts. We knew that the dreams and visions that we had and the passion that we felt were shared by many of our colleagues throughout the United States. These qualified, exceptional professionals were on the frontline, making a difference for children, many times under daunting circumstances. The work of speech-language pathologists is highly demanding, necessitating intensive, in-depth, and comprehensive preparation. Speech-language pathologists must be prepared to work with students and families who present with widely varying circumstances. Over the past 15 years, the field of speech-language pathology has changed dramatically, as has the landscape of educational institutions. Through it all, our own daily work has been spent continually dealing with the many complex and sensitive issues that surround the families and systems that deal with individuals who have disabilities.

We believe that "the schools are where children spend the majority of their day, and, therefore, the most influential place for speech pathologists to help students improve their speech, language and communication. The school setting presents unique opportunities and challenges" (Pritchard Dodge, 2000, p. ix). When working in a public school, it is important to keep in mind that school is a child's natural environment. This is the place where children spend about 13 years of their lives—almost their total childhood. In most cases, the school is integrated into the community, and children are keenly aware of what school they are attending and which school they are likely to go to for the next grades. Many nonschool speech-language pathology work settings (e.g., hospitals, private practices, and rehabilitation agencies) are quite different. Such settings are not children's natural places but are places created to assist children at particular points in their lives.

The current interest in educating all children in inclusive schools is designed to bring all children into their natural school environment, which is conducive to building friendships and academic skills. The more speech-language pathologists know about the school environment and how it works, the more effective and meaningful their contribution becomes for the students and staff there. Today, speech-language pathologists are a vital link to classroom learning for millions of American children. We look to future speech-language pathologists to carry on the work and to create any change that is needed for children, as well as for the system.

In addition, we believe that for speech-language pathologists to be successful in public schools, they must understand the "big picture" of education. They must recognize the educational issues that influence decisions and decision-makers, know and understand the laws for providing services to students and the legal basis on which they were passed, and know the field of speech-language pathology. In many cases, speech-language pathologists will be their schools' experts on etiologies of disabilities, assessment and service delivery, intervention techniques to use in the classroom, and legal matters surrounding special education. We believe that speech-language pathologists who work in public schools are able to influence children's lives not only directly through intervention but indirectly because they are an integral part of the educational system in which they work.

This project has been a work of passion about the field of speech-language pathology and the field of education. We believe that the work of school-based speech-language pathologists is unique and fulfilling. Our effort here is to capture how the blending of many disciplines makes for a challenging work setting for speech-language pathologists and how the lives of educators and students are enriched through their connections with speech-language professionals.

With this book, we bring to the next generation of speech-language pathologists a new perspective on how speech-language services and special education are considered in public schools. Our focus is broad, incorporating the whole educational system, never imagining or wanting the work of speech-language pathologists to occur in isolation. Previously, communication disorders courses about speech-language pathologists working in school-based settings presented a disability-driven service delivery model. Our intent, instead, is to broaden the focus to the total educational environment, legal and otherwise, in which we practice our craft. In addition, we have brought to the reader many "first-time" pieces of information gathered in one place for the reader's ease and reference. These include information from the American Speech-Language-Hearing Association (ASHA) School Survey, completed in 1995 and published in 1998, which replaced the last available survey from 1969; information from *Guidelines on the Roles and Responsibilities of the School-Based Speech-Language Pathologist* (ASHA, 1999c); and extracts from ASHA's technical assistance document on developing educationally relevant IEPs (Brannen et al., 2000)—in one place for your ease and reference.

A career as a speech-language pathologist in public schools is full of excitement, energy, change, and opportunity. Whether you are thinking of embarking on this career or are already employed in public schools, this book will provide a compass for your journey—one on which you will find that you can make a difference for children. This book does not describe the destination of this journey. Schools are too dynamic, education is too volatile, and the profession is evolving too rapidly for this book to be static. Additionally, this resource is not meant to be an in-depth study on any individual topic—instead it provides an overview of most of the daily issues that speech-language pathologists in public schools deal with from one moment to the next.

The intent of this book is to provide a new framework for an expanded working situation and to create a vision of the possibilities for children and professionals within legal guidelines and requirements. Public education, the profession of speech-language pathology, and the students and families we serve are constantly changing.

As the world anticipated the dawn of the twenty-first century, society took the opportunity to both look back and look forward. In this book, we will take you through a brief history of the role of speech-language pathologists in public schools; present a discussion of school reform issues; and then examine changes in federal legislation and regulations in special education, including how speech-language pathologists work as school team members for prevention, assessment, and intervention. In addition, we provide broad-based information on service delivery as it relates to children with communication disorders, including issues that speech-language pathologists frequently label "the things they never taught me in school." We know that the issues and situations surrounding the delivery of speech-language services in public schools will continue to change. Our collective experience, and the wisdom of others, leads us to the final chapter of this book, envisioning the future of speech-language services in public schools. This future will be your daily reality and work world if you become a school-based speech-language pathologist—a future connected like never before to the changes in general education.

We hope that you will be intrigued and stimulated by the readings in this book and will then understand and share in our passion for speech-language pathology. Always consider the range of student needs that must be addressed and the scope of responsibilities assigned to speech-language pathologists in schools. In doing so, you will understand our respect for how speech-language pathologists in public schools truly are making a difference for America's children. We welcome you to the field—one that we know is exceptional and one in which *you* can make a difference.

> Do not follow where the path may lead.
> Go instead where there is no path and leave a trail.
>
> —Muriel Strode

Acknowledgments

As in many of these kinds of projects, it is impossible to list all those who provided wisdom, insight, inspiration, and encouragement. We want to name a few whose special touch helped make this book better.

First, we acknowledge Julie Burns, principal at Cambridge School in Orange, California, who opened her doors to us, and the students and teachers at Cambridge School.

Also, we appreciate those at the Kathleen Muth Literacy Center at Chapman University, whose smiles symbolize our work.

We acknowledge the many school-based speech-language pathologists and professionals throughout the country who inspired us with their innovative interventions, constant energy, and total commitment to children and youth, especially:

- The speech-language pathology staff of Los Angeles Unified School District, Santa Ana Unified School District, and Fountain Valley School District, who supported Judy K. Montgomery in becoming a school-based speech-language pathologist

- Melissa Jakubowitz and Ellen Pritchard Dodge, who willingly provided honest input when it was sought

- Terry Olson and Cathen Phelps, for sharing their year-round schedules

- Beth Nishida, for always being there to discuss ideas and for providing unending support

- The 2000–2001 designated services and classroom-based speech-language pathologist team at El Rancho Unified School District, who inspires Barbara Moore-Brown daily with its amazing talent and insight

- Gina Smith, Carol Lee Huffman, Jane Moir, and Esther Myers, for sharing their outstanding forms

We extend thank-yous to Sharon Donnelly, who captured our concepts in photographs and who brought to the project her own special touch; and to Darin Barber, who helped to locate court cases and dates; and to the highly professional staff at the American Speech-Language-Hearing Association, who always provide assistance when we need it. We would also like to recognize the members of the 1999 Council of State Speech-Language-Hearing Presidents (CSAP), who eagerly shared their ideas and experiences and cheered us on.

We also acknowledge those who reviewed the early manuscripts—Nancy Creaghead, Karen Kuhn, Amy Perkins, Marie Stadler, and Elliot Weiman—and the staff at Thinking Publications, who shared excitement for this project. And finally, we extend a very special acknowledgment to Nancy McKinley, who nurtured the idea that grew into what you see here. Thank you, Nancy, for your vision, commitment, concern for the field, and trust in us.

CHAPTER 1

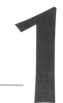

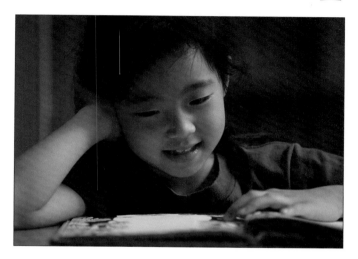

Speech-Language Services in the Educational System: Trends and Considerations

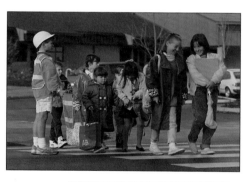

IN THIS CHAPTER

This chapter introduces the issues surrounding the educational system within which school-based speech-language pathologists work, including school reform issues for both general and special education; characteristics of children and families of the twenty-first century; and incidence of children with disabilities who are identified as needing special education (e.g., speech-language) services in the schools. The chapter concludes with consideration of predictions about school reform and the changing roles of professionals.

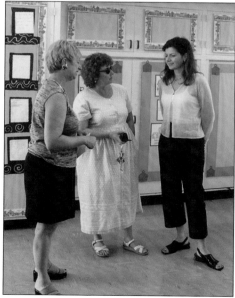

1. How has the role of the school-based speech-language pathologist changed since the late 1960s and early 1970s?

2. What is meant by "educational reforms"? Why is it important for speech-language pathologists in public schools to be aware of general and special education reforms?

3. How have school reform movements affected the delivery of speech-language services in schools?

4. Discuss why the information presented about children and their environments is important to speech-language pathologists in schools.

5. Discuss your thoughts on the consistent increases in children identified as requiring special education services.

Speech-Language Services in Public Schools

Many people participate in working to make the American educational system successful for children. Among the talented and dedicated people who make a difference for children in America's public schools are those who specialize in speech, language, and communication development and disorders: speech-language pathologists. While the discipline of communication sciences and disorders is comprised of two professions—speech-language pathology and audiology—the focus of this book will be on the practice and contributions of speech-language services in America's public schools and the difference that these services, and those who provide them, make for children whose communication needs hinder their accomplishments in reading, writing, listening, and speaking.

Speech-language services in public schools serve a vital function for students with COMMUNICATION DISORDERS, and the provision of such services has grown and evolved significantly over the past 25 to 30 years. Accordingly, the roles of speech-language pathologists in public schools are nearly unrecognizable compared to the work of speech-language pathologists in the late 1960s and early 1970s. This change is due to two simple realities. First, schools, as institutions, are not the same as they were 30 years ago. Second, the profession of speech-language pathology and the children served have different needs and bring a more diverse life experience to the school setting. For speech-language pathologists to work effectively in the public school setting, they must not only be competent in the treatment of communication disorders, delays, and disabilities, but also understand the educational system in which they work.

Communication disorders university programs previously taught that speech-language pathologists in the school setting were predominantly segmented and separate from the general education system that employed them. Such segmentation is no longer true for speech-language pathologists in schools. Educational systems (used here to refer to public school systems) are increasingly dynamic and interactive institutions. Speech-language professionals, in either preservice or in-service situations, must be able to view their work in the context of the larger dynamic, interactive, and responsive educational system. The educational system of the twenty-first century is not segmented. The work of all professionals working with children is meaningfully connected.

Educational Reforms That Shaped the Profession

The United States and Europe have a long history of programs for certain types of communication disabilities, such as deafness (Lowe, 1993; O'Connell, 1997), although such programs were generally found only in special schools. School programs to address the issue of "stammering" were first introduced into public education in 1910

(O'Connell, 1997). Teachers of English literature were frequently given some training to provide "speech correction" to their students, and between the 1920s and 1940s, university programs for specialists in the area of "speech improvement" or "speech correction" developed. Legislation was passed in 45 states to provide funding for speech and hearing programs by the mid-1960s (Neidecker, 1987; O'Connell, 1997). Between the 1960s and 2000, speech-language programs have evolved as a vital part of public school services.

From the early titles of "speech teacher" or "speech correctionist" (O'Connell, 1997), a variety of titles have since been used to describe the professional who is responsible for the treatment of communication disorders in schools: *speech-language specialist, communication specialist, speech therapist,* and *speech-language pathologist.* The title speech-language pathologist will be used in this book to refer to a specialist who operates a speech-language program addressing communication disorders in a public school setting.

The professional organization of speech-language pathologists and audiologists is the AMERICAN SPEECH-LANGUAGE-HEARING ASSOCIATION (ASHA). School-based speech-language services have received increasing recognition within ASHA since 1925, when the organization was founded under the original name of the American Society of Speech Correction. By 1969, ASHA had created a full-time staff position to focus on school and clinic affairs. Two years later, the journal *Language,*

Speech, and Hearing Services in Schools became a standing ASHA publication (Neidecker, 1987). The 1997 *ASHA Omnibus Survey Results* reported that 53 percent of ASHA members were speech-language pathologists working in schools (ASHA, 1997b).

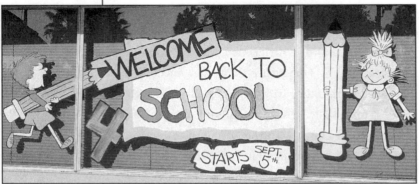

Speech-language services in schools are provided as part of the continuum of special education services, which exist through the mandates created by state and federal legislation during the wave of civil rights reforms in the 1970s. SPECIAL EDUCATION was not intended to exist in a vacuum, but rather as an extension of the general education system. Consequently, special education programs have been affected by the long history of educational reforms that have unfolded with increasing intensity since the early 1980s. As these reforms are reviewed, the reader should keep asking the question, "How do these changes affect speech-language services?"

Institutional change is a part of American culture in nearly every segment of society, responding to forces on many levels: economic, demographic, political, and social. Education reflects change in all of these areas. Reforms have been designed to adjust to the issues that occur inside and outside schools (Fullan, 1995).

In a classic example, the nation was caught off guard in the 1950s when the Soviet Union launched Sputnik, the first satellite, into space. The United States reacted by dramatically increasing the focus on science education in the early 1960s. Thus, politics, economics, and world public opinion fostered educational reform in the United States.

Current reform movements in general education began with the infamous report from the National Commission on Excellence in Education in 1983 entitled *A Nation at Risk: The Imperative for Educational Reform.* This report announced the dismal performance of America's children on reading, writing, and math testing compared to their peers from other countries. The report rocked the educational system and set off waves of reform movements in every state legislature, school district, and neighborhood school (Evans and Panacek-Howell, 1995). Since the 1980s, significant changes have occurred in how school systems are governed, instruction is delivered and measured, and business is conducted in schools across the country.

In the mid-1980s, business leaders pointed to the nation's public schools and criticized them for failing to prepare an adequate work force. As education came to the political forefront, President George Bush convened a Governors' Summit on Education in 1989, and in 1990, six national education goals were adopted by the National Governors' Association. The goals were expanded to eight (see overview of goals in sidebar) under President Bill Clinton, who signed the Goals 2000: Educate America Act to fund efforts to reach the eight goals (National Education Goals Panel [NEGP],

1999). These projects were not without controversy (Ohanian, 2000). As part of the strategy to meet these national goals, a new approach—standards-based education—came into national and statewide focus. Standards-based reform was intended to provide a systematic approach for educational improvement with the stated intent to address the needs of *all* children.

The thoughtful citizen might ask what progress has been made as a result of placing a national focus on education. Speech-language pathologists and those studying the field might also pause to consider the implications of not meeting the national goals, and also the possible impact on their CASELOADS. The NEGP annually reports on each of the goals (available at *www.negp.gov*). Progress is reported for nearly every goal, but national indicators show that all areas continue to need focused national attention.

By the 1990s, the original goal of special education, to provide access to educational services, had been "reasonably well met" (Cook, Weintraub, and Morse, 1995, p. 123). Special education reforms have taken the form of the REGULAR EDUCATION INITIATIVE (REI) and the INCLUSION movement. The REI—led by Madeline Will, Assistant Secretary for Special Education and Rehabilitative Services, with her 1986 report *Educating Students with Learning Problems: A Shared Responsibility*—criticized the dual system of general and special education and contained a set of proposals that called for general and special educators to share responsibilities for the education of students with disabilities. In the late 1980s and 1990s, the REI evolved into the Inclusion movement (Kubicek, 1994), which "referred to the integration of students with disabilities into general education classrooms" (Hocutt and McKinney, 1995, p. 51).

New/Mod. ideas to deal c̄ poor stud.

Three Waves of Educational Reforms

Educational reforms refer to policy and program changes that have been put in place to specifically address the issues of student learning identified in *A Nation at Risk* (National Commission on Excellence in Education, 1983). Educational reforms typically deal with new or modified ideas on how to address poor student achievement.

In reform discussions, the term RESTRUCTURING is often used. Restructuring refers to all aspects of reform, including the redesign of curriculum and instruction, participatory governance, site-based management, and the increasing involvement of parents and communities in the development of partnerships and networks. The goal of restructuring strategies is

---

National Education Goals for the Year 2000

Goal 1: All children in America will start school ready to learn....

Goal 2: The high school graduation rate will increase to at least 90 percent....

Goal 3: All students will leave grades 4, 8, and 12 having demonstrated competency over challenging subject matter including English, mathematics, science, foreign languages, civics and government, economics, arts, history, and geography, and every school in America will ensure that all students learn to use their minds well, so they may be prepared for responsible citizenship, further learning, and productive employment in our Nation's modern economy....

Goal 4: The Nation's teaching force will have access to programs for the continued improvement of their professional skills and the opportunity to acquire the knowledge and skills needed to instruct and prepare all American students for the next century....

Goal 5: United States students will be the first in the world in mathematics and science achievement....

Goal 6: Every adult American will be literate and will possess the knowledge and skills necessary to compete in a global economy and exercise the rights and responsibilities of citizenship....

Goal 7: Every school in the United States will be free of drugs, violence, and the unauthorized presence of firearms and alcohol and will offer a disciplined environment conducive to learning....

Goal 8: Every school will promote partnerships that will increase parental involvement and participation in promoting the social, emotional, and academic growth of children....

Source: NEGP (1999, p. 3-1)

to provide for overall school improvement, particularly in the area of student performance (Audette and Algozzine, 1992; Cook et al., 1995; Evans and Panacek-Howell, 1995; Harris and Evans, 1994; Paul and Rosselli, 1995; Paul, Yang, Adiegbola, and Morse, 1995).

The reform movements in general education in the early 1980s began with heightened concern about the skills of American students and the desire to improve their performance. The first wave of reform efforts were considered top-down initiatives. They were based on the belief that poor student performance was due to poor teaching. Wave One reform movements were characterized by increasing the support and status of the teaching profession, increasing public control of curriculum and spending, strengthening performance standards, and changing the structure of schools and classrooms. These reforms took the form of career ladders, merit pay, higher graduation requirements, tougher performance standards for teachers and students, curriculum reform, higher teacher salaries, focus on teaching time, elimination of tracking, focus on technology, and development of a relationship between businesses and schools. Wave One reform stressed the need for higher standards and greater efforts on the part of students, teachers, and administrators because a mediocre education was considered dangerous to the health of the nation.

The second wave of educational reform was characterized by bottom-up initiatives and began in the late 1980s. Focusing on changes in the teaching condition, including teacher preparation, these efforts were directed toward empowerment, COLLABORATION, and building the professionalism of teaching. They took the form of systemic changes in the organizational and governance structure of schools and the relationships of those involved in the educational process. Some examples of Wave Two changes included site-based management; shared decision making at the site level; state regulation waivers; increased union involvement and support; school choice; and partnerships between businesses, communities, and schools. Wave Two reforms focused on improvement of the school organization, school policy, and teacher competence.

The third wave of educational reform began in the late 1990s and focused on the issue of equity for children with special learning needs. Such children included those in disadvantaged learning environments, those who had dropped out of school, those who were English language learners (ELLs), those who were economically disadvantaged, and those who had disabilities. Wave Three reform seriously underscored the word *all* in the national education goal statements and called for reform at national, state, and local levels. This wave, which began at President George Bush's Governors' Summit on Education in 1989, brought the interests of general and special education together (Audette and Algozzine, 1992; Paul and Rosselli, 1995). Some legislative evidence of Wave Three reform can be seen in the 1997 federal requirements for inclusion of students with disabilities in statewide testing programs and in state actions to end social promotion at the end of the 1990s (i.e., advancing students to the next grade level if they did not meet grade-level standards).

Conflicts between General and Special Education Reforms

Reforms have occurred in both general and special education but for different reasons. Reform of general education programs was prompted by national concerns about the skills and potential competitiveness of American students in a global economy. Reform of special education programs occurred as part of the ongoing mission to seek access to general education for students with disabilities. General and special education reform movements have occurred in a parallel but not coordinated fashion, raising concern about a dual education system that cannot promote systemwide change so long as general and special education do not work together to create a unified educational system to serve all students (Audette and Algozzine, 1992; Danforth, Rhodes, and Smith, 1995; Myers and Sobehart, 1995).

While special educators and policymakers have been pushing in different directions, problems have existed with the reform movements themselves. These problems have not arisen because of a philosophical disagreement within the field of education, but due to the lack of connection between general and special education reforms (Gartner and Lipsky, 1987; Sailor, 1991).

A wide chasm has long existed between special and general education, leading to separate, parallel reform efforts. The division is hardly surprising, given that the special education system has emerged as a separate educational subsystem—not as a set of services within an overall educational framework. Over

the years, general and special education have evolved independently, with separate funding streams, administrative structures, accountability demands, curricula, personnel, certification requirements, and even separate facilities. (Cooley, 1995, p. 1)

The early reform movements of general education did not address children with disabilities (Hocutt and McKinney, 1995; Paul and Evans, 1995; Paul and Rosselli, 1995). Anderson (1992) charged that general education reform movements only dealt with 90 percent of America's children as the 10 percent receiving special education were left out. The lack of reference to children with disabilities in general education reform movement was even referred to as "deafening" (Hocutt as cited in Hocutt and McKinney, 1995, p. 50). The National Council on Disability (NCD, 1993) reported to President Clinton, "Students with disabilities have been largely forgotten by the mainstream of our educational system and by reformers of that system" (p. 82).

Even though the special education reform movement was called the Regular Education Initiative (REI), it did not connect with the general education reform movements. Hocutt and McKinney (1995) identified the following discrepancies:

- The REI was occurring at the same time reform was being called for in general education.

- The general education reform movements eventually led to the National Governors'

Summit on Education in 1989, which eventually led to Goals 2000: Educate America Act.

- Goals 2000 referred to all children, though there was no specific reference to children with disabilities.

- The REI called for greater integration of students with special needs at a time when general education reform was pushing for a commitment to excellence, which typically meant more time in school, more standards, more courses, and more homework.

- The REI came from special education and was discussed in special education circles with no input from general education.

Hocutt and McKinney (1995) further commented that both the REI and the Inclusion movement came from special education. These authors noted that these movements were neither being addressed in general education reform discussions, nor did general education seem to be "clamoring" (p. 57) to teach students with disabilities, especially if the students had behavioral problems.

The Interface between General and Special Education Reforms

Since special education operates within the general education system, reform must occur within that context. Paul et al. (1995) recommended

↓ not reform, but...

using *transformation,* "inventing a different kind of educational system for tomorrow," rather than *reform,* "improving the schools of today" (p. 11). An article by Audette and Algozzine (1997) entitled *Re-Inventing Government? Let's Re-Invent Special Education* was highly critical of any special education system that did not serve children or other participants (e.g., teachers and parents) well. They called on the federal government to use information on human development and learning, be creative, and support partnerships between general and special education to preserve the vision intended in special education laws.

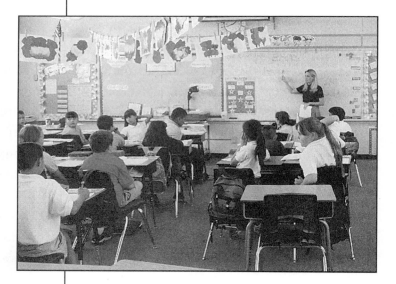

A key point for *all* educators and citizens is to agree on the true purpose of education. General educators tend to believe that the purpose of education is to have strong academic achievement; special educators tend to believe that the purpose of education is to produce productive members of society (Mulkerne, 1992). Paul et al. (1995) argued that the extent to which public education is open to all children will depend on the critical decisions we make based on our beliefs about the purpose of education. Another consideration critical to this discussion is that building special education on a medical model contributes to the belief that special treatment, or a separate system, is needed (Lipsky and Gartner, 1996). The interface between general and special education has historically focused on access, but "as reforms raise the demand for excellence (standards), special education cries foul and stresses equity. The difficulty with many of the debates on reform is that they seek to accommodate incompatible goals and values" (Paul et al., 1995, p. 11)

Education can play a unique role in the transmission and perpetuation of values that seek to rectify political and social inequalities. Schools have the opportunity to demonstrate how educators and students can live in a world of diversity. The education of individuals with disabilities has been portrayed as educating a diverse population of students (Danforth et al., 1995; Sailor and Skrtic, 1995). Therefore, to serve these students who have special needs in a public school system, specialists and other educators must rectify the complications of a dual system and develop partnerships, practices, and relationships that address the needs of students through access, equity, and goals while aspiring to standards of excellence for all students (Cook et al., 1995; Paul et al., 1995).

According to Lipsky and Gartner (1996), the heart of the special education reform issue was to deal with the nature of the dual system, that the implications and consequences were

significant, and that the work to be done was "extensive" (p. 791). They reminded educators that this issue was not just about mainstreaming, inclusion, or test scores. Instead they asserted that the issues were about social justice and building a diverse, democratic, and inclusive society. What Lipsky and Gartner envisioned would be the realization of Wave Three reform, which focused on educational equity for *all* children.

Change in schools is frequently considered slow and difficult. Understanding change and change processes is critical (Hall and Hord, 1987). "Delivering special education supports to all students with disabilities in a manner that begins with the assumption of regular class PLACEMENT represents a fundamental change for many schools in this country" (McGregor and Vogelsberg, 1998, p. 7). Congress stated that implementation of special education has "been impeded by low expectations" (INDIVIDUALS WITH DISABILITIES EDUCATION ACT [IDEA] AMENDMENTS, 1997, § 687) for students with disabilities. Professionals must work to "break down barriers" (McGregor and Vogelsberg, p. 11) between general and special education and engage in inclusive schooling practices, which "lead to the creation of supportive educational communities" (McGregor and Vogelsberg, p. 11).

In January 2000, the executive director of the National Association of Secondary School Principals (NASSP), Gerald Tirozzi, spoke at the National Association of State Directors of Special Education's 62nd Annual Conference, stating, "We need to find a common ground, a partnership. Previously, regular educators have not really been involved in the development of the IDEA and special educators in the ESEA [Elementary and Secondary Education Act]" ("Break Down Barriers," 2000, p. 9). To bridge the gap between general and special education, he proposed consideration of these key questions ("Break Down Barriers," 2000):

- "How do we evaluate the impact of special education programs on students?"

- "How do we approach testing in schools?"

- "How will we continue to label students?"

- "How will we be held responsible for fiscal resources?" (p. 9)

These are the questions that speech-language pathologists, special educators, administrators, and general educators need to address. A key change in practice that should facilitate these outcomes is a new requirement for special education teachers and specialists to link their students' INDIVIDUALIZED EDUCATION PROGRAM (IEP) goals to the general education curriculum. According to Thomas Hehir (1999), former director of the Office of Special Education and Rehabilitative Services (OSERS), "The fundamental principle here is simple: children with disabilities should be learning the same content as other children and schools must be held accountable for the results" (p. 6). McLaughlin (1999) noted that the 1997 IEP requirements and procedures "have the potential to alter the nature of 'special education' services," and that "new assessment and accountability provisions

> **Children with disabilities should be learning the same content as other children and schools must be held accountable for the results.**
>
> **(Hehir, 1999, p. 6)**

signal a clear presumption that students with disabilities should have access to the general curriculum and to the same opportunity to learn challenging and important content that is offered to all other students irrespective of the setting in which they receive their instruction" (p. 9).

Goal setting is the center component to the IEP plan for students in special education (see Chapter 4 for a discussion of IEP goal development). The shift toward building from curriculum as the basis for goals written in IEPs began to bridge the gap between the dual systems of general and special education. Special educators have not always looked to core curriculum for the basis of writing goals for their students' IEPs, so students were not presented with these expectations or challenges, widening the difference between what was mastered by their peers and what was mastered by students in specialized programs. Moore-Brown's 1998 dissertation study examined these questions: "What is the degree to which IEP goals, written for students receiving Resource Specialist Programs (RSP) and speech-language services, compare/relate to subject area content standards [which set forth what students need to learn at each grade level]," and "What educational areas are being addressed in the development of IEPs for students receiving RSP and speech-language services?" The findings indicated that most IEP goals matched skills identified in subject area content standards, but most often these were the lowest level skills or skills for much younger grade levels. These findings were reported as being similar to Shriner, Kim, Thurlow, and Ysseldyke (1993) who found that goals written for students in the area of math were not written to develop higher level skills. These researchers

> posed the concern that students with disabilities will not do well on statewide accountability measures if they are not taught higher level skills. IEPs are developed by teams comprised of educators and parents.
>
> Content standards are intended to lay forth a variety of complex skills. IEP teams must become familiar with the gradation and expectations of the standards. If the IEP is meant to be a procedural accountability tool and if access is a key concern in special education, then IEP team members must realize how a student is being denied access if his goals are focusing on lower level skill development. In addition, the dream of improved outcomes for children with disabilities will not be realized if goals are set too low (Moore-Brown, 1998, p. 91).

There are many commonalties in the reform movements of general and special education on which a unified system can be built. The challenge is transformation, the inventing of a different kind of educational system for the future (Paul et al., 1995). The call is to build on the commonalties and resolve the differences, not as general or special educators, but as educators of *all* children. As speech-language pathologists provide services within school settings, understanding the issues of reform (see Chapter 2)

and the demands of the educational system (see Chapter 5) is necessary to support students within the context of reform programs. To this end, the U.S. Department of Education (1999) reported to Congress:

> Joint participation and leadership of general and special educators in curriculum and standards development, professional development, resource allocation, and instruction are critical in helping students with disabilities access the general education curriculum and acquire skills that will better prepare them for life after school. (p. ii)

Children and Families in the Twenty-First Century

In the early decades of television, the traditional nuclear family was frequently portrayed as two parents and two children, usually one boy and one girl. Not surprisingly, educators often came to expect that children in their classes came from such a family. The realities of children and families in the twenty-first century are that not only has the family structure changed, but the circumstances of families have changed as well. No longer does only one member of the family serve as the breadwinner, as was often characterized by television shows like *Ozzie and Harriet* or the *Brady Bunch*. And perhaps more importantly, the economic conditions of families were different in the late 1990s, entering the twenty-first century.

Indicators of Children's Well-Being

Despite media characterizations, even in 1950, only 47% of children in the United States lived in traditional families; by 1990, this number had shifted to a mere 17.9% of children living in families in which the father worked full-time and the mother was not in the work force. A difference also existed between White and Black families. In the 1940s to 1960s, 45 to 50% of White children and less than 30% of Black children lived in traditional families. These numbers shifted to only 20% for White children and only 5% for Black children in 1990 (U.S. Department of Commerce, 1993).

An awareness of the conditions of the families in a community and in the country is important for speech-language pathologists and other educators, especially when school teams are asked to consider children's learning challenges. Consider the information reported by the Federal Interagency Forum on Child and Family Statistics (1999). When reviewing the statistics in the sidebar, think of the impact each condition might have on normal child development, including language that affects learning.

Profiling America's Children:
Selected Key Indicators of Well-Being

Number of Children in the United States

- In 1998, there were 69.9 million children in the United States, 0.3 million more than in 1997. This number is projected to increase to 77.6 million in 2020.

- The number of children under 18 has grown during the last half-century, increasing about half again in size since 1950. (p. 3)

Children as a Proportion of the Population

- Children are projected to remain a fairly stable percentage of the total population. They are expected to comprise 24 percent of the population in 2020.

- Together, children and senior citizens make up the "dependent population": those persons who, because of their age, are less likely to be employed than others. In 1950, children made up 79 percent of the dependent population; by 1998, they made up 67 percent. That percentage is expected to continue to decrease, to 59% in 2020. (p. 4)

Racial and Ethnic Composition

• In 1998, 65 percent of U.S. children were White, non-Hispanic; 15 percent were Black, non-Hispanic; 15 percent were Hispanic; 4 percent were Asian/Pacific Islander; and 1 percent were American Indian/Alaska Native.

• The percentage of children who are white, non-Hispanic has decreased from 74 percent in 1980 to 65 percent in 1998.

• The number of Hispanic children increased faster than that of any other racial and ethnic group, growing from 9 percent of the child population in 1980 to 15 percent in 1998. By 2020, it is projected that more than 1 in 5 children in the United States will be of Hispanic origin. (p. 5)

Difficulty Speaking English

• The number of school-age children (ages 5 to 17) who spoke a language other than English at home and who had difficulty speaking English was 2.4 million in 1995, up from 1.3 million in 1979. This was 5% of all school-age children in the U.S.

• The percentage of children who speak English with difficulty varies by region of the country, from 2 percent of children in the Midwest to 11 percent of children in the West.

• Likewise, the percentage of children who speak another language at home (with or without difficulty speaking English) varies by region of the country, from 6 percent of children in the Midwest to 26% percent in the West. This difference was due to differing concentrations of immigrants and their descendants in the regions. (p. 6)

Child Poverty and Family Income

• In 1997, 19 percent of American children lived in families with cash incomes below the poverty line.

• The percentage of children in poverty has stayed near or slightly above 20 percent since 1981.

• Children under age 6 are more often found in families with incomes below the poverty line than children ages 6 to 17. In 1997, 22 percent of children under age 6 lived in poverty, compared to 18% of older children.

• Children in married-couple families are much less likely to be living in poverty than children living only with their mothers. In 1997, 10 percent of children in married-couple families were living in poverty, compared to 49 percent in female-householder families. (p. 12)

General Health Status

- Child's health varies by family income. As family income increases, the percentage of children in very good or excellent health increases. In 1996, about 65 percent of children in families below the poverty line were in very good or excellent health, compared with 84 percent of children in families living at or above the poverty line.

- The percentage of children in very good or excellent health remained stable between 1984 and 1996. The health gap between children below and those at or above the poverty line also did not change during the time period; each year, children at or above the poverty line were about 20 percent points more likely to be in very good or excellent health than children below poverty. (p. 23)

Activity Limitation

- Children whose activities are limited by one or more chronic health conditions may need more specialized health care than children without such limitations. Their medical costs are generally higher; they are more likely to miss days from school; and they may require special education services.

- In 1996, 8 percent of children ages 5 to 17 were limited in their activities because of one or more chronic health conditions, compared to 3 percent of children younger than 5…. Children and youth ages 5 to 17 had much higher rates of activity limitation than younger children, possibly because some chronic conditions were not diagnosed until children enter school.

- Children and youth in families living below the poverty line have significantly higher rates of activity limitation than children in more affluent families. Among children and youth ages 5 to 17, 12 percent of children living below poverty had activity limitation due to chronic conditions, whereas 7 percent of children in families at or above poverty had a limitation in 1996. (p. 24)

Low Birthweight

- The percent of infants born of low birthweight was 7.5 percent in 1997, up slightly from 7.4 percent in 1996…. The 1997 rate was the highest level reported since 1973.

- About 1.4% of infants were born with very low birthweight (less than 1,500 grams) in 1996 and 1997, up from 1.3 percent in each year, 1989–95, and 1.2 percent in each year, 1981–88. (p. 25)

Family Reading to Young Children

- In 1996, 57 percent of children ages 3 to 5 were read aloud to by a family member every day in the last week, up slightly from 53 percent in 1993.

- As a mother's education increases, so does the likelihood that her child is read to every day. In 1996, about three-quarters (77 percent) of children whose mothers were college graduates were read aloud to every day. In comparison, daily reading aloud occurred for 62 percent of children whose mothers had some postsecondary education, 49 percent whose mothers had completed high school but had no education beyond that, and 37 percent whose mothers had not completed high school.

- White, non-Hispanic children were more likely to be read aloud to every day than either black, non-Hispanic or Hispanic children. Sixty-four percent of white, non-Hispanic children, 44 percent of black, non-Hispanic children, and 39 percent of Hispanic children were read to every day.

- Children in families with incomes below the poverty line are less likely to be read to every day than are children in families with incomes at or above the poverty line. Forty-six percent of children in families in poverty were read to every day in 1996, compared to 61 percent of children in families at or above the poverty line.

- Children living with two parents are more likely to be read aloud to every day than are children who live with one or no parent. Sixty-one percent of children in two-parent households were read to every day in 1996, compared to 46 percent of children living with one or no parent. (p. 45)

Early Childhood Education

- In 1997, 48 percent of children ages 3 to 4 yet to enter kindergarten attended preschool, a substantial increase from the 30 percent who attended preschool in 1980, an increase from 45 percent in 1996. (p. 46)

- Children with more highly educated mothers are more likely to attend an early childhood center than others. Seventy-one percent of children whose mothers had completed college attended such programs in 1996, compared to 37 percent whose mothers had less than a high school education. (p. 47)

- Black, non-Hispanic children were somewhat more likely than white, non-Hispanic children and much more likely than Hispanic children to attend an early childhood center. In 1996, 63 percent of black, non-Hispanic children ages 3 to 4 attended such programs, compared to 54 percent of white, non-Hispanic children and 37 percent of Hispanic children. (p. 47)

Source: Federal Interagency Forum on Child and Family Statistics (1999, pp. 3–6, 12, 23–25, 45–47)

Significance of Child and Family Statistics

Why should speech-language pathologists attend to statistics such as these? Simply put, language and other learning issues that arise out of conditions mentioned above strongly influence which children are more likely to be referred for special education services (IDEA, 1997). Concerns were raised by Congress in the IDEA reauthorization about the rate of increase in the number of racial and ethnic minority students who were identified as requiring special education services. Between 1980 and 1990, the rates of special education identification grew 53% for Hispanic children, 13.2% for African American children, and 107.8% for Asian children. This compared to an increase of 6% for White children. The *Twentieth Annual Report to Congress on the Implementation of the Individuals with Disabilities Education Act* (U.S. Department of Education, 1998) remarked on what educators know:

> The disproportionate representation of racial and ethnic minorities in special education is a highly complex issue because it is difficult to isolate the effects of poverty, limited English proficiency, residence in inner cities, and race/ethnicity on special education eligibility. (pp. II-20–II-21)

The experience of a child's upbringing can significantly affect classroom performance. Language growth and development depend on many factors, both constitutional (nature) and experiential (nurture). Cognitive development, working memory, and vocabulary size all influ-

ence success in the classroom (Biemiller, 1999; Erickson and Kopenhaver, 1995; Merritt and Culatta, 1998). Oral language development, which occurs from infancy on, lays the foundation for reading, writing, and other school experiences. Speech-language pathologists in schools must understand the implications of differences in the language development experiences of children from all types of backgrounds and experiences (Langdon, 2000).

Referencing several studies, Biemiller (1999) noted that children from low-income families had been found to have "smaller vocabularies and less advanced language development than their more advantaged peers" (p. 13). In a longitudinal study of the language and achievement differences between advantaged and disadvantaged children, Hart and Risley (as cited in Biemiller, 1999) found that "advantaged children were found to have twice the vocabulary of welfare children, and were adding vocabulary at twice the rate" (p. 14). Intriguingly, Hart and Risley (1995) reported:

> The longitudinal data showed that in the everyday interactions at home, the average (rounded) number of words children heard per hour was 2,150 in the professional families, 1,250 in the working-class families, and 620 in the welfare families.... Given the consistency we saw in the data, we might venture to extrapolate to the first 3 years of life. By age 3 the children in professional families would have heard more than 30 million words, the children in working-class families 20 million, and the children in welfare families 10 million. (p. 132)

Children who come to school with a primary language other than English or from a different cultural background will also bring different linguistic experiences. These experiences can be varied, from realizing the benefits of bilingualism to having limited opportunities to develop language skills and school-type experiences (Biemiller, 1999; Menyuk, 1999; Ripich and Creaghead, 1994).

The linguistic abilities that a child brings to school lay the foundation on which the child will build his or her academic knowledge. As members of a building, district, or regional support team, speech-language pathologists will be called on to build strong schoolwide programs that will help to develop the linguistic, cognitive, academic, and behavioral skills of students with and without disabilities. Speech-language pathologists are in a unique position to work as members of multidisciplinary teams that serve children schoolwide in order to develop the language and communication skills needed for school success.

Incidence of Children with Disabilities

The federal law that provides for special education is the Individuals with Disabilities Education Act or IDEA. The official title of the 1997 revision of the law is the Individuals with Disabilities Education Act Amendments of 1997. (See Chapter 2 for a discussion of the development of IDEA.) Annually, the U.S. Department of Education reports to Congress on the latest issues and information about the children served under IDEA. The following data were taken from the 1998 and 1999 reports of the U.S. Department of Education. Note that summary data for these reports are typically from three to five years prior. For this reason, most of the data reported here are from the 1996 and 1997 or 1997 and 1998 school years. Also note that the reports are typically released to the public the year following the actual date on the report. For example, the 1999 report was released in March 2000.

IDEA (1997) requires that services be provided to children who are identified as having a disability from birth to 21 years of age. By December 1997, the number of infants and toddlers (ages 0–3) who received services was 197,376. The number rose from 165,351 in 1994, representing a 19% increase in the number of infants and toddlers served. They were most frequently served at home (55.3%) in 1996–97 or an early intervention classroom (25.6%). Between 1992 and 1993 and 1997 and 1998, the number of preschool children (ages 3–6) served rose 25% from 455,449 to 571,049. Over 50% of these children were served in general education classes.

The Executive Summary of the *Twenty-First Annual Report to Congress on the Implementation of the Individuals with Disabilities Education Act* (U.S. Department of Education, 1999) reported, "The number of students with disabilities served under IDEA continues to increase at a rate higher than both the general population and school enrollment" (p. iv). Increases were found between 1988 and 1989 and 1997 and 1998 at the following rates: ages 6–11, 24.31% increase; ages 12–17, 37.58% increase; and ages 18–21, 15.85% increase (p. II-39). Of these children, 90% were identified with disabilities in one of four categories in

1996–97: LEARNING DISABILITIES (51.1% or 2,676,299 children), speech or language impairments (20.1% or 1,050,975 children), mental retardation (11.4% or 594,025 children), and emotional disturbance (8.6% or 447,426 children).

As mentioned previously, the *Twentieth Annual Report to Congress on the Implementation of the Individuals with Disabilities Education Act* (U.S. Department of Education, 1998) discussed concerns related to the disproportionate representation of children in poverty and from racial and ethnic minorities who are served under IDEA (1997). The complexity of issues such as poverty, language proficiency, and environmental deprivation contribute to difficulties in appropriate identification of children with disabilities.

The statistics and numbers reported here, both in terms of the conditions in which children live and the identified number of children served through special education programs, give a sense of the sometimes daunting nature of the issues that are faced and must be considered by school-based speech-language pathologists. Throughout a student's training program in communication disorders and throughout a speech-language pathologist's working career, it will be critical to have refined clinical skills in all areas of the field. However, when working with children in a school setting, one of the foremost tasks is to understand the circumstances in which a child lives. Speech-language pathologists must seek information regarding a student's living situation and then understand the ecological impact this has on his or her language and learning development in order to design appropriate diagnostic practices, intervention protocols, or both. This awareness marks the beginning of seeing the student as a whole child and as a member of a family, classroom, and school community.

> [O]ne of the foremost tasks is to understand the circumstances in which a child lives.

Predictions for the Future

This first chapter has presented a broad view of the issues facing educational systems, particularly as they apply to the education of children with disabilities and the provision of special education, specifically speech-language services, in the public schools. While reading the chapters in this book, consider the application of points of law or the provision of assessment and intervention services within the context of the forces and issues that affect the educational system and the children and families served. Also consider the evolving roles for speech-language pathologists in schools. Consider how this role evolution embraces system change and allows speech-language pathologists to be a part of building the systems of the future while providing services to students and working in concert with educators and interested others.

In order for these reforms to be successful, O'Shea and O'Shea (1997) offer:

Regardless of the impediments that currently block forward thinking, local collaboration is a cornerstone of effective school reform.... Although past assessments, interventions, and service delivery models often worked effectively for twentieth-century programming, reform approaches now require new thinking to achieve education-related service delivery that is appropriate to life in the next century. The following twenty-first century predictions emanate from research on the need for school reform, national goals, federal legislation, and local school reform efforts. These predictions may help advocacy groups, community agency representatives, educational personnel, parents, and researchers seeking collaborative models to guide their forward thinking. (p. 454)

As you proceed through this book, consider the predictions of O'Shea and O'Shea (1997) and how these might affect each topic area considered in each chapter and the overall educational system:

1. "Interagency processes will become more prominent" (p. 454).

2. "Despite new collaborative and collective visions, legal and ethical issues, political issues, administrative structures, and educational practices will continue to shape assessment and programming in learning support" (p. 455).

3. "Preservice training agendas will change in order to address school restructuring and service delivery systems" (p. 455).

4. "School reform will affect experienced teachers" (p. 457).

5. "Learning settings will expand" (p. 458).

6. "Technology will shape the collaboration format" (p. 458).

7. "The effects of parent and community advocacy groups will increase in prominence" (p. 459).

8. "Family diversity will change professionals' roles" (p. 459).

9. "Student diversity will affect professionals' roles" (p. 459).

10. "Local groups will shape local school structures" (p. 460).

Speech-language pathologists working in public schools will be a part of the realizations toward, or shifts away from, these predictions. Ask yourself, "What role will I play?" and "How will these programs, initiatives, movements, and predictions influence my work?" While you consider these questions, let us say, "Welcome to the public schools!"

CHAPTER 2

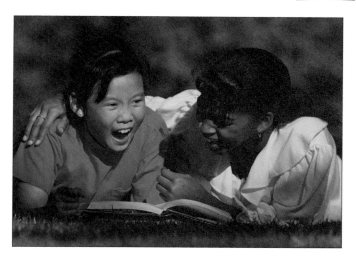

Legislative Foundation of Special Education

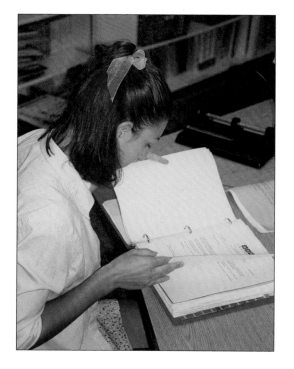

IN THIS CHAPTER

This chapter provides an overview of the legislative history of special education in the United States; describes the foundations of the law; reviews the development of special education legislation, and describes issues which exist under IDEA (1997), including the implications of standards-based reform. This chapter introduces the foundation concepts of free appropriate public education (FAPE) and least restrictive environment (LRE) and discusses the relevance of these for speech-language services in schools.

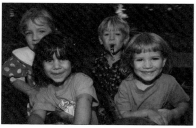

CHAPTER QUESTIONS

1. Explain how the legislative history of special education led to laws that are considered to be civil rights protections.

2. Discuss how the concepts of FAPE and LRE apply to speech and language programs.

3. Review some of the significant changes in IDEA (1997). Discuss why you think these changes are now required in federal law.

4. Consider what challenges might exist for speech-language pathologists when accessing standards and core curriculum for their students.

Legislative History of Special Education

On June 4, 1997, President Bill Clinton signed into law the reauthorization of the 1990 INDIVIDUALS WITH DISABILITIES EDUCATION ACT (IDEA). IDEA (1997) included amendments revising its provisions and extending appropriations for IDEA programs until fiscal year 2002. The road to this ceremony on the South Lawn of the White House was long, beginning before the implementation of the EDUCATION FOR ALL HANDICAPPED CHILDREN ACT (EAHCA) in 1975, which established the framework for SPECIAL EDUCATION as it is known today.

The history of special education has been characterized by controversy encountering debate ranging from philosophical to fiscal issues. Critics of special education, including general educators and politicians, have become increasingly vocal about their concerns regarding expense (see "Funding" in Chapter 9), lack of adequate results (see "Including Children with Disabilities in Assessments, Performance Goals, and Reports to the Public" [beginning on page 43]), and a dual system for disciplining students (see "Behavior and Student Discipline" in Chapter 8).

Perhaps in response to some of these critics, IDEA (1997) strongly reaffirmed the national mandate regarding the education of students with disabilities, especially with the statement of findings in the introduction to the bill (see sidebar on next page). Congress acknowledged the impressive history that led to the establishment of special education and not only emphasized that

these issues should not be forgotten, but also presented the challenge to educators and those involved with students with disabilities to improve educational results for these children. Speech-language pathologists and other special educators who work under IDEA (1997) should understand the long battle and historic events that have led to the current special education system.

The federal government played virtually no role in the education of children with disabilities until well into the 1960s, with the exception of providing some assistance between the 1820s and 1870s in creating special schools for children who were blind, DEAF, or mentally ill (Martin, Martin, and Terman, 1996; Turnbull, 1993). Most of the responsibility for educating children with disabilities previously fell to states or to private individuals and organizations.

According to the Council for Exceptional Children (CEC, 1997b), by 1911, a United States Bureau of Education survey found "6% of cities reporting special classes…, 11% for gifted; 25% for backward; 10% for physically exceptional (non-English speaking); and 17% for morally exceptional, delinquent, and incorrigible" (p. 11).

In 1930, "the White House Conference on Special Education reported the following statistics of handicapped children in the United States: 300,000 crippled; 18,212 deaf; 3,000,000 hard of hearing; 14,000 blind; 50,000 partially seeing; 1,000,000 defective speech; 450,000 mentally retarded; and 1,500,000 gifted" (CEC, 1997b, p. 20).

After both World War I and World War II, the U.S. government recognized the need for vocational-type training for veterans, especially those who returned with disabilities from war. Federal involvement in the education of children with disabilities was slow to follow. Some states provided education to students who entered public education with a variety of difficulties, including mental retardation. Notably, states such as Illinois, New York, Florida, California, and Wisconsin implemented programs that followed functionally based (called *occupational* or *vocational education*) curricula, focusing on job skills, community skills, living skills, and some academically related skills. The need for federal involvement in mandating and regulating the education of children with disabilities began to emerge with a growing parent movement and with the assistance of President John F. Kennedy, who established the President's Committee on Mental Retardation

---

IDEA (1997) Statements of Findings

The Congress finds the following:

(1) Disability is a natural part of the human experience and in no way diminishes the right of individuals to participate in or contribute to society. Improving educational results for children with disabilities is an essential element of our national policy of ensuring equality of opportunity, full participation, independent living, and economic self-sufficiency for individuals with disabilities.

(2) Before the enactment of the Education for All Handicapped Children Act of 1975 (Public Law 94-142) (A) the special educational needs of children with disabilities in the United States were not being fully met; (B) more than one-half of the children with disabilities in the United States did not receive appropriate educational services that would enable such children to have full equality of opportunity; (C) 1,000,000 of the children with disabilities in the United States were excluded entirely from the public school system and did not go through the educational process with their peers; (D) there were many children with disabilities throughout the United States participating in regular school programs whose disabilities prevented such children from having a successful educational experience because their disabilities were undetected; and (E) because of the lack of adequate services within the public school system, families were often forced to find services outside the public school system, often at great distance from their residence and at their own expense.

(3) Since the enactment and implementation of the Education for All Handicapped Children Act of 1975, this Act has been successful in ensuring children with disabilities and the families of such children have access to a free appropriate public education and in improving educational results for children with disabilities.

(4) However, the implementation of this Act has been impeded by low expectations, and an insufficient focus on applying replicable research on proven methods of teaching and learning for children with disabilities.

Source: IDEA (1997 § 601 [c])

in the early 1960s (CEC, 1997b; Neubert, 1997; Turnbull, 1993).

In 1958, President Dwight D. Eisenhower signed Public Law 85-926, the Education of Mentally Retarded Children Act, which was a bill that provided financial assistance to colleges educating teachers of children with mental retardation. The first direct subsidy for services to special populations, including children with disabilities, came in 1966, the second year of the Elementary and Secondary Education Act (ESEA), Public Law 89-10. This act established the system of remedial education for economically disadvantaged students, known as TITLE I, and provided some entitlements to state-supported or state-operated schools "for the handicapped" *[sic]* (Martin et al., 1996, p. 27).

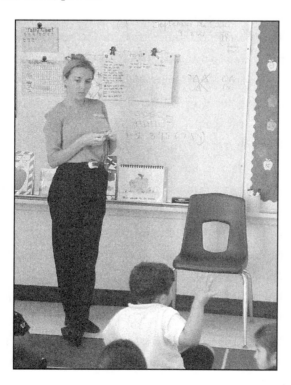

Roots of Special Education in Civil Rights Legal Action

The lack of federal assistance was not just apparent in the education of children with disabilities, but also in terms of other educational issues. The Supreme Court case that changed all of this was *Brown v. Board of Education* (1954). The Supreme Court ruled unanimously that the doctrine of "separate but equal" was inherently unequal and therefore unconstitutional. While *Brown* specifically dealt with racial segregation, it laid the foundation for the education of children with disabilities and other groups because the right-to-education issue was argued on the principles of equal protection under the law for all citizens.

In *Brown* it was proven *[sic]* that although the U.S. Constitution never once refers to a public education, its principles of equal protection and due process under the Fifth and Fourteenth Amendments have a significant effect on public education. Nowhere is this fact clearer than in the right-to-education cases. This is significant because, as noted, the federal Constitution does not guarantee the right to an education. State constitutions guarantee it. But if a state denies (as many had) an education to some students, usually those with disabilities, but provides it to others, the state violates the equal protection doctrine of the federal Constitution and, depending on the provisions of the state's constitution, its own constitution as well. The essential point of *Brown*, however, is that the states were violating the equal protection clause of the federal Constitution. (Turnbull, 1993, p. 8)

Equal protection and DUE PROCESS have continued to be critical to special education law. Two major court cases solidified the connection between equal protection and due process under the FOURTEENTH AMENDMENT: *Pennsylvania Association for Retarded Children (PARC) v. Commonwealth of Pennsylvania* and *Mills v. D.C. Board of Education.*

The *PARC* case (1971) challenged a state law in Pennsylvania that allowed public schools to deny an education to children whom examiners determined to be below the MENTAL AGE of five. *PARC* was settled on a consent decree that (1) provided full access to an education for children with mental retardation, (2) established the standard of appropriateness, and (3) established a standard for least restrictive environment.

On the heels of the *PARC* case, *Mills v. D.C. Board of Education* (1972) was a case brought by students with varying types of disabilities who had been excluded from school and denied an education in the District of Columbia schools. The basis of their exclusion from school was due to the disabilities of these children.

> The U.S. District Court ruled that school districts were constitutionally prohibited from deciding that they had inadequate resources to serve children with disabilities because the equal protection clause of the Fourteenth Amendment would not allow the burden of insufficient funding to fall more heavily on children with disabilities than on other children. (Martin et al., 1996, p. 28)

With the strength of *Brown, PARC,* and *Mills,* court cases continued to be brought forward, yet estimates showed that millions of children with disabilities still were not receiving a public education. Most states had some form of special education programs, but these varied dramatically from state to state. Ultimately, during the 1970s, states joined with existing advocacy groups to seek federal legislation that would provide financial assistance and guidance for the provision of education to children with disabilities (Martin et al., 1996; Turnbull, 1993).

Legislative Response: Special Education as a Federal Mandate

In 1970, Congress passed the EDUCATION OF THE HANDICAPPED ACT (EHA, Public Law 91-230). This law established minimum requirements for states to follow to receive federal assistance. Following *PARC* and *Mills,* Congress acted by passing laws in the area of nondiscrimination and funding. In SECTION 504 of the REHABILITATION ACT OF 1973 (Public Law 93-112), discrimination against those with disabilities was prohibited in any system that received federal funding (see "Parental Notification and Involvement" in Chapter 8). Additional federal financial assistance for states came in the Education Amendments of 1974 (Public Law 93-380) for provision of special education allowing for "full educational opportunities for all handicapped children" (Turnbull, 1993, pp. 13–14). In 1975, Congress amended the EHA by passing the EAHCA (Public Law 94-142). This law established special education as it is known today, with requirements for the provision of services, procedural safeguards, and funding mechanisms to support the programs. The federal mandate for special education has been revised and updated several times since 1975. The 1990 amendments (Public Law 101-476) renamed the law to be the "Individuals with Disabilities Education Act" commonly referred to as IDEA, which is how the law is now known. In addition, the AMERICANS WITH DISABILITIES ACT (ADA, Public Law 101-336) was signed into law by President George Bush in 1990, further expanding the scope of discriminatory practices identified as illegal in all public accommodations. The 1997 amendments to IDEA kept the name IDEA, but resulted in a new public law number: 105-17.

Federal mandates, including those for special education, provide guidance through legislation, but then require states to develop their own programs to implement the federal regulations. It is for this reason that the provision of services may look different from state to state. Monitoring how states implement their special education programs is done by the Office of Special Education Programs (OSEP). OSEP works closely with the STATE EDUCATIONAL AGENCIES (SEAs) to insure that federal requirements are being met in each state (U.S. Department of Education, 1999) and uses a continuous improvement monitoring model that focuses on student outcomes.

States work hard to maintain their own identity in the provision of special education services. Issues such as provision of FREE APPROPRIATE PUBLIC EDUCATION (FAPE), LEAST RESTRICTIVE ENVIRONMENT (LRE), student discipline, funding, and SERVICE DELIVERY to students in correctional facilities have provided arenas for the struggle between state and federal interpretations of special education procedures. The history of special education shows a recurring pattern of a series of legal cases, followed by revisions to the law, followed by another series of legal cases that interpret the revisions.

The Education for All Handicapped Children Act (EAHCA)

In 1975, the EAHCA put into place the system under which special education has operated since its origination. The act described a complex set of procedures designed to rectify the issues that had been brought forward by the courts, parents, educators, and states. Congress was concerned with the number of children who remained unserved by the public school systems, so "CHILD FIND," a mandate that LOCAL EDUCATIONAL AGENCIES (LEAs) be proactive in finding children with disabilities, was instituted as an important requirement under this new law. The history of court decisions leading up to the establishment of the EAHCA was reflected in the law's key components, including:

- Providing federal funding for special education programs

- Establishing procedures to insure the provision of special education services

- Establishing conceptual parameters under which the procedures were to be followed, including free appropriate public education, least restrictive environment, and zero reject

- Requiring the provision of services to children ages 0–21, identified through child-find activities, resulting in an evaluation process and qualifying according to certain ELIGIBILITY criteria

Following the passage of EAHCA in 1975, states were allowed three years to put into place a state plan for the implementation of the law. The federal law gave the outline of a process for developing an INDIVIDUALIZED EDUCATION PROGRAM (IEP) that would be based on evaluation to determine the child's eligibility for the program (see Chapter 4 for a full description of IEP processes and procedures including eligibility requirements).

One of the most critical features of the EAHCA (1975) was the institution of due process protection for children and parents, which provided full partnership for parents in the decision-making processes in special education. When used in special education, *due process* refers to the procedural rights, protections, and safeguards for parents and children and also refers to procedures involving hearings and mediation. Procedural safeguards provide (1) timelines for evaluations, (2) access to and review of records, (3) parental involvement and consent, (4) parental input into program development, and (5) procedures for complaints and disagreements. If parents and school districts are unable to agree on identification, evaluation, or any other aspects of the IEP program or PLACEMENT (including GOALS and SHORT-TERM OBJECTIVES or BENCHMARKS), then either party may request a DUE PROCESS HEARING. A due process hearing involves presentation of evidence by both parties before an impartial hearing officer. Prior to the hearing, mediation may be requested or required. (See Chapter 8 "Mediation, Due Process Hearings, and State IDEA Complaints.")

Over the years, several amendments have been added to the EAHCA (1975), increasing the requirements under this law. Two important changes occurred in 1986. First came the PRESCHOOL AMENDMENTS TO THE EDUCATION OF THE HANDICAPPED ACT (Public Law 99-457). Part H was added to extend the age of eligibility to include infants and toddlers who qualified for services under less-intensive eligibility criteria. This change came as a result of professionals and parents lobbying Congress to fund early intervention services, with the belief that early intervention would prevent or reduce the need for lifelong special services. The other significant addition to the law in 1986 came with the passage of the HANDICAPPED CHILDREN'S PROTECTION ACT (known as the Attorneys' Fees Bill, Public Law 99-372). This act authorized awarding attorneys' fees to families who prevailed in lawsuits under the due process provisions of the law.

The Individuals with Disabilities Education Act (IDEA): EAHCA Revised

The 1990 revisions to the 1975 EAHCA included a new name: the Individuals with Disabilities Education Act (IDEA). This name reflected the consciousness of the "People First" movement, which emphasized that persons with disabilities should be recognized as individuals first, replacing the label as a name (see sidebars below and on page 30).

The following modifications to the 1975 EAHCA in the IDEA (1990) provisions (summarized from the works of McEllistrem, Roth, and Cox, 1998; Martin et al., 1996; Neubert, 1997; Turnbull, 1993) reflected further changes in the communities of persons with disabilities and special education:

• The addition of two new eligibility categories: traumatic brain injury (TBI) and AUTISM. Children with these conditions were certainly eligible for special education previously, but were usually identified under other categories that did not fully describe the disability. By 1990, medical technology enabled higher survival rates from accidents, evidenced by an increase in students with TBI in schools. These children showed a different

pattern of recovery, in that their special needs did not result from a developmental condition as did all other eligibility areas. Identifying these students under the categories of speech or language impairment, mental retardation, and/or other health impairment did not accurately identify the learning needs of these students.

By 1990, much controversy existed regarding the education of students with autism. Again, identification under categories such as speech and language or mental retardation did not accurately describe characteristics that were unique to children with autism. Therefore, autism was added to the list of eligibility categories.

• Inclusion of a requirement for TRANSITION planning beginning at the age of 16. This requirement came out of findings that most students who had been receiving special education and RELATED SERVICES

American Psychological Association's (APA's) Guidelines for "People First" Language

The guiding principle for "nonhandicapping" language is to maintain the integrity of individuals as human beings. Avoid language that equates persons with their condition (e.g., *neurotics, the disabled)*; that has superfluous, negative overtones (e.g., stroke *victim);* or that is regarded as a slur (e.g., *cripple)*....Use *disability* to refer to an attribute of a person [e.g., child with a learning disability] and *handicap* to refer to the source of limitations, which may include attitudinal, legal, and architectural barriers as well as the disability itself (e.g., steps and curbs handicap people who require the use of a ramp [and severe visual impairment is a handicap to drivers])....As a general rule, "person with _____," "person living with _____," and "person who has _____" are neutral and preferred forms of description.

From *Publication Manual of the American Psychological Association* (4th ed., p. 53), by the American Psychological Association (APA), 1994, Washington, DC: Author. © 1994 by the APA.

"People First" Language

person with a disability	individual without speech
speech of children with language impairment	man with cerebral palsy
child who has autism	person with Down syndrome
person who has quadriplegia	person who uses a wheelchair
persons who stutter	children with normally developing speech

Sources: Folkins (1999); Parent Advocacy Coalition for Educational Rights (PACER) Center (1989)

---

were not successful in the world of work. It became apparent that as part of their special education services, IEP teams needed to specifically address the development of skills that students needed to master to hold a job. As a result, a statement of needed transition services, often called an INDIVIDUAL TRANSITION PLAN (ITP), was required for students beginning at the age of 16 (changed to age 14 under IDEA [1997]).

• A renewed focus on students with severe disabilities and on the integration of these students into their communities and schools. This focus was consistent with the REGULAR EDUCATION INITIATIVE (REI) and the INCLUSION movement (discussed in "Educational Reforms That Shaped the Profession" in Chapter 1) that fought against the isolation and segregation of students with disabilities. The new requirements under IDEA (1990) called for greater integration of students with even the most significant disabilities.

• The clarification that ASSISTIVE TECHNOLOGY (AT) devices should be considered as part of a student's IEP. This requirement mandated consideration and purchase of assistive technology devices if the IEP team finds that the student is in need of such services.

Free Appropriate Public Education (FAPE) and Least Restrictive Environment (LRE)

The intent of Congress to provide free appropriate public education (FAPE) was set forth in 1975 under the EAHCA and has been reinforced through subsequent amendments. State educational agencies (SEAs, e.g., State Departments of Education) and local educational agencies (LEAs, e.g., school districts) are required to establish policies and procedures to ensure that each child with a disability has available free appropriate public education through both procedural and regulatory conditions. These are designed to avoid the possibility of functional exclusion when students are unintentionally excluded from services or "fall through the cracks."

First, *appropriate* [italics added] is defined generally in terms of the procedure schools must use: (1) The child must be furnished with an individualized education program, (2) must be evaluated on a nondiscriminatory basis, (3) and is entitled to a due process hearing if the appropriateness of his or her education is in doubt, (4) the parents are entitled to be included in the development of their child's individualized education program, (5) the child is entitled to appropriately and adequately trained teachers, (6) has the right of access to his or her school records, (7) is entitled to a barrier-free school environment, (8) and may be included in preschool programs; and (9) the child's representatives (parents or other) are entitled to participate in and be given notice of school actions affecting special education programs and the child's own education. Although separately provided for by the IDEA, as a whole these requirements are intended to answer the problem of functional exclusion and to assure an appropriate education.

Second, Sections 300.4 and 300.300–.307 of the regulations defined *free appropriate education* to mean special education and related services that

(1) are provided at public expense, under public supervision and direction, and without charge; (2) meet the standards of the SEA, including requirements of the IDEA; (3) include preschool, elementary, and secondary school education in the state involved; and (4) are provided in conformity with the child's individualized education program. (Turnbull, 1993, p. 47)

Martin et al. (1996) clarify that the lengthy list of entitlements and rights is not a blank check for an ideal program:

In general, the standard for judging appropriateness is whether the child's educational program is (1) related to the child's learning capacity, (2) specially designed for the child's unique needs and not merely what is offered to others, and (3) reasonably calculated to confer educational benefit. However, the entitlement is not open-ended: the child is not entitled to every service that could conceivably offer a benefit. (p. 34)

IDEA (1997 § 602 [8]) reinforces that students with disabilities have available to them free appropriate public education, meaning special education and related services that:

(A) have been provided at public expense, under public supervision and direction, and (B) without charge;

A. meet the standards of the State education agency;

B. include an appropriate preschool, elementary, or secondary school education in the State involved; and

C. are provided in conformity with the individualized education program required under section 6124 (d).

Designing an educational program that meets the requirements of FAPE falls to the team that develops the individualized program for the student (i.e., the IEP team). In designing the IEP, the team considers the student's identified needs and what programming and services are necessary in order to assist the child in meeting goals and short-term objectives or benchmarks (see Chapter 4 "Development of Goals and Short-Term Objectives or Benchmarks" for further discussion). Functionally, FAPE means that students receive the services they need but not more than they need.

Like FAPE, the interpretation of least restrictive environment (LRE) has varied widely. The regulations require:

LRE

01. that to the maximum extent appropriate, children with disabilities, including children in public or private institutions or other care facilities, are educated with children who are not disabled; and 2. that special classes, separate schooling, or other removal of children with disabilities from the regular education environment occurs only when the nature or severity of the handicap is such that education in regular classes with the use of supplementary aids and services cannot be achieved satisfactorily. (34 CODE OF FEDERAL REGULATIONS [C.F.R.] § 300.550)

The underlying principle of LRE is that children with disabilities will be, to the fullest extent possible, educated alongside their peers who are not disabled. Before federal legislation, it was common practice to segregate children with disabilities from their nondisabled peers.

The concept of LRE also calls for a continuum of alternative placements for children who are in need of special education and related services. Under the provisions of FAPE, these program options, if needed, would be provided at no cost to children or their families.

The LRE principle is "inextricably tied to the notion of appropriateness, which makes it all the more complex because appropriate education itself is difficult to define" (Turnbull, 1993, p. 174). LRE, then, provides for education with peers who are not disabled in an integrated setting, except when that is not appropriate for the individual child. Because the law was not specific about what constituted appropriateness, the courts were left to clarify interpretation.

The realization of the concepts of FAPE and LRE means that individuals with disabilities should be treated and have the same opportunities—including education—as those without disabilities. The presence in mainstream society of individuals with disabilities has ultimately influenced the greater integration of society (Turnbull, 1993).

Landmark Court Decisions Regarding FAPE and LRE

The Rowley Standard

The first special education case heard by the United States Supreme Court was a 1982 case out of New York: *Board of Education v. Rowley*. This case set the standard for defining an appropriate program. Amy Rowley was a student who was deaf and attending a general first-grade class, following a successful kindergarten year. School authorities provided Amy with an FM wireless ASSISTIVE LISTENING DEVICE for amplification of the teacher's voice in the classroom. She was to receive additional support from tutors and her parents. Amy's parents requested that the school also provide Amy with a sign language interpreter. The school district denied their request, because a trial period with a sign language interpreter had demonstrated to the district that this service was unnecessary since Amy learned just as well without the interpreter. The Supreme Court ruling in this case held that Congress did not intend for schools to develop maximum potential for children with disabilities; rather, Congress intended to open the school house doors and provide students with an educational opportunity to benefit (Martin et al., 1996; Osborne, 1988).

The standard for FAPE was that a student would have "access to a basic floor of opportunity in which the student receives some educational benefit" (Albanese, 2000, p. 1). The *Rowley* case reinforced the importance of the IEP process in defining appropriate education. The standard for educational benefit, and not maximum development, was upheld by the courts in later rulings (Martin et al., 1996; Osborne, 1988; Turnbull, 1993). States establish their standards for FAPE. The *Rowley* interpretation of a

> [T]he IEP should be designed so that it results in educational advancement or meaningful educational benefit.

floor, not ceiling, of opportunities is upheld in most states.

Initially, lower courts strictly applied the *Rowley* standard to other court cases. However, later courts struggled with the distinction between "some" educational benefit being more than just "trivial" benefit. Courts later moved to a less strict interpretation and extended the *Rowley* standard to that of "meaningful" educational benefit. Special educators must understand that the IEP should be designed so that it results in educational advancement or meaningful educational benefit that the student can reasonably be expected to achieve (Osborne, 1992).

Early Cases

While the Regular Education Initiative (REI) and the Inclusion movement may have advocated for normalizing the setting and methods for providing services to children with disabilities (see "Conflicts between General and Special Education Reforms" in Chapter 1), the courts are where clarification occurred in terms of what would be acceptable settings and methods. The procedural safeguards afforded to parents allowed for either parents or school districts to request a due process hearing or mediation if there was a disagreement on any issue dealing with the identification, evaluation, educational placement, or provision of FAPE to a child, including issues arising in the IEP process (see "Mediation, Due Process Hearings, and State IDEA Complaints" in Chapter 8 for full discussion). The ruling of an administrative law judge or impartial hearing officer stands as the final decision, unless the decision is appealed. Appeals in these cases may be heard as a civil action in federal court or may be heard in a state court of competent jurisdiction. As in most other legal proceedings, complainants in due process proceedings are required to exhaust administrative remedies before filing a court action.

Following *Rowley,* three major court actions reinterpreted LRE in terms of "inclusion," or placement of a child with disabilities into a general education classroom. These cases were all heard first at the level of due process hearing and then worked their way to the court system.

Daniel R.R. v. State Board of Education

Daniel was an elementary school student with Down syndrome. His parents wanted Daniel included in a regular classroom, but the school district denied the placement (Martin et al., 1996; Martin and Weatherly, 1996; U.S. Courts Affirm, 1996). Noting a strong congressional preference for MAIN-STREAMING, in 1989 the Fifth Circuit Court created a two-part inquiry for determination of placement:

> First, the school must determine whether placement in the regular classroom, with supplementary services, could be achieved satisfactorily. To make that determination, the school must ask the following questions:

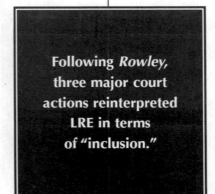

Following *Rowley,* three major court actions reinterpreted LRE in terms of "inclusion."

- Has the school taken steps to provide supplementary aids and services to modify the regular education program to suit the needs of the disabled child?

- Once modifications are made, can the child receive an educational benefit from regular education?

- What effects will the disabled child's presence have on the regular classroom environment and, thus, on the education the other students are receiving?

> Second, if the decision is made to remove the child from the regular classroom for all or part of the day, then the school must also ask whether the child has been mainstreamed (spending some time in the regular classroom) to the maximum extent possible. (Martin et al., 1996, p. 35)

Oberti v. Board of Education of Borough of Clementon School District

In *Oberti v. Board of Education of Borough of Clementon School District* (1993), the Third Circuit Court ruled that the school district bore the burden of proof in LRE cases and that mere token attempts at inclusion on the part of the district were not satisfactory to meet the requirement. Rafael Oberti was a student with Down syndrome placed in a developmental kindergarten class in New Jersey school district. He was reported to show disruptive behaviors and was difficult for the teacher to manage. The Findings of Fact in this case chronicled that the school district did not provide enough support, or even effort, to make the placement work. The court concluded that the preference for mainstreaming was so strong that the argument in favor of the placement could be rebutted only if the school district could prove any of the following: (1) that the student would receive little or no benefit from the inclusion placement, (2) that the student would be so disruptive that other students' learning would be impaired, or (3) that the cost of providing services in the regular classroom would have a negative effect on other students. The court found that, in this case, additional teacher training might have eliminated any potential disruption to the classroom and that the necessity to modify the curriculum was not a reason for exclusion (Martin and Weatherly, 1996; Osborne and DiMattia, 1995; Pennsylvania Department of Education, 1999; Price, Mayfield, McFadden, and Marsh, 2000; Schnaiberg, 1996; Winget, Boyle, and Reynolds, 1994).

Sacramento City Unified School District v. Rachel H.

Sacramento City Unified School District v. Rachel H. (1994) case involved a child with mental retardation whose parents wanted her fully included in a regular classroom. In the *Rachel H.* case, the Ninth Circuit Court established a four-factor balancing test to consider in determining appropriate placement (Martin and Weatherly, 1996; Martin et al., 1996). Winget et al. (1994) reported the test identified by the court:

1. The educational benefits of full-time placement in a regular class

2. The nonacademic benefits of such a placement

3. The effects of the student on the teacher and other children in the class

4. The cost of a regular education placement with appropriate supplementary aids and services (p. 1:14)

Later Cases: A Shift toward Restriction with Justification

In the above-referenced cases, the courts set forth criteria that subsequently assisted IEP teams in making decisions about placement in the least restrictive environment. School districts bear the responsibility of demonstrating that a less restrictive environment could not work, rather than arguing for more restrictive placement without first attempting the less restrictive. Three later decisions involving inclusion reflected some shift in the courts' interpretation of LRE.

Poolaw v. Bishop

Poolaw v. Bishop (1995) was a Ninth Circuit Court decision that affirmed an Arizona District Court decision in favor of placing a 13-year-old student with significant communication needs requiring intensive instruction in American Sign Language at the state school for the deaf. Notably, the Ninth Circuit (as cited in Maloney and Pitasky, 1996) commented on IDEA's (1997) LRE requirement:

In some cases, such as where the child's handicap is particularly severe, it will be impossible to provide any meaningful education to the student in a mainstream environment. In these situations, continued mainstreaming would be inappropriate and educators may recommend placing the child in a special education environment. (p. iv)

McWhirt by McWhirt v. Williamson County School

McWhirt by McWhirt v. Williamson County School (1994) is a Sixth Circuit Court inclusion decision that a fourth-grade student with multiple disabilities be placed appropriately in a comprehensive special education class with partial mainstreaming rather than in the less restrictive resource room desired by her parents. The Sixth Circuit found that the severe nature of the student's disabilities prevented her from "functioning constructively in regular education" (Maloney and Pitasky, 1996, p. v).

Kari H. v. Franklin Special School District

The Sixth Circuit Court later relied on its authority in *McWhirt by McWhirt v. Williamson County School* in its ruling on *Kari H. v. Franklin Special School District* (1995). In this case, the inappropriate behaviors of the student in previous mainstream placements, as well as the functional gains she could realize in a special education classroom, were determined by the court to outweigh any minimal benefit she might realize from placement in the regular classroom (Maloney and Pitasky, 1996).

The above rulings are significant in terms of an apparent conflict between FAPE and LRE. FAPE may not be possible in inclusive settings for some students, and FAPE can prevail over LRE when the two do conflict. The message of the courts appears to be that FAPE and LRE are most adequately maintained with a continuum of services (Maloney and Pitasky, 1996; U.S. Courts Affirm, 1996).

Court cases may seem like they are remote and removed from the daily work of speech-language pathologists in public schools. These cases do, however, strongly influence the direction given by administrators to IEP teams so that current rulings are reflected in decision making. Table 2.1 illustrates the effect of the above-mentioned cases on the practice of speech-language pathologists.

Determining Meaningful Benefit from FAPE

The 1997 IDEA reauthorization added new elements to the interpretation of FAPE. The 1999 C.F.R. identified the focus of special education as extending beyond high school by emphasizing FUNCTIONAL OUTCOMES for successful adulthood: "To ensure that all children with disabilities have available to them a free appropriate public education that emphasizes special education and related services designed to meet their unique needs and prepare them for employment and independent living" (34 C.F.R. § 300.1 [a]). When considering that the federal definition of FAPE now extends until after high school (until a student's 22nd birthday), and that Congress has focused on improving results for students

Table 2.1

A Summary of Key Court Cases and Their Effect on the Practice of Speech-Language Pathologists

Court Case	Court Direction	Effect on Speech-Language Pathologists' Practice
Board of Education v. Rowley (1982) (State of New York; Supreme Court Decision)	• Set standard for determination of FAPE • Ruled a goal of special education is not to maximize potential • Ruled a goal of special education is access to educational benefit	Influences decisions for recommendations for therapy
Daniel R.R. v. State Board of Education (1989) (State of Texas; Fifth Circuit Court of Appeals)	• Set guidelines for determination of provision of supplementary aids and services to modify the regular classroom in order for the child to receive educational benefit • Considered the influence of the child with a disability on the education of other children in the class	Influences the need for speech-language services to be provided either in the general education classroom or in conjunction with the work of the classroom (i.e., the curriculum)
Oberti v. Board of Education of Borough of Clementon School District (1993) (State of New Jersey; Third Circuit Court of Appeals)	• Placed the burden of proof on the school district to demonstrate that the student would receive no educational benefit from educational placement in a regular classroom • Recommended teacher training to deal with potential problems • Ruled a need to modify the curriculum was not a reason for exclusion	Influences the need to work with families and requests for services in the regular classroom; must attempt and prove a type of service delivery does not work
Sacramento City USD v. Rachel H. (1994) (State of California; Ninth Circuit Court of Appeals)	• Established four-factor balancing test to determine FAPE • Considered educational and nonacademic benefits	Means educational and nonacademic benefit must be basis of placement considerations
Poolaw v. Bishop (1995) (State of Arizona; Ninth Circuit Court of Appeals)	• Found that in certain cases, the severity of the student's disability may require a more restrictive environment to provide the child educational benefit	Allows for consideration of specialized communication needs
McWhirt by McWhirt v. Williamson County School (1994) (State of Tennessee; Sixth Circuit Court of Appeals) and Kari H. v. Frankin Special School District (1995) (State of Tennessee; Sixth Circuit U.S. District Court)	• Determined that the severe nature of a student's disability can prevent the student from receiving educational benefit in a regular classroom	When working as part of an individualized education program team, one considers the complexities of the disability for program service decisions

with disabilities, speech-language pathologists and all educators can see that FAPE decisions must focus on the concept of meaningful benefit.

Meaningful benefit must be defined through the IEP goals, which are outcome-oriented and address the student's needs from a functional point of view. Specifically, IEP goals must be designed to teach skills that will make students functional in the general education environment and in their vocational and social roles after receiving a high school diploma. (See Chapter 4 for further discussion of IEP goal development.)

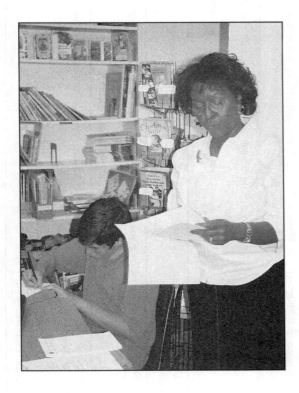

Court cases will decide the ultimate definition of this new standard of meaningful benefit to determine FAPE (Albanese, 2000). This change in the law will continue to have effects on students, professionals, and parents. Speech-language pathologists and educators will need to work to this standard as they develop goals for their students' IEPs.

Application of FAPE and LRE to Speech-Language Services

Educators feel the impact of legislative and judicial decisions on their daily work (Montgomery, 1994a). In 1995, Putnam, Spiegel, and Bruininks surveyed educators with special education expertise to identify trends they believed were both desirable and likely to occur by the year 2000. The educators' expectations included the following:

- Inclusionary practices would increase

- Use of categorical labeling would be gradually reduced

- Students with moderate and mild disabilities would be educated primarily in the regular classroom

- Integration would be more likely to occur at elementary than secondary levels

- Educators would need to increase their instructional methods to accommodate greater student diversity

- Personnel preparation would include training in teamwork, group process, and communication skills with a focus on instructional categories (e.g., math and reading) rather than student categories (i.e., disability areas)

- Technology would take a more predominant role in education

- Shifts in societal values would more greatly influence service trends than research

Trends in economics, society, and education are no longer identified on a 5- to 10-year projection, but rather on a 2- to 3-year projection. The influence of technology and the rapid pace of the information society are familiar to us. When examining the predictions noted above, however, the educators surveyed seemed to have an accurate view of the future for education, special education, and the working world of speech-language pathologists. The above trends demonstrate the evolution of the foundational concepts of FAPE and LRE.

Speech-language programs must comply with FAPE and LRE guidelines. To ensure that all children receive FAPE, "the services and placement needed by each child with a disability to receive FAPE must be based on the child's unique needs and not on the child's disability" (34 C.F.R. § 300.300 [3] [ii]). To ensure that LRE is achieved, states are required to provide a "continuum of alternative placements to meet the unique needs of each child with a disability" (34 C.F.R. § 300.130; 300.551). Speech-language pathologists need to provide a continuum of services using several different service delivery models, which may include COLLABORATION, co-teaching, direct/pull-out services, CONSULTATION, and others. A one-size-fits-all model might have been typical of service delivery in the early 1970s, but is not in the spirit of FAPE and LRE.

The continuum of special education programs in schools must also be broad. This means that not only will the continuum of placements be extensive (i.e., resource room, special class, related services, special school), but also that the service delivery models of each will be varied. In working with other members of the IEP team, speech-language pathologists will need to coordinate their services with the continua and delivery models of other service providers. These new and evolving applications of FAPE and LRE can provide rich rewards for students and service providers (see Chapter 5 for a further discussion of service delivery).

Requirements of IDEA 1997

Special education and other educational programs are governed by a combination of federal, state, and local laws and regulations. Special education laws are extensive and encompass broad requirements. At the federal level, IDEA (1997) sets forth a framework of what is required. This law is then interpreted and administered by the Department of Education, which sets forth federal rules, known as the Code of Federal Regulations (C.F.R.). States then pass legislation that incorporates their interpretation of the federal law and regulations. Counties, administrative units, and school districts can adopt detailed procedures directing their implementation of state and federal laws. State laws may grant greater rights to children with disabilities and their parents than federal laws do, but they must at least meet the federal requirements. In some cases, the federal law leaves procedures to be set by states and local entities.

With the reauthorization of IDEA in 1997, Congress identified the lack of positive educational results as a major concern for the education of students with disabilities. IDEA shifted the focus of special education from educational access to accountability for educational results. According to Cernosia (1999), new requirements reflected this significant shift in the law with four main themes:

IDEA

1. Strengthening parental participation in the educational process

2. Accountability for student's participation and success in the general education curriculum and mastery of IEP goals/objectives

3. Remediation and disciplinary actions addressing behavior problems at school and in the classroom

4. Responsiveness to the growing needs of an increasingly more diverse society (p. 1)

According to the Office of Special Education and Rehabilitative Services (OSERS, 1999), while acknowledging that the mandate for special education had resulted in progress, Congress (IDEA, 1997) stated that there was a need to do much more. In order to accomplish this, reauthorization focused on the following five areas (OSERS, 1999). Each of these areas will be discussed in the sections that follow.

1. Raising expectations for children with disabilities

2. Increasing parental involvement in the education of their children

3. Ensuring that regular education teachers are involved in planning and assessing children's progress

4. Including children with disabilities in assessments, performance goals, and reports to the public

5. Supporting quality professional development for all personnel who are involved in educating children with disabilities

Raising Expectations for Children with Disabilities

Under IDEA (1997), IEP procedures contained several requirements for describing how the student would access the general education curriculum and identifying how the student's disability affected his or her ability to be successful in the curriculum. For speech-language pathologists, this requirement clearly pointed to the necessity of knowing and understanding the demands of the curriculum at all grade levels and across school, district, and state requirements (see Chapter 4 for specific regulations). Students are to participate in school-wide testing and demonstrate that they are making progress in the general education curriculum. Accommodations for a student's disability cannot be allowed to water down the curriculum or slow the pace of learning. The goal of achieving general education expectations challenges special educators to identify methods that will allow them to access the curriculum (Bateman and Linden, 1998; McLaughlin, Nolet, Morando Rhim, and Henderson, 1999).

> IDEA shifted the focus of special education from educational access to accountability for educational results.

Increasing Parental Involvement in the Education of Their Children

The history of special education—the denial of services to children and unilateral decision-making on the part of school personnel prior to the passage of EAHCA (1975)—led to the establishment of comprehensive procedural safeguards to ensure parent participation in the design of an IEP for their child. IDEA (1997) called for even greater parent involvement:

> The parents of a child with a disability are expected to be equal participants along with school personnel, in developing, reviewing, and revising the IEP for their child. This is an active role in which the parents (1) provide critical information regarding the strengths of their child and express their concerns for enhancing the education of their child; (2) participate in discussions about the child's need for special education and related services and supplementary aids and services; and (3) join with the other participants in deciding how the child will be involved in and progress in the general curriculum, how the child will participate in State- and district-wide assessments, and what services the agency will provide to the child and in what setting of those services. (34 C.F.R. Part 300, Appendix A, Question 5)

How to include parents as partners is described throughout IDEA (1997). For example, in defining who must participate in an IEP meeting, the federal law now identifies the parents of the child first on the list of required IEP meeting participants (34 C.F.R. § 300.344). The CFR contains several requirements designed to guarantee parent participation, including notifying parents with adequate time so that they have the opportunity to attend an IEP meeting;

Avenues to Improve Accountability in Special Education

Congress targeted these issues to address the concerns raised during the IDEA (1997) reauthorization process:

1. Improving scholastic performance
2. Accessing the general education curriculum
3. Supporting successful transitions
4. Providing placement in the Least Restrictive Environment (LRE)
5. Preventing school dropouts
6. Addressing children's behavioral problems effectively
7. Coordinating services for children and families
8. Supporting full family participation in children's education
9. Resolving disputes through mediation

Source: U.S. Department of Education (1999, pp. IV–2)

scheduling a meeting at a mutually agreed on time and place; involving students when appropriate; and documenting phone calls, correspondence, home visits, and all efforts to include parents (34 C.F.R. § 300.345).

Additional regulations clarified that while the parents have the right to participate in meetings regarding their child, this does not include:

> Informal or unscheduled conversations involving public agency personnel and conversations on issues such as teaching coordination of service provision if those issues are not addressed in the child's IEP. A meeting also does not include preparatory activities that public agency personnel engage in to develop a proposal or response to a parent proposal or response to a parent proposal that will be discussed at a later meeting. (34 C.F.R. § 301.501 [b] [2])

This specific provision is important for speech-language pathologists and other special educators because historically parents have raised the question about predetermination of eligibility and services if staff met to discuss the student in an informal meeting.

One additional requirement includes parental input in the review of education data for evaluation purposes (34 C.F.R. § 300.533). While this requirement was specific to an initial evaluation, GOOD PRACTICE would direct the speech-language pathologist to include parent input in each speech-language diagnostic assessment.

Working with parents as partners in the IEP process can be both rewarding and chal-

lenging. Speech-language pathologists of the future must have well-developed skills in many different areas to work with parents, both as participants in the IEP and evaluation processes and as partners in the intervention for identified children.

Ensuring That Regular Education Teachers Are Involved in Planning and Assessing Children's Progress

Regular education teachers must participate in the development, review, and revision of IEPs.

> Very often, regular education teachers play a central role in the education of children with disabilities and have important expertise regarding the general curriculum and the general education environment. Further, with the emphasis on involvement and progress in the general curriculum added by the IDEA Amendments of 1997, regular education teachers have an increasingly critical role (together with special education and related services personnel) in implementing the program of FAPE for most children with disabilities, as described in their IEPs. (34 C.F.R. Part 300, Appendix A, Question 1)

IDEA (1997) requires the following for the participation of general education teachers in the IEP process:

- The student's teachers must have access to the IEP document (34 C.F.R. § 300.342 [b]).

- Teachers must be informed of their specific responsibilities related to implementing the IEP (34 C.F.R. § 300.342 [b]).

- Teachers must be informed of the specific modifications, and supports that must be provided to the student (34 C.F.R. § 300.342 [b]).

- Teachers must participate in the development, review and revision of the IEP, including assisting in developing positive behavioral interventions and determining supplementary aids and services and program modifications (34 C.F.R. § 300.346 [d]).

> [S]peech-language pathologists must know the workings of the general education classroom and the expectations for teachers and students, in order to provide support to both.

- Services to assist the teacher, such as consultation or training, can be included under supplemental aids and services (34 C.F.R. § 300.347 [a] [3]).

- Attendance and participation of a regular education teacher is required if the student is, or may be, participating in the regular education environment (34 C.F.R. § 300.344 [a] [2]).

The intent of these regulations is to guarantee that special education is not a "place," or a separate system, but rather a support to general education. Consequently, speech-language pathologists must know the workings of the general education classroom and the expectations for teachers and students, in order to provide support to both.

The requirement for participation of general education teachers on IEP teams brings a new dimension to the IEP. For professionals, it reinforces the reality that children on their CASELOAD are part of a school system. The services provided by the speech-language pathologist or any other special educator must be designed to assist the child in benefiting from the core curriculum. The general education teacher brings this focus to the IEP team. General education teachers will need guidance in terms of their role and responsibilities as team members and at IEP meetings. Chapters 5, 6, and 7 offer ideas that might help the general education teacher be prepared to participate on the IEP team.

Including Children with Disabilities in Assessments, Performance Goals, and Reports to the Public

Children with disabilities had traditionally been excluded from statewide academic assessments, often known as high-stakes testing (Allington and McGill-Franzen, 1992; Chard, 1999; Gartner and Lipsky, 1987; McGill-Franzen and Allington, 1993; McGrew, Thurlow, Shriner, and Spiegel, 1992; Thurlow and Thompson, 1999; Ysseldyke, Thurlow, McGrew, and Shriner, 1994). Such testing would include any achievement testing done on a large scale (e.g., schoolwide, gradewide, districtwide, statewide). Examples of statewide testing are the Stanford 9 or the Iowa Test of Basic Skills. Frequently the results of such testing are reported in the newspapers; posted on the Internet; and, more recently, used to determine if a school or school district should have state-assisted intervention to improve student performance at a particular classroom, school, or district (Raber, Roach, and Fraser, 1998).

Students with disabilities were typically excluded from statewide assessments until the mid-1990s, when reform movements in both general and special education called for educational systems to be responsible and accountable for the learning of all students. Under IDEA (1997), states are now required to include students with disabilities in statewide and districtwide assessment programs (34 C.F.R. § 300.347; § 300.138; § 300.347). For students who cannot participate in the state or districtwide assessment programs, alternate assessments must track the progress of these students.

> For students who cannot participate in the state or districtwide assessment programs, alternate assessments must track the progress of these students.

In addition to including students with disabilities in the statewide and districtwide accountability program, IDEA (1997) also requires states to have performance goals and indicators established for children with disabilities. These goals must be consistent to the maximum extent appropriate with the performance goals and standards for children without disabilities.

Supporting Quality Professional Development for All Personnel Who Are Involved in Educating Children with Disabilities

IDEA (1997) requires each state to maintain a Comprehensive System of Personnel Development (CSPD). Professional development is provided in a variety of different ways. Among these are workshops, conferences, specialized trainings, mentoring, staff meetings, professional study groups, professional journals, and others. Individuals may obtain professional development from professional associations, such as the AMERICAN SPEECH-LANGUAGE-HEARING ASSOCIATION'S (ASHA's) or state-level speech and hearing associations' meetings, or from other agencies that provide workshops and trainings. Increasingly, LEAs are taking on the responsibility of staff development. These trainings might focus on an identified need area in the school or district. State and regional trainings might also be available to both general and special education professionals.

Under IDEA (1997), states are responsible for ensuring an adequate supply of qualified special education, general education, and related services personnel, as well as paraprofessionals who are prepared to work with children with disabilities. The state is also responsible to implement practices for recruitment, preparation, and retention of qualified personnel. As much as any other requirement, the need for fully qualified staff is at the center of implementing special education programs that will enable students to be successful.

Once individuals are hired into the system, employing agencies have an obligation to continue to ensure the professional growth of their staff. At one time, school districts held that this was a professional's personal responsibility, a perspective shared by the authors (see "Continuing Education" in Chapter 9). However, due to the need for districts to attract and retain qualified staff, as well as increased demands and the need to insure that professionals are utilizing researched-based strategies with students, employers are viewing provision of staff development opportunities as part of a their ongoing responsibilities and necessities.

Offers of professional development can be a key to recruitment of skilled staff. Following through with those offers can be key to retention. Many agencies find recruitment and retention to be a staggering task, due to documented shortages, which exist for a variety of reasons. Because of the short supply of speech-language pathologists, employing agencies must support their existing staff. Encouraging and providing professional development is one way to accomplish this.

Due to the comprehensive shortage of special education and related services staff (of which speech-language pathologists are a part), a shift has occurred in the employment of other-than-fully-qualified staff. It is not unusual for individuals to be working in special education, general education, or related service areas before completing the requirements for that position. Due to this situation in the late 1990s, school districts and local regionalized areas took on training and staff development in new and creative ways, including using mentor teachers or coaches and other methods for assisting educators in their classroom or direct service situations.

Teacher shortages may also create collateral, albeit unintentional, consequences on existing staff. One is that caseload size could be increased due to an inability of a district or LEA to fill vacant positions. Another issue is that the fully trained speech-language pathologist (or other education specialist) is likely to be working with team members who did not have the necessary training for their job. Speech-language pathologists, due to a greater level of education, were frequently called on to provide leadership in these situations in the 1990s. Although often a taxing situation, expanded opportunities for leadership and skill development have evolved for school-based speech-language pathologists.

The issue of "Developing a Highly Trained Teacher Workforce" is addressed in the *Twenty-First Annual Report to Congress on the Implementation of the Individuals with Disabilities Education Act* (U.S. Department of Education, 1999). Although reforms have been ongoing since the 1980s (see Chapter 1 for a discussion of the three waves of educational reform), the report states that teacher preparation programs have remained "virtually unchanged" (p. I-33). Well-prepared teachers are critical to the success of any reform movement. "[T]he critical link between teaching practice and student achievement" (p. I-33) is evident, but had previously been ignored. Educators entering the workforce must come in prepared to meet the many challenges waiting for them in the classroom. Effective preservice training is a key beginning to educating skilled professionals.

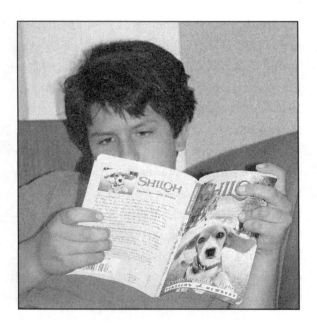

Including Students with Disabilities in Standards-Based Reform

Three waves of educational reform are discussed in Chapter 1. Wave Three reform was described as the reform movement that would join the forces of general and special education in setting high standards to improve educational results for *all* children, including those with disabilities. Standards-based reform has been evident since the early 1990s. According to the

Twentieth Annual Report to Congress on the Implementation of the Individuals with Disabilities Act (U.S. Department of Education, 1998), standards-based reform was built on four concepts:

1. Establishing high standards, both in terms of what students are expected to know (rigor), but also in terms of the level of performance at which this is to be demonstrated

2. Accountability to students and the educational system

3. The implementation of consequences, including sanctions and rewards, as part of the accountability system

4. The use of assessments to measure the performance and progress of students toward meeting the standards

To realize these four concepts, federal and state agencies will mandate and watch for the involvement of individuals with disabilities in various activities, including: "(1) involvement of special education in State-based reform activities, (2) current practices and policies in statewide assessments, (3) reporting of the performance of students with disabilities, and (4) research findings relevant to standards-based reform" (U.S. Department of Education, 1998, p. IV-3).

Standards-based reform relies on a philosophy of having a systematic method of measuring student achievement. Standards were meant to apply to all students. In terms of students with disabilities, this approach represented a significant shift in the thinking about student learning and programming. Special education was built on the design of an individualized plan for each learner, that is an individualized education program, or IEP. Individualized determinations were made for each student. Previously, "neither the federal nor any state statute has attempted to specify *what* children with disabilities could or should learn" (McDonnell, McLaughlin, and Morison, 1997, p. 53). IDEA (1997) called for a shift from access to quality education; sitting in a classroom with nondisabled peers was no longer considered enough for students with disabilities. These students must learn and the system must be responsible. In a system seeking results, individualized performance was no longer the only consideration for students with disabilities. How special education students performed alongside the other learners in the school was equally considered. "From the perspective of standards-based reform, however, the issue is not *where* students with disabilities receive their education, but whether they have access to a challenging curriculum and high-quality instruction consistent with state and local standards" (McDonnell et al., 1997, p. 60).

Broadening the view toward the bigger picture of the educational system will be no small task for some special educators. Speech-language pathologists must realize how the philosophy of standards-based reform will shape their own view of the task they undertake when working with students. To this end, speech-language pathologists must consider their role as one who is knowledgeable in language development and disorders, as well as knowledgeable in curriculum:

Curriculum and instruction are the meat of the educational process. Real change in education comes with changes in the content that teachers teach and students learn and in the instructional methods that teachers use. Both curriculum and instruction in turn are shaped by expectations about the kinds of educational outcomes that students should manifest by the time they graduate from high school.

Standards-based reform has been built around a specific set of assumptions about curriculum and instructions, embodied in the content and performance standards that are central to the reforms. Special education, for its part, has been built around a set of assumptions about valued post-school outcomes, curricula, and instruction that reflect the diversity of students with disabilities and their educational needs. Whether students with disabilities will participate successfully in standards-based reform will depend largely on the degree of alignment between these two sets of assumptions." (McDonnell et al., 1997, p. 113)

Requirements were put in place that reflected the expansion of these new considerations (34 C.F.R. § 300.347). Speech-language pathologists and other special educators must address the following areas when developing IEPs for students:

- PRESENT LEVELS OF EDUCATIONAL PERFORM-ANCE, including how the disability affects involvement and progress in the general education curriculum

- Measurable annual goals, including benchmarks or short-term objectives related to enabling the student to be involved and progress in the general curriculum and to meet other educational needs

- Program modifications or supports for school personnel that will be provided for the child to advance toward annual goals; to be involved and progress in the general curriculum and in extracurricular and nonacademic activities; to be educated and participate with disabled and nondisabled peers

- Explanation of reasons and the degree to which students will not participate with nondisabled peers in the general education classroom and nonacademic activities

- IEP reports (at least as often as general education)

The ever-changing and evolving world of education requires the school-based speech-language pathologist to change as well. ASHA's *Guidelines for the Roles and Responsibilities of the School-Based Speech-Language Pathologist* (1999c) described the evolution of the role of the school-based speech-language pathologist from "speech correctionist" to speech-language pathologist, who serves an extremely complex caseload in a variety of service delivery models.

School-based speech-language pathologists' roles and responsibilities have evolved. They now include preparing students for academic success and the communication demands of the work force in the 21st century as well as alleviating handicapping conditions [sic] of speech and language disorders. (ASHA as cited in ASHA, 1999c, p. 12)

Students with and without disabilities are being educated in an environment of standards-based reform. Speech-language pathologists must know and understand the demands of the curriculum at various grade levels. They must know and understand the content and performance standards put in place for the students they serve. In order to provide services that will assist students in mastering curriculum and demonstrating achievement of benchmarks, speech-language pathologists need to design intervention with these goals in mind. In many cases, standards will be the link for the students. By using standards in IEP planning, benchmark setting, and intervention activities, speech-language pathologists will make meaningful connections to the classroom for teachers, parents, and students.

The history of special education has followed an evolutionary path. When the EAHCA was passed in 1975, the law focused on "child find," development of IEPs after a multidisciplinary assessment, and provision of an education in proximity to nondisabled peers. After more than 25 years of special education mandates, the law is now focused on the provision of a quality education with demonstration of progress in the general education curriculum. Making this happen requires the work of a team, of which the speech-language pathologist is a critical member.

CHAPTER 3

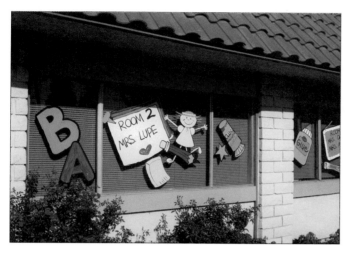

Referral and Assessment

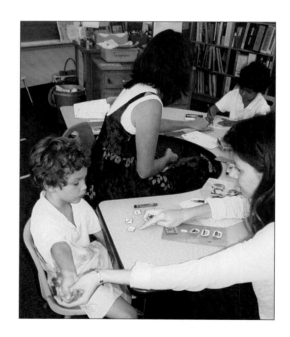

IN THIS CHAPTER

This chapter will describe the process that results in a student being identified as requiring special education services and placed in a special education program. The chapter will examine prereferral requirements and the referral and assessment process. Assessment methods considered to be good practice for speech-language services are highlighted. Procedural timelines are very important in educational programs.

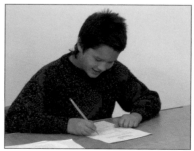

CHAPTER QUESTIONS

1. What is the difference between screening and assessment? Under what circumstances should the speech-language pathologist screen a student? How do the parent's rights differ for each activity and why?

2. Discuss the role of the speech-language pathologist in the prevention/intervention process in schools.

3. What are some of the classroom behaviors that should trigger a teacher to make a referral for a speech-language evaluation?

4. What are the three types of test protocols that speech-language pathologists should use for assessment and why are they all necessary?

Avenues to Referral

Not all children come to school having the same background and opportunities. Children come to school from homes in which English is the primary language and homes in which English is not the primary language; homes with hundreds of books and homes with no books; homes in which bedtime stories are read every night and homes in which no one has the LITERACY skills to help children with homework. Regardless of their background, public education in the United States greets all of these children and more.

Teachers and other educators are under a considerable amount of pressure at the beginning of the twenty-first century to provide a high quality education to students, developing youngsters who will become productive workers in an economy that promises to be dramatically different from that which the teachers knew. Children who do not successfully develop skills in math, language, reading, and problem solving will have great difficulty securing employment in an information work world. The economic reality of the widening gap between what is needed in the future work world and the potential for success for individuals who do not secure a solid education is cause for concern. Educators must face the weighty burden of dealing with each and every child who does not bring to the classroom the tools and circumstances that typically spell success. The situation is not new to schools. What is new is the high-profile focus on school reform, the keen societal interest in test scores and student performance, and the reality of an economic future that will not have vocational jobs for an unskilled labor force.

Students with speech, language, and hearing difficulties may be identified through individual REFERRAL, SCREENING, or both. These are two distinct activities with different purposes. Individual referrals are addressed as they arise throughout the school year. Screening, however, is part of an organized early observation process for some school districts scheduled at a specific time during the year in response to specific events (e.g., a child moves into the school district).

Referral

Screening Procedures

Some school districts ask speech-language pathologists to screen each year to identify students with communication difficulties who may not be referred by teachers, other professionals, or parents. Screening refers to a rapid pass/fail procedure used by speech-language pathologists to record communicative behaviors of all students of a particular grade level, category, or class and identify candidates for formal evaluation. The speech-language pathologist may, for example, screen all kindergartners, all third graders, all new students (see Figure 3.1 for an example from Charlotte-Mecklenburg Schools), all children at risk, or all children in the first quartile in reading achievement.

Screening usually employs a short face-to-face interview with the child, but screening may also include a teacher interview. The speech-language pathologist engages each child in a series of questions, a conversation, or both, to decide if more in-depth observation or

---

Figure 3.1

K–1 New Student Information

(after group screenings)

| To be completed by the classroom teacher and submitted to the SLP |

The following student has enrolled in my classroom:

Student: _____   Teacher: _____

Enrollment Date: _____   Enrolled From: _____

Please check records for hearing and speech / language screening information (health card or screening form)

Has this student had a hearing screening THIS year? _____   Date: _____

Has this student ever had a speech/language screening? _____   Date: _____

From *Handbook for Speech-Language Pathologists*, (p. 37), by the Charlotte-Mecklenburg Schools, Exceptional Children Department, 2000, Charlotte, NC: Author. © 2000 by the Charlotte-Mecklenburg Schools. Reprinted with permission.

assessment is necessary. Parental permission is not necessary at the screening level, since it is conducted with all children in a target population, is not a special education service, and is not diagnostic. Some districts keep documentation of screening as one of their CHILD FIND procedures required in the INDIVIDUALS WITH DISABILITIES ACT (IDEA) AMENDMENTS of 1997 (see Figure 3.2).

If the speech-language pathologist conducts a screening program, his or her responsibilities are to:

- Select screening measures with technical adequacy

- Administer and/or interpret a speech-language screening

- Administer and/or interpret a hearing screening in accordance with state and

local policy, procedures, and staffing patterns (American Speech-Language-Hearing Association [ASHA], 1997c).

Under direct supervision, support personnel may assist the speech-language pathologist to conduct screening programs. According to ASHA (1998b) guidelines, trained support personnel may administer a screening test, but not interpret it. (See Chapter 9 for further explanations of duties and limitations of support personnel.)

In some cases, formal or informal screening tasks are used by speech-language pathologists to observe a child in a classroom before holding a discussion with the STUDENT STUDY TEAM (SST) or similar school-based team. These teams meet regularly to problem-solve regarding students, recommend in-class modifications, or make referrals for special services. Parental permission is not required for observing at this level.

Figure 3.2

Speech-Language-Hearing Screening Results

Teacher: _____ Grade: _____ School Year: _____

Student Name	Date	Hearing Screening			Date	Speech/Language Screening				Comments
		R	L	HC		A	L	V	F	

Key

Hearing Screening: R = Right Ear   S/L Screening: A = Articulation
L = Left Ear   L = Language
HC = Health Card Marked   V = Voice
F = Fluency

Key for Marking Results

P = Passed Screening   **F** = Failed Screening   **M** = Monitor

From *Handbook for Speech-Language Pathologists* (p. 38), by the Charlotte-Mecklenburg Schools, Exceptional Children Department, 2000, Charlotte, NC: Author. © 2000 by the Charlotte-Mecklenburg Schools. Reprinted with permission.

Some districts do not conduct any screening, preferring to rely on referrals as more likely to correspond with adverse educational impact. Screening is a permissive activity determined by each school district, which means that procedures are established at the local level and can vary widely. Each speech-language pathologist needs to follow the policies and procedures of his or her employing district.

The AMERICAN SPEECH-LANGUAGE-HEARING ASSOCIATION (ASHA) has approved PREFERRED PRACTICE PATTERNS (1997c) for the Profession of Speech-Language Pathology in speech screening and language screening (see Appendix A) and in intervention (see Appendix B) to guide the speech-language pathologist. The screening patterns use the same elements as the assessment guidelines discussed later in this chapter (see "Preferred Practice Patterns in Assessment," page 75).

The Prereferral → Prevention
Prevention/Intervention Process

Long before a specialist becomes involved with a student for CONSULTATION or service, a teacher typically encounters the child in his or her classroom. Observant general education teachers immediately assist children if they begin to struggle with classroom demands. Such assistance might include providing individualized instruction, assigning the child an instructional aide, changing or modifying the materials or mode of presentation, using peer or cross-age tutoring, changing the child's seating position in the classroom, or making a variety of other adjustments to the classroom instructional program. All of these approaches constitute good teaching and are usually appropriate and effective, though such strategies may need to be reintroduced several times during the year when progress or motivation is lacking. Children receiving such support are not likely to need outside assistance. However, if left unassisted, these children may continue to struggle and eventually be referred to the special education system.

Traditionally, speech-language pathologists in public schools only dealt with identification of and remediation for students with COMMUNICATION DISORDERS. Today, however, speech-language pathologists are also engaged in prevention and prereferral activities. According to ASHA (1999c), the speech-language pathologist's role in prevention of communication disorders is "important" and "expanding" in three different ways:

Primary Prevention: The elimination or inhibition of the onset and development of a communication disorder by altering susceptibility or reducing exposure for susceptible persons. (p. 16)

Secondary Prevention: The early detection and treatment of communication disorders. Early detection and treatment may lead to the elimination of the disorder or the retardation of the disorder's progress, thereby preventing further complications. (p. 16)

Tertiary Prevention: The reduction of a disability by attempting to restore effective functioning. The major approach is rehabilitation of the disabled individual who has realized some residual problems as a result of the disorder. (p. 17)

The Student Study Team (SST)

Nearly all schools have a formalized process designed to support students who are struggling (see Figure 3.3). This prevention/intervention process may be commonly referred to as the Student Study Team (SST), Child Study Team (CST), Student Assistance Team (SAT), or

Figure 3.3

School-Based Prereferral Process

> Parent, teacher, or staff member observes that student has difficult, different, or delayed communication skills.

> Educator, in consultation with the parent, attempts own modifications and/or consults with other staff to assist the student.

> If student continues to struggle after modifications in place for a reasonable length of time (i.e., 6 weeks), an educator may:

Consult with the SLP who will:

1. Recommend additional modifications.

2. Provide follow-up consultation.

3. Observe and/or screen student.

4. Review results of modifications, screening, or consultation.

5. Recommend referral to SST.

6. Recommend referral for assessment.

Refer to the Student Study Team (SST) who will:

1. Recommend additional modifications to the teacher(s).

2. Recommend screening and/or consultation by SLP.

3. Discuss with the SLP.

4. Recommend a referral to SLP for assessment.

Student Success Team (SST) process. The name of this process varies in different parts of the country. For the purposes of this book, Student Study Team (SST) process will be used. The SST is a general education process intended to help any student in the school who is having difficulties in the classroom, as well as his or her teachers and family. The team usually consists of general education teachers from different grade levels, an administrator or counselor, a special education representative, and possibly the school psychologist or speech-language pathologist. The parents, and child if appropriate, are invited to the SST meeting.

The SST usually appoints a facilitator and a recorder. The facilitator will lead the team in a problem-solving discussion about the student, following a familiar, two-part process, such as:

1. Gathering Known Information

   • What are the student's strengths?

   • What do we know about the student?

   • What are the concerns?

   • What intervention strategies (i.e., accommodations and modifications) have been attempted? What were the results?

2. Troubleshooting

   • Brainstorm ideas for assistance.

   • Select what to try next and assign responsibility.

• Schedule when to meet again to report on progress.

Depending on the school and the district, the SST varies in its effectiveness and sophistication. Documented attempts to modify the general education program prior to referral for special educator evaluation are critical to determining if a student has a disability and if the student is in need of SPECIAL EDUCATION. Some states, such as California, require such documentation. The prevention/intervention process is intended to be an extension of the general education program and is not intended to be organized or facilitated by an individual from the special education program. Many schools, however, find that the speech-language pathologists and other specialists serving their sites have much to offer and so they invite them to be a part of the SST.

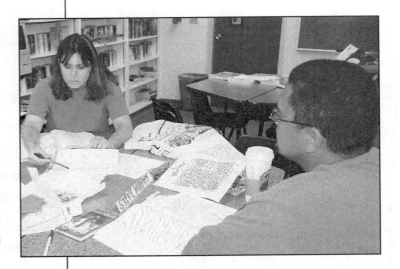

A frequent criticism of the SST process is that teachers (and sometimes parents) view the process as a delay to special education identification. In fact, the intent of the SST process is to provide adjustments to the instructional program to facilitate a student's learning. Not all children who are struggling in school have disabilities. Students who are considered "at risk" for educational failure (i.e., teen parents, children with low achievement or poor attendance, students involved with drug or alcohol, or delinquent behavior) or students who are educationally disadvantaged (e.g., children from homes with poverty or cultural/linguistical differences) may struggle in the classroom (Hardman, Drew, and Egan, 1999). These students should not necessarily be identified as disabled learners, who require special education and RELATED SERVICES. In fact, in IDEA (1997), Congress specifically addressed the problem of overidentification of minority children as being disabled, stating, "Greater efforts are needed to prevent the intensification of problems connected with mislabeling and high dropout rates among minority children with disabilities" (§ 601 [c] [8] [A]). This is one reason why many districts and states require several intervention strategies to be documented before referral to special education. Clearly these learners need assistance, but not necessarily special education.

The SST process enables educators to provide assistance to students before beginning a process of possible identification of a disability. The intention is to provide early support for children and families, but the SST process can also serve as part of the required child-find system for special education. The members of the SST ensure that meaningful modifications and interventions (not simply a shortening of assignments or changing in seating) have been attempted over a reasonable period of time prior to a referral for special education assessment.

Another reason that a formal prevention/intervention process is necessary is that once a student has been evaluated, the MULTIDISCIPLINARY ASSESSMENT TEAM must determine not only that the student has a disability, but also that the student is in need of special education and related services. If modifications to the general education program have not already been made, it will be difficult to document a need for special education.

The Speech-Language Pathologist's Role in the SST

The speech-language pathologist can contribute in several ways to the prevention/intervention process, including inservice training, consultation with parents and teachers, ideas for prereferral interventions, and screenings (ASHA, 1999c). Being an active member of the SST may also serve to prevent inappropriate referrals for speech-language services. Participation on this team can have collateral benefits of marketing the skills of speech-language pathologists, as they demonstrate their knowledge and expertise to parents, teachers, and administrators.

> As SLPs, we should function as regular members of a prereferral/referral committee. Decisions are made within this committee that directly affect our caseload. Speech-language-impaired students *[sic]* often have academic issues as well as speech-language concerns that need to be addressed before making a referral decision.
>
> Completion of interventions before screening referral ensure *[sic]* that a student's prob-

lems are not situational. There are times when we can avoid the evaluation process by observing in the classroom and consulting with the teacher. (Homer, 2000b, p. 3)

Children with perceived "speech only" problems are often referred directly to the speech-language pathologist, bypassing the SST process. These children may have articulation, fluency, or voice disorders. The benefit of using the SST process, instead of going directly to referral for assessment, is to ensure that other academic or social issues are not also affecting the student. Whether the need is speech or language, concern about academic impact must be considered. For example, as knowledge of the impact of phonemic awareness on literacy development has become more evident, a student with an articulation disorder should also be considered by the team in terms of reading skills. Utilizing the SST guarantees that the team reviews the student's progress in all learning areas. As a result of the speech-language pathologist's participation on the SST, other team members will develop awareness about the relationship of speech-language skills to academic performance.

After a teacher has attempted a variety of modifications for accommodations for a student and such adjustments are not successful, the teacher or parent can refer the student into a process designed for prevention of school failure and/or identification of needed intervention services.

The Referral Process

Some professionals who work with children are legally required to refer a child with a suspected disability to the school district. These professionals include physicians, nurses, teachers at state or county residential facilities, psychologists, social workers, or administrators of social agencies. Before making the referral, the professional must inform the parent that the referral will be made. The referral must be in writing and must include the reason why the child is believed to have a disability. Classroom behaviors that may be indications of possible communication problems and lead to referral include:

- Difficulty with reading
- Difficulty with spelling and writing
- Difficulty being understood when speaking in class
- Vague or evasive answers
- Frequent absences or avoidance of school
- Inability to attend or stay focused
- Rubbing ears or complaining of pain in ears
- Unusual vocal quality or recurrent hoarseness
- Avoiding making eye contact with teachers or others (not culturally based)
- Unwillingness to speak in front of the class

If speech-language pathologists provide an inservice for teachers on how and when to refer students, teachers will be more skillful observers and this method of identifying students can be very effective. Schulman (as cited in Campbell, 1999a) observed that teachers could accurately identify students with possible communication disorders in their classes, especially if the teachers had received training from a speech-language pathologist. Referral of a student by a teacher usually initiates an individual screening and a teacher interview by the speech-language pathologist or a referral to the SST.

Referrals for assessment may come from many sources: parents, teachers, school psychologists, physicians, and students themselves. If parents ask the school to assess their child, speech-language pathologists, as members of the team, must address this request immediately. Referral by a teacher requires general education interventions before a formal assessment is undertaken. Written permission from parents is necessary to continue further in the formal assessment process for determination of special education ELIGIBILITY.

Initial Assessment for Speech and Language Disabilities

Once a referral is received, the speech-language pathologist gathers information from the referring source; consults with the parents; observes the student formally, informally, or both; and then decides what diagnostic testing is necessary. Written parent permission is required before diagnostic testing is begun. Several team members' activities depend upon the speech-language pathologists' actions. In some cases, parents need reassurance. Psychologists may need corroborating data for a diagnosis that

includes a communication component. General educators may be totally unaware of the academic impact of a hearing loss or AUDITORY PROCESSING problems and will need guidance during this information-collection stage.

Speech-language pathologists need to exercise careful judgement to move to the stage of formally testing a child. In-depth testing utilizes a state's "battery of tests" if there is one, the speech-language pathologist's choice of supplementary tests, plus the anecdotal records and comments from others in the child's circle of acquaintances.

A child may be referred for a speech-language evaluation in a variety of ways. Most typically, the student will be referred from either the SST or the child's parents. Referrals may also come directly from classroom teachers, mass-screening coordinators, and medical or mental health professionals. Some school districts have received referrals from judges who order assessments to be completed in child custody or other types of situations. If a referral of this nature is received, special education administration should be consulted by the team or individual receiving the referral. Districts and states may choose a variety of ways to respond to such a referral. While the majority of referrals for assessment will come through the SST, the speech-language pathologist and other educators should never ignore any request for assessment. These professionals must have a complete understanding of the process and procedures for dealing with referrals from all sources other than SST.

No child may be provided special education and related services until an evaluation is completed (34 CODE OF FEDERAL REGULATIONS [C.F.R.] § 300.531). This is a critical part of the law. "Comprehensive assessment (data collection) and evaluation (interpretation of that data) enable the speech-language pathologist to identify students with significant communication disorders that are educationally relevant" (ASHA, 1999c, p. 32).

Conducting an evaluation before providing services is a logical course of events. The potential difficulty for a speech-language pathologist may arise if a parent, teacher, or administrator tries to pressure the speech-language pathologist to "just put Johnny in speech class. He only needs a little bit of help with his speech." Students must be evaluated and then determined eligible because of a disability requiring special education services. Any attempt to circumvent this process is considered a violation of the student's DUE PROCESS rights. Additionally, evaluation allows for a thorough assessment of the student's learning strengths and needs.

> The importance of an accurate and thorough evaluation cannot be overstated. The evaluation is the key to detecting the existence of a student's disability or disabilities, and it sets the parameters for the course of special education and related services that will follow if the student is determined to be eligible. (Gorn, 1997b, p. 2:1)

Team Approach

An efficient and effective assessment of a student's communication skills facilitates the work of the team in identifying needs of the student and family. The steps necessary for an initial assessment for a communication disability are outlined in Figure 3.4.

The speech-language pathologist alone does not determine eligibility for special education services; all evaluations must be multidisciplinary. Once a referral is received, the MULTIDISCIPLINARY TEAM (MDT) must develop an ASSESSMENT PLAN and obtain parental consent. The assessment plan must include an evaluation of the child in "all areas related to the suspected disability including, if appropriate, health, vision, hearing, social and emotional status, general intelligence, academic performance, communicative status, and motor abilities" (34 C.F.R. § 300.532 [g]). State law will dictate the timelines required for presentation of the assessment plan, generally ranging from 10 to 15 days. In both California and New Jersey, for example, the MDT has 15 calendar days, following a request for assessment, to present the parent with an assessment plan.

Often the SST or similar schoolwide decision-making group suggests that a communication problem could be contributing to a student's poor achievement. The student may be referred to the speech-language pathologist for assessment due to an academic problem noticed by the team. When approached this way, the second condition of the identification process, adverse educational impact, has already been noted and the speech-language pathologist needs to investigate possible speech- and

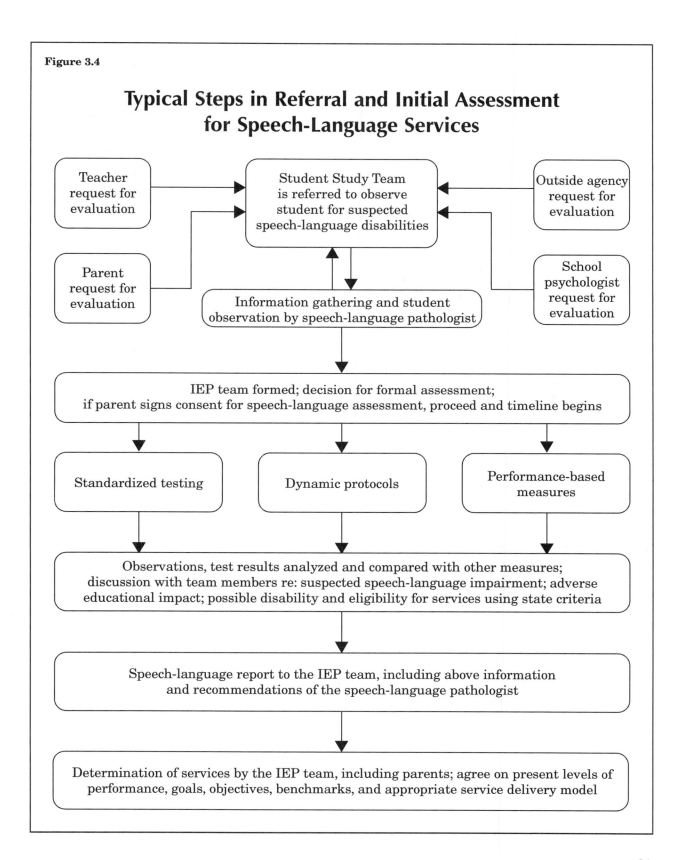

Figure 3.4

Typical Steps in Referral and Initial Assessment for Speech-Language Services

Teacher request for evaluation

Parent request for evaluation

Outside agency request for evaluation

School psychologist request for evaluation

Student Study Team is referred to observe student for suspected speech-language disabilities

Information gathering and student observation by speech-language pathologist

IEP team formed; decision for formal assessment; if parent signs consent for speech-language assessment, proceed and timeline begins

Standardized testing

Dynamic protocols

Performance-based measures

Observations, test results analyzed and compared with other measures; discussion with team members re: suspected speech-language impairment; adverse educational impact; possible disability and eligibility for services using state criteria

Speech-language report to the IEP team, including above information and recommendations of the speech-language pathologist

Determination of services by the IEP team, including parents; agree on present levels of performance, goals, objectives, benchmarks, and appropriate service delivery model language-related causes. The speech-language pathologist, as a member of the SST or similar school assistance team, may already be familiar with the student's learning challenges. If the student is not known to the speech-language pathologist, a discussion with the team is the first step. Involvement with the SST may be part of the prereferral process, required by IDEA (1997) and described in professional documents on speech-language assessment (ASHA, 1989a, 1999c). Prereferral activities assure the speech-language pathologist and other team members that modifications and non-special education interventions have been attempted before the student is referred for possible assessment.

Parent Consent

Informed parent consent is one of the most important procedural safeguards afforded to parents, ensuring their participation in the process and that they have been informed that their child is suspected of having a disability. (Chapter 8 provides a full discussion of procedural safeguards in "Parental Notification and Involvement.")

(1) Informed parent consent must be obtained before—

    (i) Conducting an initial evaluation or reevaluation; and

    (ii) Initial provision of special education and related services to a child with a disability.

(2) Consent for initial evaluation may not be construed as consent for initial placement... (34 C.F.R. § 300.505)

Consent means that—

(i) The parent has been fully informed of all information relevant to the activity for which his or her consent is sought, in his or her native language, or other mode of communication;

(ii) The parent understands and agrees in writing to the carrying out of the activity for which his or her consent is sought, and the consent describes that activity and lists the records (if any) that will be released and to whom; and

(iii) (A) The parent understands that granting of consent is voluntary on the part of the parent and may be revoked at anytime. (34 C.F.R. § 300.500)

An initial assessment must not begin until a parent returns a consent form. The speech-language pathologist, as a member of the SST may have already informally observed the child. When the consent form is sent to a parent or guardian, notification of parent and child rights must be sent as well. (See the example cover letter in Figure 3.5 and the example consent form in Figure 3.6.) The parent must agree in writing to the assessment. During the assessment, parents should be interviewed by the speech-language pathologist as IDEA (1997) requires parent input to the assessment process.

Figure 3.5

Cover Letter to Accompany Consent Form

Dear Parent:

   Your child has been referred to the Multidisciplinary Team for a speech/language evaluation. In order to evaluate your child's speech/language skills, we need your consent. Our goal is to provide your child with the best possible education to meet his or her needs.

   Enclosed is a consent form for you to sign and a Handbook of Parents' Rights to give you more information about the Exceptional Children's Services. Please sign the enclosed form and return the white copy to school tomorrow. You may keep the yellow copy and the Handbook for your records.

   Remember, speech and language skills are very important for reading and writing. If you have any questions about the speech/language evaluation, please don't hesitate to call. We will contact you soon to schedule a conference to discuss the evaluation results.

Sincerely,

_____

Speech/Language Pathologist

_____

Phone Number   Date

From *Handbook for Speech-Language Pathologists* (p. 29), by the Charlotte-Mecklenburg Schools, Exceptional Children Department, 2000, Charlotte, NC: Author. © 2000 by the Charlotte-Mecklenburg Schools. Reprinted with permission.

The initial assessment is the first of several times that parents must be informed of their procedural rights. Members of the evaluation team must make sure that parents and students understand their rights. The speech-language pathologist is often responsible for providing a copy of the rights to parents, and it is important to document that a copy of the parent/child rights were given to the parents. (See Chapter 8 for a further discussion of parent and child rights.)

Parents sometimes refuse to give their consent for assessment. If school district personnel believe that a child has a disability, the school district may need to request mediation or a DUE PROCESS HEARING on the issues (34 C.F.R. § 300.505 [b]), depending on state law. In California, for example, state law requires that school districts file for (i.e., request) a due process hearing if the parent's actions do not afford the child access to FREE APPROPRIATE PUBLIC EDUCATION (FAPE). The C.F.R. also directs school districts that "A public agency may not use a parent's refusal to consent to one service or activity…to deny the parent or child any other service, benefit, or activity of the public agency" (34 C.F.R. § 300.505 [e]). Generally, school districts are not allowed to simply agree to or ignore a refusal of consent, because it may not be in the best interest of the child. Speech-language pathologists should always consult a special education administrator when these questions or issues arise.

The majority of the time, parents consent to the proposed assessment. The CASE MANAGER

Figure 3.6

Notice and Consent Regarding Need to Conduct Additional Tests

Name of child (last, first, middle)	Date of birth	District of Residence

Dear _____ Date _____

Previously you were notified of the school district's intent to evaluate your child to determine whether he/she has a disability (impairment and need for special education). The individualized education program (IEP) team is responsible for this evaluation. You are a participant on the IEP team. The IEP team considered the following existing evaluation procedures, tests, records or reports:

The IEP team has determined that additional tests or other evaluation materials are needed to determine whether your child has a disability.

☐ You participated in making this decision.

☐ You did not participate and the school district made 3 attempts to involve you as follows:

The school district needs your written consent (permission) before it can administer tests or other evaluation materials to your child. With your consent the following tests of other evaluation materials will be administered.

The following tests or other evaluation materials will be administered:

Areas to be Evaluated	Description of tests and other evaluation materials and titles, if known	Qualifications to Evaluate	Name, if known

Other evaluation options considered, if any, and reasons rejected and a description of any other factors relevant to the proposed evaluation of this child:

❑ None

Following the administration of these tests or other evaluation materials the IEP team will meet to review the results of these tests and other evaluation materials as well as other existing information available on your child, including information provided by you. Each IEP team participant who administered additional tests or other evaluation materials will have prepared, based upon his/her evaluation, a written summary of findings that will assist with program planning. A copy of each of these participant's summary of findings will be made available to all IEP team participants at an IEP team meeting. Using the results of these tests or other evaluation materials along with other available information, the IEP team will make a determination of whether your child has a disability. As a participant on the IEP team, you will be involved in this determination. Upon completion of the evaluation, the IEP team will prepare an evaluation report which will include documentation of your child's eligibility for special education. If the IEP team determines that your child is a child with a disability, the team will develop an IEP to meet your child's needs and determine a placement to carry out the IEP.

If at any point during an IEP team meeting to determine your child's eligibility for special education, develop an IEP, or determine a placement, you or other IEP team participants believe that additional time is needed to permit your meaningful involvement, additional time will be provided. This IEP team process may be concluded in one meeting or may require more than one meeting depending on individual circumstances.

At the beginning of any meeting to address the evaluation, IEP, or placement of your child, the school district must discuss with you your right to have additional time as described above and of your right to have a copy of the IEP team's evaluation report prior to developing an IEP and placement. Upon request you and the other IEP team participants may receive a copy of the team's evaluation report prior to continuing with the development of your child's IEP and placement. If you have not requested a copy of the team's evaluation report the school district will give you a copy of the report when you receive a notice of your child's placement or notice that your child is not a child with a disability.

You and your child have protection under the procedural safeguards (rights) of special education law. Previously you received a copy of your procedural safeguard rights in a brochure about parent and child rights. If you would like another copy of this brochure, please contact the school district at the telephone number above. In addition to district staff, you may also contact _____ at _____ if you have questions about your rights.

_____
(Name and Title of District Contact Person)

PARENT CONSENT/PERMISSION TO ADMINISTER TESTS AND OTHER EVALUATION MATERIALS AS PART OF AN INITIAL EVALUATION

I understand my consent is voluntary and may be revoked at any time during the administration of tests or other evaluation materials. I also understand that if I do not consent for the school district to administer these tests or other evaluation materials, the school district may request mediation or initiate a due process hearing regarding whether those tests or other evaluation materials should be administered. I understand the action proposed by the school district and

❑ I give my consent for the school district to administer these tests or other evaluation materials described above to my child as part of an initial evaluation.

❑ I do not give my consent for the school district to administer these tests or other evaluation materials described above to my child as part of an initial evaluation.

_____   _____
(Signature of parent or legal guardian or adult student)   (Date)

From *Revised Sample Special Education Forms* (pp. 10–12) [Microsoft Word Format], by the Wisconsin Department of Public Instruction, 2000, Madison, WI: Author.

should always note on the assessment plan the date that the signed plan was returned to school. Sometimes parents forget to return the paper. If this should happen, a phone call or note home is generally enough of a reminder.

Timelines

Once the assessment plan is received, the MDT has a certain period of time in which to complete the assessment. IDEA (1997) requires that the district complete the evaluation and make services available within "a reasonable period of time following the agency's receipt of parental consent to an initial evaluation of a child" (34 C.F.R. § 300.343 [b]). Specific timelines vary from state to state. Generally, the timeline is between 30 and 60 days. Some examples include Michigan: 30 days, New York: 40 days, California: 50 days, and Illinois: 60 days.

Diagnostic testing may take upwards of 6 hours, a scheduling challenge for many speech-language pathologists with large CASELOADS and long lists of students to assess. Timelines for the assessment process, such as the sample in Table 3.1, are designed by many states and school districts to aid special educators in meeting the IDEA (1997) requirements. Such timelines may vary from state to state. Note that the speech-language pathologist must respond to the parents within 15 days when an assessment is requested, and have the results of the assessment within 50 days after the date of permission to assess is received. In some school districts, one or more speech-language pathologists rotate from school to school to assist with testing so that timelines can be maintained. It is important

for the speech-language pathologist to notify a supervisor if help is needed, as violations of timelines are considered serious problems with repercussions at local, district, and state levels.

State-imposed timelines refer to the number of calendar days (not school or work days) the MDT has between the time the family returns the assessment plan and an IEP meeting is convened (Gorn, 1997b). A one- or two-month wait for a team decision and the possible start of services can be difficult for parents, students, and teachers. Table 3.2 illustrates critical timelines for evaluation and IEP activity.

The regulations, timelines, documentation, and procedures of special education are all tightly regulated and businesslike. Families who are from cultures other than that of mainstream America, or who are struggling with issues of daily living, may not always be responsive to the important timelines and deadlines in special education. Some speech-language pathologists have experienced working with refugee families who are fearful of authority, due to the oppression in the countries they fled. In other situations, cultural parameters value oral, not written, communication, so meeting notices go unheeded, but visits to the home are welcomed. Individuals may also operate on a different value system regarding time. The team may find that the family arrives for a meeting (sometimes with many family members) either several hours early or several hours late. Transportation issues may also prevent families from coming to a meeting; for example, a family may not have the resources to access transportation services that might be available to them.

Table 3.1

Procedural Timeline for a State Special Education Program Designed to Meet IDEA (1997) Requirements

Identification, Screening, Referral, Assessment, Planning, Instruction, Review

Time Frame	Task
15 calender days	Referral of individual with exceptional needs and parents contacted. Assessment plan developed. Parents receive written rights and safeguards. Notification of assessment is written.
15 calender days	Parents have this amount of time to decide and provide written consent if they wish to proceed.
20 calender days	Students who transfer into a district may be placed in a comparable program for this length of time before additional assessment or previous records are obtained.
50 calender days	Assessment is conducted by multidisciplinary assessment team. Parent receives written notice of IEP team planning meeting. Meeting is held and eligibility is determined.
30 calender days	An interim placement determined by the IEP team.
Immediately or within a few days	Parent consents in writing to the IEP. The plan is implemented.
One year (sooner if requested)	Review of the IEP is completed.
Three years (sooner if requested)	Reassessment, as needed or at parent request, and determination if student continues special education services.

Source: California Department of Education (1999c)

Table 3.2

Evaluation Action Timelines

Action	Timelines	Notes
Request for assessment received	10–15 days to present parent with an assessment plan (AP)	If parent does not return AP signed, follow-up is needed
Signed assessment plan received	Team has specified days (30–60) to complete assessment	All days indicated are calendar days
IEP meeting held	Meeting notice sent 1–15 days prior to meeting date	Completed reports presented

Sometimes, issues created as a result of cultural difference become the responsibility of the IEP team. Helping families with these issues, and respecting their challenges, will help the student in the long run. Speech-language pathologists must utilize their own cultural competence to know and understand when paperwork and compliance with the legal parameters of the special education process are overwhelming or outside of the purview of the student's family. In these situations, assistance of a very different nature may be necessary.

Selecting the Appropriate Measurements

Selecting appropriate assessment tools is the next step in the process. Speech-language disabilities can be assessed using many different methods or a combination of methods. There are basically three methods for assessing students: STANDARDIZED TESTS; performance-based measures, including curriculum-based measures;

and dynamic protocols. Each method helps speech-language pathologists to gather information in a different way. Speech-language pathologists need to know each method, appropriate tools for that method, and when to use them.

Guidelines for assessment can be found in professional documents, graduate school textbooks (Damico, Secord, and Wiig, 1992), and state departments of education regulations. IDEA defines each eligible disability category including a speech-language disability (see Chapter 4 "Federal Eligibility Criteria for Special Education"). This section discusses what constitutes GOOD PRACTICE in communication assessment, and gives guidance in identifying a speech-language disability. States may specify what instruments to use, and local school districts may also specify particular approaches and tools for the speech-language pathologist. The sidebar provides examples of methods of assessment, which are commonly used in school settings. A second sidebar on page 72 lists initial evaluation requirements as specified within the C.F.R.

Methods of Assessment Commonly Used in School Settings

I. Standardized tests for each ability area
- Speech
- Language
- Voice
- Fluency
- Reading and writing skills
- Vocabulary
- Memory
- Word retrieval
- Perception
- Statewide achievement tests

II. Performance-based measures, including curriculum-based tests
- Video- or audiotaping
- Physiological functioning—vital capacity, oral motor examinations
- Checklists and scales of learning
- Local proficiency tests
- Unit tests
- Fine motor skills
- Self-help skills
- Social-emotional skills

III. Dynamic tests
- Cognitive tasks in nonstandardized format
- Floor-time
- Checklist with levels of support

Additional Methods of Assessment

I. Screening tests
- Speech-language
- Hearing

II. Observations
- Classroom
- Playground
- Home

III. Interviews
- Parents
- Teachers
- Other educators

IV. Review of student products
- Oral
- Written
- Technology based

Standardized Tests

Norm-referenced tests are produced by commercial publishers and are standardized on large populations of students. Such tests divide language and speech into components that are probed with a series of questions or tasks. Examiners must administer the tests in a standardized format, and only re-administer a test in the prescribed manner. The student's correct answers are tallied and this raw score is converted to a score on a statistical scale, which can be compared to the table of norms or average scores for other children of the same age. If the student's score is significantly lower than age expectations, he or she is judged to have a deficit in that area. Standardized tests are static measures. They take a "snapshot" of the student at one point in time, using one set of criteria, and administered in a prescribed way.

Standardized tests are used primarily to identify speech impairments, LANGUAGE DISORDERS, auditory perceptual problems, and academic achievement. There is a norm, or expected performance, for each tested skill at different ages. Students' abilities can be compared to other students of the same age across the country.

Standardized tests are constructed to account for the amount of growth expected within a year for a typical student, reflected in the scaled or standard score. After a student has taken a standardized test, retesting a year later is likely to show approximately the same standard score or lower. If a student made one year's growth in one year, his or her standard score would stay the same. If he or she made less than one year's growth—common for many students with disabilities who learn at a slower rate—his or her standard score would be lower than the initial testing because the standard score compares his or her growth with the expected growth for that period of time for students in the sample.

This statistical representation of growth is the reason that many thoughtful speech-language pathologists do not use standardized tests to measure change. If a student is making month-for-month progress, there will be no apparent improvement in the score. If a student makes less than one year's progress in one year, his or her skills will appear to decline because of the lower score. A student's standard score will increase only if he or she makes exceptionally fast progress and surpassed the rate of growth in the norming sample. Therefore, standardized tests are the most useful the first time they are given, especially for identification and initial assessment purposes, and they become less useful each time they are given thereafter. In some cases, students will show improvement on a standardized test, but the next two types of assessment procedures discussed are more reliable for this purpose.

Items on standardized tests are assumed to be appropriate for all children, though they are often normed on a population sample that does not reflect the cultural and linguistic diversity found in today's schools. Many of these tools are biased toward children in the economic, cultural, and linguistic mainstream. They assume that all students have the same experiences, language opportunities and styles of learning. For this reason, such tests must be selected and interpreted with care.

A standardized test should always be given in its entirety. Using subtests, or parts of tests, means standard scores do not apply and cannot be reported. Subtest tasks are viewed as performance indicators, not test scores. A few standardized tests are actually a battery of tests, and those subtests can be given independently. Speech-language pathologists need be completely familiar with the administration and technical manuals of the standardized tests they use. It is unwise to use standardized tests in nonstandardized ways at any time. Doing so prevents speech-language pathologists from administering a valid test at a later date, since the student's performance would be affected by familiarity with the items.

Performance-Based Assessments

Performance-based assessments are another form of static testing. Students are required to demonstrate knowledge and skills in either artificially created or authentic situations. Speech-language pathologists may engage students in conversation to assess, for example, topic maintenance, focus, vocabulary, fluency, or degree of dysarthria. Students may be asked to write, draw, explain, persuade, summarize, read a passage in a book, or retell a story. The process of collecting and analyzing a language sample is an example of performance-based assessment (Miller, 1999). The tasks are in real time and reveal the actual performance of the student.

Student products, rather than student behavior, may also be analyzed in performance-based testing. Speech-language pathologists may look at journal writing, artwork, term papers, homework, or school projects. Students may be observed participating in class or communicating with peers. Some speech-language pathologists use video- or audiotape to record the performance of a student for later, often team, analysis.

Recording physiological functioning—vital capacity, oral peripheral examinations, hearing acuity tests, monitoring of throat clearing—are other examples of performance-based assessments familiar to speech-language pathologists. Assessing a person with highly dysarthric speech, swallowing problems, a hearing loss, or English as a second language requires speech-language pathologists to interact with the individual rather than to ask questions from a formal test (Arvedson, 2000; Homer, Bickerton, Hill, Parham, and Taylor, 2000; Pena and Gillam, in press; Ukrainetz, Harpell, Walsh, and Coyle, 2000). AUGMENTATIVE AND ALTERNATIVE COMMUNICATION (AAC) users should be assessed on performance-based measures, because speech-language pathologists are interested in how well the AAC users communicate their ideas, and how they physically and linguistically create and transmit their message. Speech-language pathologists often want to determine if a student initiates and responds to communication in a natural setting, or want to measure COMMUNICATIVE INTENT.

Performance-based measures are not typically prepared commercially, although speech-language pathologists may be familiar with some tools that require students to make, create, or do something that is suggested on a checklist. The examiner is instructed to watch the child perform the activity and to record how a problem

---

Requirements for Initial Evaluations

- Evaluation materials are selected and administered so as not to be discriminatory on a racial or cultural basis

- Evaluation materials are in the child's native language or mode of communication as much as feasible

- Materials and procedures minimize the effect of English language skills for students with limited English proficiency

- A variety of tools and strategies gather relevant functional and developmental information

- Information from parents must be included

- Information must be included related to enabling the child to be involved in and progress in the general curriculum or appropriate preschool activities

- Information must assist in determining whether this is a child with a disability and what the contents of the IEP should be

- Standardized tests are valid for the purpose, and administered by trained and knowledgeable personnel according to directions

- Any nonstandard uses of tests are reported

- Evaluation materials include those tailored to assess specific areas of educational need, not just a single general intelligence quotient

- Tests are selected and administered to minimize effects of impaired sensory, manual or speaking skills

- No single procedure is used as the sole criterion for determining if this is a child with a disability or determining an appropriate program

- The child is assessed in all areas related to the suspected disability including, if appropriate, health, vision, hearing, social and emotional status, general intelligence, academic performance, communicative status, and motor abilities

- Comprehensive assessment identifies all special education and related service needs, whether or not these are commonly linked with the disability area identified with the child

- Technically sound instruments are used which may assess the relative contribution of cognitive and behavioral factors, in addition to physical or developmental factors

Source: (34 C.F.R. § 300.532)

---

is solved, an object is described, or a barrier is surmounted. Speech-language pathologists commonly use protocols to record the performance when instrumentation is used (e.g., audiometers, nasometers, or tape recorders). Speech-language pathologists may begin or end an assessment with performance-based tasks, making notes on students' SYNTAX, fluency, word choice, or eye contact without the restrictions of standardized questions, time limits, or uniform administration of items.

Performance-based testing is not informal assessment, although it is conducted informally. It is based on what students do in various situations, not on how they respond to an examiner's topic through standardized questioning. A student's skills are not compared to other students' skills, or found superior, average, lacking, or deficient. Rather, student performance is described, recorded, analyzed, and evaluated as a way of understanding what a student has learned and how he or she communicates.

Dynamic Testing

Dynamic testing is the observation of language or learning during the mediation process (Cole, Dale, and Thal, 1998; Lidz, 1991). Dynamic testing is not a static method of assessment; rather than taking a snapshot of performance (as standardized tests do) or analyzing a student's behavior, work, or functioning (as performance-based assessments do), dynamic testing looks for a description of behavior under varying conditions. The examiner is actively engaged in the task with the student, using a process-oriented approach that looks at the child as a learner (Ukrainetz et al., 2000). "Dynamic assessment is an interactive approach to the assessment process based on intervention, and it yields information that typically is limited in traditional (static) testing: predictive and prescriptive information" (Pena, 1996, p. 281).

Dynamic testing uses a test-teach-retest approach. A task is presented to the student who is then supported by the speech-language

pathologist, in all manner of ways, to accomplish the task. In this way, the speech-language pathologist can ascertain what type and degree of assistance is needed for the student to be successful. "One important assumption of dynamic testing is that all children are capable of learning" (Pena, 1996, p. 282). The examiner continues to provide assistance to the student until the student can perform. The examiner's role is interactive, not passive as it is in static testing. DYNAMIC ASSESSMENTS emphasize the learning process the child is using, not the products of past learning (Haywood, Brown, and Wingenfeld, 1990; Lidz, 1991; Pena, Miller, and Gillam, 1999; Wetherby and Prizant, 1998).

Known as process-oriented testing, dynamic assessment is based on the early twentieth-century work of Vygotsky (1978). He demonstrated that children achieved more when their teachers varied the learning tasks in deliberate ways. He considered intellectual development as a socially created phenomenon that could be manipulated by the adults in a child's world. Dynamic testing is used as the method to find out what types and amount of manipulation are helpful to student learning. This assessment information leads directly to intervention planning. Student success is measured by how much less mediation is needed to get the same result after intervention.

Dynamic testing does not result in scores. Instead, this method requires speech-language pathologists to record the student's level of performance, along with the type and degree of assistance that was most helpful as a starting point for the intervention process. *Modifiability* is the term used to describe the degree of assistance the student needs to be successful (Pena, 2000; Ukrainetz et al., 2000). Dynamic protocols can be used for assessing articulatory behaviors, voice abnormalities, pragmatics, and stuttering. Determining a student's specific phoneme stimulability is a dynamic assessment technique. Choosing phonological processing targets by cycling through all the phonemes is a dynamic process as well. There is limited research on applications for assessing language disorders dynamically (Pena, 1996; Pena, Quinn, and Iglesias, 1992). Widespread use of this approach is anticipated in the future (Butler, 1997; Secord and Damico, 1998; Wetherby, 1998). There are no set items or materials to conduct the assessment, and any conducive environment may be used.

Successful applications of dynamic assessment have included the assessment of children who are CULTURALLY/LINGUISTICALLY DIVERSE (CLD); preschool children (Moore-Brown, 2000; Pena et al., 1992; Schraeder, Quinn, Stockman, and Miller, 1999); and students with severe disabilities (Blackstone, 2000; Erickson and Koppenhaver, 1995; Wetherby, 1998). Speech-language pathologists in some school districts with culturally diverse populations have been taught to use dynamic assessment methods. Preliminary investigations of the assessment of Native American kindergartners have provided support for the further development of dynamic assessment as a less biased evaluation procedure than other testing protocols (Ukrainetz et al., 2000). Speech-language pathologists who have been trained to use dynamic assessment have reported increased confidence in their ability to diagnose difference from disorder in second-language learners (Pena et al., 1992).

Quality-of-Life Issues

Speech-language pathologists have few outcome measurements to help identify a student's level of participation in their life activities. FUNCTIONAL OUTCOMES refer to meaningful activities in one's life, which is a very large territory to assess. Quality of life should be measured using scales, inventories, and even wellness measures (WHO, 1980). For example, secondary-level students with speech-language challenges might be asked to respond to such questions as:

- Are you happy about your life?

- Do you enjoy what you are doing?

- Do you have friends? Can you communicate with them when you wish?

- Can you practice your religious faith or spiritual beliefs?

- Do you have a meaningful job?

- Are you making money for yourself and others? Are you paying taxes?

Elementary-level students might have a more limited range of quality-of-life statements. They could appear as:

- Are you happy almost every day?

- Do you enjoy school? Can you get what you need and want each day?

- Do you have friends? Can you talk to them easily?

- Can you receive help if you need it at school? At home?

- Do you have a hobby or favorite thing to do? Can you do it in your leisure time?

Students with communication disabilities should be able to have a typical quality of life.

School-based speech-language pathologists are responsible for determining if students' communication disabilities impede their learning, so assessments should always include functional outcomes. It is important to know the differences among *impairment, disability,* and *handicap* and how each is assessed to assure that eligibility is determined by both impairment and disability. These three terms are discussed in detail in Chapter 4 under "Federal Eligibility Criteria for Special Education." The term *handicap* will soon be replaced by *participation,* indicating the level of involvement the person experiences in a positive sense, rather than the negative statement, handicap (Threats, 2000).

A student's year-to-year growth is measured functionally in interpersonal, emotional, and academic disability areas, not by retesting to see if the impairment remains. In some cases, an impairment will not change, while a disability will be drastically reduced. For example, Zua had a hearing loss that resulted in significant academic, social, and language disabilities. After two years of therapy, she made notable growth in academic, conversational, and dis-course skills. Her hearing loss was no longer a disability, but she still had the same impairment—a hearing loss. Likewise, students with cerebral palsy or AUTISM SPECTRUM DISORDER who make great communication strides during therapy will be less disabled, but will have the same impairment. Again, it is important to measure the year-to-year growth in the disability area, not solely in the impairment area.

Preferred Practice Patterns in Assessment

The three methods of assessing youngsters just described use the principles of assessment found in ASHA's *Preferred Practice Patterns for the Profession of Speech-Language Pathology* (1997c). Each of the preferred assessment patterns are listed in Appendix A, separated by disorder. School-based speech-language pathologists should follow these guidelines in their work setting. Although school districts' or states' criteria for determining eligibility for services may differ, the elements of a professional speech-language assessment remain constant. The elements to consider when performing an assessment are listed in the sidebar.

---

10 Common Elements of Assessment for Communication Disabilities

1. Overall statement of purpose

2. Professionals who perform the procedures

3. Role, if any, of support personnel in this procedure

4. Expected outcomes

5. Clinical indications

6. Clinical process

7. Setting and equipment specifications

8. Safety and health precautions

9. Documentation

10. ASHA policy and related references

Source: ASHA (1997c)

Following ASHA's Preferred Practice Patterns helps ensure that speech-language assessments performed in schools will be qualitatively similar to those performed in other settings. These guidelines may also be used as an educational tool for related professionals, consumers, and policy makers.

The Assessment Report

The speech-language assessment should give an overall picture of the child as a communicator in the school setting. Framing statements about the child as a student in his or her class is very important. If terms like *pragmatics, syntax,* or *lexicon* are used, the speech-language pathologist should give curriculum-related examples so that educators and family members can comprehend the impact of problems in these areas.

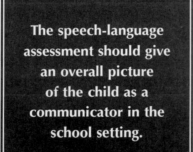

The speech-language assessment should give an overall picture of the child as a communicator in the school setting.

Student assessment is conducted during the school day, by arranging with the teacher suitable periods of time that the student may leave class. The student needs to be assessed in the areas identified by the referral. Testing, observation, checklists, and other forms of assessment can take many hours to complete, depending on the child's age, attention, and skill level. With very young children, especially if autism spectrum disorder is a consideration, discussions with parents or caregivers and communication development checklists can provide more information for diagnosis than interactions with the child can (Wetherby, 1998).

The speech-language pathologist should meet with other team members to compare and validate his or her findings. The report should describe the presenting problem, describe the nature of the assessment including purpose and results of tests, and include recommendations for intervention or support services.

Speech-language pathologists should use good judgment when interpreting behaviors or interactions and have sufficient documentation for conclusions. Ideally, the report should be two pages or less in length and available at the meeting to all team members. Parents may request to see the report before the IEP meeting. A prompt short report is much more helpful to the team than a long comprehensive one that may take much longer to compose and be read. School-based speech-language pathologists need to become skilled at writing brief but complete reports, using descriptions understood by team members representing other disciplines. Speech-language pathologists may need to write a longer, more comprehensive report if there are extenuating circumstances.

Speech-language pathologists may be able to use a comprehensive format to present all the information about a student's assessment and functioning level. Using one format is particularly helpful for students with complex medical needs or developmental disabilities in which large amounts of evidence and observational information must be conveyed to the team. Speech-language pathologists in schools who use performance-based assessments appreciate the convenience of the "Communication Profile" in Appendix C. This approach is particularly helpful for recording observations and comments to use as an assessment report. The profile form can streamline the effort of all team members when students have complicated behaviors.

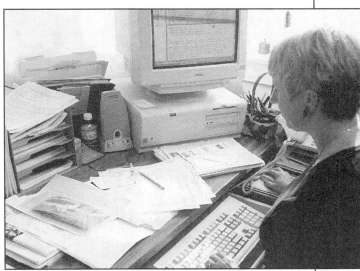

As the speech-language pathologist works with a group of educators over time, team members are likely to learn speech-language terminology, diagnoses, and corresponding interventions. In schools, unlike health-care or private practice settings, the speech-language pathologist is often the only person in the building who is a professional in this field. Speech-language pathologists should consider how to increase the knowledge base of all the other team members each time they assess a student, write a report, or work with an educator or family. Educating colleagues about speech-language pathology is a challenge in school programs, but well worth the effort.

Assessment is a critical aspect of working in the school setting. Unlike intervention, which may be carried out by teachers, aides, family members, assistants, bus drivers, and others under the supervision or direction of the speech-language pathologist, assessment is carried out solely by the speech-language pathologist.

Finding a base line of student abilities, recognizing the value and limits of standardized tests, and determining present levels of communication performance allows the educational team to make the best decisions about the student's eligibility for services. A well-crafted report is vital to the family, the student, and the team.

Independent Educational Evaluation

From time to time, a parent may disagree with the school team's findings and feel that an outside evaluator would arrive at a different conclusion or recommendations. Typically the parent is seeking a conclusion that includes an intervention program at school different from that desired or recommended by the school IEP team members.

If parents do not agree with an evaluation completed by school district personnel, they have the right to have an independent evaluation conducted by a qualified examiner at public expense. In these types of cases, the school district will generally present the parents with a list of two or three choices of qualified evaluators. Parents choose from this list, and the district is responsible for the cost, as well as for re-convening an IEP meeting to consider the results of the independent assessment.

In situations where parents seek or present the school district with an independent evaluation that they obtained at their own expense, the school district is still required to convene an IEP meeting to consider the results of the evaluation. Parents who seek reimbursement for an evaluation obtained at their own expense should be referred to the administrator in charge of the special education program, as this would not be determined by the speech-language pathologist. Immediate attention to such requests is critical, however, so the speech-language pathologist should contact the special education administrator immediately upon receiving such a request.

Needless to say, speech-language pathologists in schools try to avoid these confrontations when-ever possible. If the state's eligibility criteria are adhered to, and the speech-language pathologist's assessment is complete and well administered, the school district should be on solid ground. The school-based speech-language pathologist must know and agree to work within the federal, state, and local parameters of "a speech or language disability" as defined by IDEA (1997) rather than the broader definitions that might be available within other work settings. Working with legal and procedural safeguards, setting and maintaining timelines, and making team decisions are all part of the daily experience of a speech-language pathologist and can require great flexibility. Working closely with one's mentors and supervisors in the schools is advisable should any conflicts arise. (See also Chapter 8, "Independent Educational Evaluation (IEE).")

CHAPTER 4

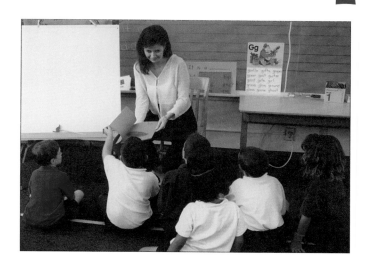

The IEP Process and Procedures

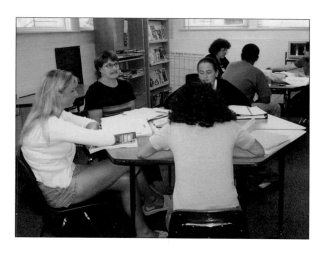

IN THIS CHAPTER

This chapter explains the who, when, and what of the IEP meeting. It highlights federal and state eligibility criteria for speech-language services in schools. Finally, the chapter integrates the procedures for determining a student's need for services with procedures for determining successful completion of services. This integrated approach increases accountability and assists families. This chapter pertains to the IEP meeting process required by IDEA (1997), as opposed to the methodologies involved in speech-language assessments, which can be found in Chapter 3.

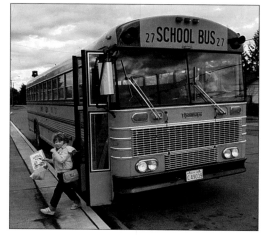

1. Examine a text from any core subject and consider the information about universal design. Does this text lend itself to the precepts of universal design? How could you use this text for individuals with speech or language impairments?

2. What is the difference between eligibility and placement? Why is this distinction important?

3. Describe the World Health Organization (WHO) chart in your own words and why it is so valuable in the school setting.

4. Explain the educational relevance of a communication disorder and why the federal government requires that "adverse educational affect" must be documented for speech and language services.

5. Discuss why you think that definitions and criteria for language impairment and services vary so much from state to state. Is this an advantage or a disadvantage? Explain your answer.

6. Examine content and performance standards from your state or district. Select areas that could be used as benchmarks or objectives for students with communication disorders.

7. Describe the precautions you must take in documentation and record keeping.

8. What is the purpose of triennial assessment?

9. When should a speech-language pathologist decide on dismissal criteria? Why?

The IEP Meeting Process

The language that describes INDIVIDUALIZED EDUCATION PROGRAMS (IEPs) is sometimes confusing due to the acronyms and dual meanings for some of the terminology used. An IEP may refer to "a written statement for a child with a disability that is developed, reviewed, and revised in a meeting" (34 CODE OF FEDERAL REGULATIONS [C.F.R.] § 300.340). Common vernacular also uses IEP to refer to the process of the meeting or to the meeting itself.

For children 2 years of age and younger, an INDIVIDUALIZED FAMILY SERVICE PLAN (IFSP) is developed in place of an IEP as the written document resulting from the IEP meeting. For children 3–5 years, the INDIVIDUALS WITH DISABILITIES EDUCATION ACT (IDEA) AMENDMENTS OF 1997 permit states to use an IFSP to meet IEP requirements if using that plan is agreed by the LOCAL EDUCATIONAL AGENCY (LEA) and the parents (34 C.F.R. § 300.342 [c]). See Chapter 6 for further discussion of preschool-age children.

Printed IEP forms include all the required components of the IEP. These components are more than just lines on a page or an intent to create burdensome paperwork. Each of these areas relates to a specific requirement of the federal or state special education law. The forms guide the IEP team through the steps of the IEP meeting process. The sections that follow describe this process.

Who Comprises the IEP Team?

The C.F.R. (34 C.F.R. § 300.344 [a]) specifies that the members of the IEP team include the following:

(1) The parents of the child;

(2) At least one regular education teacher of the child (if the child is, or may be, participating in the regular education environment);

(3) At least one special education teacher of the child, or if appropriate, at least one special education provider of the child;

(4) A representative of the public agency who—

(i) Is qualified to provide, or supervise the provision of, specially designed instruction to meet the unique needs of children with disabilities;

(ii) Is knowledgeable about the general curriculum; and

(iii) Is knowledgeable about the availability of resources of the public agency;

(5) An individual who can interpret the instructional implications of evaluation results, who may be another member of the team described in paragraphs (2) through (6) of this section;

(6) At the discretion of the parent or the agency, other individuals who have knowledge or special expertise regarding the child, including related services personnel as appropriate; and

(7) If appropriate, the child.

Others may also attend the IEP meeting. Parents or the district may bring anyone to an IEP meeting who they determine has knowledge or special "expertise" regarding their child. Often a friend or relative can give parents some support for the meeting. A notable exception is if a parent intends to bring an attorney to the IEP meeting. (See "Impartial Due Process Hearings" in Chapter 8.) School district participants may be only individuals who have a legitimate educational interest in the purpose of the IEP meeting. The confines of confidentiality apply to such meetings. (See "Record Keeping and Documentation," page 111, for a discussion on confidentiality.) Individuals such as union representatives or secretaries may not attend IEP meetings if their purpose for being there is not related to the development of the IEP for the child. Individuals attending IEP meetings must possess the required "knowledge or special expertise" about the child [34 C.F.R. Part 300,

Appendix A, Question 28], so outside individuals may not attend.

Note that the members of the MULTIDISCIPLINARY TEAM (MDT) may also be members of the IEP team. Certain MDT members, such as a psychologist, may not be able to attend all IEP meetings. Table 4.1 compares the three teams discussed in this chapter. Team responsibilities are an important part of the speech-language pathologist's role in schools.

Parent participation in IEP meetings was given renewed emphasis under IDEA (1997) (see sidebar). Lack of parent interest or the inconvenience of scheduling IEP meetings are

Table 4.1

School Team Members

Student Study Team (SST)	Multidisciplinary Team (MDT)	IEP Team
General Ed Teacher(s)	Speech-Language Pathologist	Parent
Special Ed Teacher	Psychologist	Local Education Agency Representative (Administrator)
School Administrator	Nurse	General Ed Teacher
Counselor	General Ed Teacher	Special Ed Teacher
Parent	Special Ed Teacher	Members of the MDT if reviewing assessment results
Student (if appropriate)	Parent	
Specialist(s) (Optional) *psychologist *speech-language pathologist *LD Teacher	Other Specialists* (if necessary) *occupational therapist *physical therapist *teacher of hearing impaired	Student (if appropriate)
School counselor (MS/HS)	*teacher of visually impaired	Individuals invited by parent or school district
Nurse (if necessary)	*behavior specialist	

*Specialists who potentially might be team members

Parent Participation in IEPs

(a) Public agency responsibility—general.

Each public agency shall take steps to ensure that one or both of the parents of a child with a disability are present at each IEP meeting or are afforded the opportunity to participate, including—

 (1) Notifying parents of the meeting early enough to ensure that they will have an opportunity to attend; and

 (2) Scheduling the meeting at a mutually agreed on time and place.

(b) Information provided to parents.

 (1) The notice required under paragraph (a)(1) of this section must—

   (i) Indicate the purpose, time, and location of the meeting and who will be in attendance; and

   (ii) Inform the parents of the provisions in Sec. 300.344(a)(6) and (c) (relating to the participation of other individuals on the IEP team who have knowledge or special expertise about the child).

 (2) For a student with a disability beginning at age 14, or younger, if appropriate, the notice must also—

   (i) Indicate that a purpose of the meeting will be the development of a statement of the transition services needs of the student required in Sec. 300.347(b)(1); and

   (ii) Indicate that the agency will invite the student.

 (3) For a student with a disability beginning at age 16, or younger, if appropriate, the notice must—

   (i) Indicate that a purpose of the meeting is the consideration of needed transition services for the student required in Sec. 300.347 (b)(2);

   (ii) Indicate that the agency will invite the student; and

   (iii) Identify any other agency that will be invited to send a representative.

(c) Other methods to ensure parent participation.

If neither parent can attend, the public agency shall use other methods to ensure parent participation, including individual or conference telephone calls.

(d) Conducting an IEP meeting without a parent in attendance.

A meeting may be conducted without a parent in attendance if the public agency is unable to convince the parents that they should attend. In this case the public agency must have a record of its attempts to arrange a mutually agreed on time and place, such as--

 (1) Detailed records of telephone calls made or attempted and the results of those calls;

 (2) Copies of correspondence sent to the parents and any responses received; and

 (3) Detailed records of visits made to the parent's home or place of employment and the results of those visits.

(e) Use of interpreters or other action, as appropriate.

The public agency shall take whatever action is necessary to ensure that the parent understands the proceedings at the IEP meeting, including arranging for an interpreter for parents with deafness or whose native language is other than English.

(f) Parent copy of child's IEP.

The public agency shall give the parent a copy of the child's IEP at no cost to the parent.

Source: 34 C.F.R. § 300.345

common frustrations for school personnel. School-based professionals need to pay particular attention to the requirements for involving families, including the requirements for documenting attempts at scheduling the IEP meeting at a mutually agreed upon time and place (which may be a conference call if attendance is not possible). Holding meetings before or after the speech-language pathologist's work hours may have legal, safety, and union ramifications. These considerations can be arranged with the administrator and require flexibility on everyone's part.

When Are IEP Meetings Held?

An IEP meeting must be held at least once each year (known as an annual review) and when a re-evaluation is completed. Re-evaluations can be completed for different reasons: because it is time for a triennial re-evaluation (also known as a three-year evaluation) as required by IDEA (1997), because of requests from the student's parents or teachers, or because the school district determined re-evaluation was warranted (34 C.F.R. § 300.536 [b]). (See "Annual and Triennial Assessments," on page 113, for more details.) IDEA (1997) requires that an IEP meeting must be held within 30 days of a determination that a student needs SPECIAL EDUCATION and RELATED SERVICES (34 C.F.R. § 300.343 [b] [2]).

An IEP meeting should also be held any time new factors that affect the student's program are introduced. Such examples include when a student is not making anticipated progress on GOALS; when a student is having difficulties in school (e.g., behavior problems or failing a class); when a new service is being considered; or when any member of the IEP team, including the parent or teacher, requests a meeting. At the IEP meeting, the team develops the student's individualized education program (IEP), which constitutes the basics of the student's specially designed program. Additional meetings held during the year to revise the IEP may be held as an addendum to the existing program. Local practice dictates how this process is handled.

Who Is Responsible for Sending the IEP Meeting Notice?

The responsibility for sending out the notice of an IEP meeting varies from district to district and may depend on the nature of the meeting. Generally, a CASE MANAGER is responsible for sending the IEP meeting notice, since he or she coordinates the special education program for the student. Most often, the case manager is the person who is the student's primary service provider. If the speech-language pathologist is the only service provider, then he or she is likely to be the one responsible for sending out the meeting notice. Federal regulations require that parents be notified of the meeting early enough to ensure that they will have an opportunity to attend (34 C.F.R. § 300.345 [a] [1]). States vary in terms of the days required for notifying parents; for example, in New Jersey, a 15-day notice is required and in Kansas, a 10-day notice is required.

What Must Be Considered at an IEP Meeting?

In developing each child's IEP, the IEP team shall consider—

(i) The strengths of the child and the concerns of the parents for enhancing the education of their child;

(ii) The results of the initial evaluation or most recent evaluation of the child; and

(iii) As appropriate, the results of the child's performance on any general State or district-wide assessment programs. (34 C.F.R. § 300.346)

The same section of the C.F.R. specifies that the IEP team must also consider special factors, such as:

- Behavior impeding the child's learning or the learning of others, and the need for positive behavioral supports

- In the case of a child who is blind or visually impaired, instruction in Braille and the use of Braille

- The communication needs of the child (for a child who is DEAF or hard of hearing, the child's language and communication mode)

- Assistive technology devices and services (including an intervention, accommodation, or other program modification needed by the student in order to learn or use the device or service)

The IEP team should also take into consideration the language needs for children with limited English proficiency, as those needs relate to the child's IEP. Speech-language pathologists must differentiate between a language difference and a LANGUAGE DISORDER. Speech-language pathologists must have knowledge and expertise in the normal developmental process for second-language acquisition, since some of these processes may present like a language disorder. The sidebar on page 86 highlights other skills needed by speech-language pathologists working with diverse student populations.

Federal and state laws for special education specifically deny ELIGIBILITY if the reason for the child's learning problem is due to the environment, second-language acquisition, or lack of school attendance. A checklist of eligibility guidelines for English language learners can be seen in Appendix D. The demands of a student population that is increasingly diverse necessitates that speech-language pathologists be culturally competent (Wolf and Calderon, 1999) and aware of the issues outside of school (e.g., mobility, poverty, LITERACY, access to education, access to health care, variability of language/cultural upbringing, and parental participation in the child's education) that may be affecting the school performance of students from diverse backgrounds (Moore-Brown, 1999a, 1999b). The need for trained, competent, fully certificated staff will continue to permeate the work world of schools to deal with this population.

There are many sources of guidance for serving students from diverse backgrounds. The AMERICAN SPEECH-LANGUAGE-HEARING ASSOCIATION'S (ASHA's) Multi-Cultural Affairs Division may be of assistance to members. State departments of education may also offer resources or handbooks (e.g., *Guidelines for Language, Academic, and Special Education*

> **Skills Needed by Speech-Language Pathologists Serving Diverse Student Populations**
>
> - Skills for diagnostics; intervention
> - Ability to provide differential diagnosis
> - Understanding of new roles in team membership
> - Ability to use and supervise support personnel (e.g., speech-language pathology assistants)
> - Assurance of appropriate provision of services
> - Flexibility in service delivery model
> - Ability to serving multicultural student populations in an environment of school reform
> - Demonstration of treatment outcomes
> - Application of the role of the speech-language pathologist in literacy
> - Knowledge of the curriculum
> - Ability to advocate for students and the professions
>
> From *Multicultural Issues for the Professions*, by B. Moore-Brown, 1999a. Presentation at the Fourth Annual Communication Disorders Multicultural Conference of the National Student Speech-Language-Hearing Association, Fullerton, CA. © 1999 by B. Moore-Brown. Adapted with permission.

Services Required for Limited-English-Proficient Students in California Public Schools, K–12 (California Department of Education, 1997). State association projects and reference books in the field will also provide guidance for serving students from diverse backgrounds (Langdon, 1999, 2000; Langdon and Cheng, in press; Langdon and Saenz, 1996) (see sidebars and Chapter 7).

What Are the Steps in the IEP Meeting Process?

IEP forms should guide the IEP team through the procedural requirements of the IEP. When developing an IEP, following a particular process is very important. The recommended process will not only guarantee that the requirements of IDEA (1997) are followed, but will also ensure that each member of the team can follow along and assist in building a program for the child that will provide FREE APPROPRIATE PUBLIC EDUCATION (FAPE).

When developing an IEP, think of the process and resulting document as a road map to the student's education. The IEP meeting process has three parts: (1) determination of PRESENT LEVELS OF EDUCATIONAL PERFORMANCE; (2) development of goals and SHORT-TERM OBJECTIVES or BENCHMARKS; and (3) determination of program, PLACEMENT, and services. Following this three-step process at every IEP meeting will allow for information to be shared and the resulting decisions to be made based on the requisite information.

Determination of Present Levels of Educational Performance

The first step in the IEP meeting process is determining PRESENT LEVELS OF EDUCATIONAL

Information Knowledge Needed by Speech-Language Pathologists
Serving Diverse Student Populations

Speech-language pathologists in public schools need to know the following to best serve all students, but particularly students from diverse backgrounds.

The curriculum, including requirements for
- High school exit exam
- Social promotion and retention
- Statewide assessment
- Multiple measures

The other categorical programs, including
- Federal program: Title I
- State program: Economic Impact Aid/Limited English Proficient (EIA/LEP)

The district/county/state resources
- Watch for training sessions and attend them with a general educator

The processes for helping/assisting students in your school/district
- Student Success Teams
- Local intervention programs
- Other categorical programs
- Alternative education programs (including adult education)

From *Multicultural Issues for the Professions,* by B. Moore-Brown, 1999a. Presentation at the Fourth Annual Communication Disorders Multicultural Conference of the National Student Speech-Language-Hearing Association, Fullerton, CA. © 1999 by B. Moore-Brown. Adapted with permission.

PERFORMANCE. Depending on the type of meeting being held, present levels of educational performance are considered by any and all of the following methods:

- Reviewing assessment(s), including statewide, schoolwide or classroom, as well as specialist or psychoeducational
- Reviewing classroom work
- Reviewing grade reports
- Teacher or specialist report (oral or written)
- Parent and student information and interests
- Review of the previous year's goals and the progress made
- Consideration of new information brought forth by any member of the team
- Report on student progress and behavior by service providers
- Discipline and behavioral information

The new IDEA (1997) regulations require that all IEPs include a statement of the child's present levels of educational performance, including:

Positive Statements of Present Levels of Educational Performance

After completing an assessment and focusing on a student's areas of need, it can be difficult to restate them in terms of what he or she is able to do. When describing present levels of educational performance, discuss the student's strengths and state needs in positive terms.

Negative

- Can't understand what he says
- Doesn't use words
- Doesn't know his alphabet

- Has not mastered sound/symbol relationships

Positive

- Able to produce 5 single words intelligibly
- Uses gestures to communicate intent
- Able to distinguish between letters and numbers
- Identifies words that begin with the same sound 60% of the time

---

(i) How the child's disability affects the child's involvement and progress in the general curriculum (i.e., the same curriculum as for nondisabled children); or

(ii) For preschool children, as appropriate, how the disability affects the child's participation in appropriate activities (34 C.F.R. § 300.347)

Conducting intervention with curriculum goals in mind is not a new concept in the speech-language field (Hoskins, 1990; Montgomery, 1994b; Moore-Brown, 1992; Nelson, 1990; Nelson, 1992), but the new IDEA requirement puts the conceptual practice into law (Brannen et al., 2000). Speech-language pathologists in public schools must be able to integrate knowledge of COMMUNICATION DISORDERS with knowledge of the scope and developmental sequence of curriculum.

Classroom curriculums are built on taxonomies that reflect the developmental levels of children in each grade. Children who are delayed or disordered will most certainly have challenges with the curriculum of the classroom. State or local standards for learning describe the instructional concepts that must be mastered at each grade level. These documents must be available to all teachers in a school district, and should be available to specialists as well. If speech-language pathologists do not have a copy of the district's adopted standards, they should contact the principal or the district's administrator of educational services. Speech-language pathologists must know what the expectations are of students in each grade in order to assist the child in his or her interaction with the curriculum.

As an IEP team member, the speech-language pathologist will need to go beyond sharing the results of standardized or nonstandardized assessments of communication skills. He or she must be able to interpret how those results are related to what happens in the classroom and design intervention to meet curriculum-based goals or outcomes.

Speech-language pathologists new to the field might wonder why this requirement is emphasized so strongly. The U.S. Department of Education (1999) addressed Congress regarding the issue of shifting the focus from physical access to access to the general education curriculum:

> [F]or a growing number of students with disabilities, special education today is not preparing them for increasingly rigorous graduation requirements and career skills that are based on problem solving, COLLABORATION, and technology. Why is this? Special education has typically been viewed as an intervention of remediation.... As we approach the 21st century, the challenge for educators is to provide students with disabilities meaningful access to instruction that is aligned with high-level standards and supported by special education interventions. (p. I–21)

Since special educators were rarely involved in the development of the curriculum under the dual educational system described in Chapter 1, adapting the curriculum to the special needs of students was left to individual educators. To meet the mandate for access to the general education curriculum, curricula that have students' specialized learning needs in mind need to be developed, as described by Orkwis and McLane (1998):

Access to the curriculum begins with a student being able to interact with it to learn. ...[T]he curriculum must be delivered with an array of supports for the student. The barriers to access must be removed, but importantly, the curriculum has to continue to challenge them [students]. (pp. 6–7)

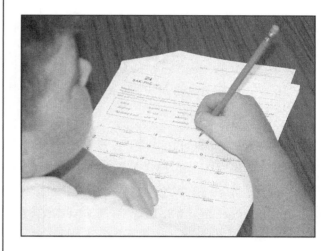

The method for removing barriers is UNIVERSAL DESIGN. According to Orkwis and McLane (1998):

> In terms of learning, universal design means the design of instructional materials and activities that allows the learning goals to be achievable by individuals with wide differences in their abilities to see, hear, speak, move, read, write, understand English, attend, organize, engage, and remember. Universal design for learning is achieved by means of flexible curricular materials and activities that provide alternatives for students with disparities in abilities and backgrounds. These alternatives

should be built into the instructional design and operating systems of educational materials—they should not have to be added on later. (p. 9)

For school districts and local curriculum committees, the U.S. Department of Education (1999) recommended the following considerations to guide curriculum selection:

- "Does the curriculum provide multiple means of presentation of content?"

- "Does the curriculum provide multiple and flexible means of student engagement or participation?"

- "Does the curriculum provide multiple means of student responses? (p. I–26)"

The U.S. Department of Education was concerned that special educators were often not involved in the development of curriculum, at either a state or local level. Additionally, the U.S. Department of Education noted that standards and universal design would only be effective if educators were trained in pedagogy, understanding how to make the curriculum concepts meaningful to all students. A need for instructional materials that are accessible to students through a variety of formats and in multiple presentation modes was identified by the U.S. Department of Education.

Finally, instructional strategies must be intense, frequent, explicit, and individually referenced for the student(s) so that students will "acquire skills that will better prepare them for life after school" (U.S. Department of Education, 1999, p. I–30). California is one example of a state that has included information on univer-

sal design in its framework in order to assist educators in developing curriculum (California Department of Education, 1999d). Further, IDEA (1997) requires that the LEA representative on the IEP team is knowledgeable about the general curriculum (34 C.F.R. § 300.344 [a] [4] [ii]) to direct the linkage between the special education program and the general education curriculum and setting.

Federal Eligibility Criteria for Special Education

If the purpose of the IEP meeting is to review initial assessments (see Chapter 3 for a discussion of the initial assessment process), then present levels of educational performance will be determined when eligibility is considered. If the purpose of the IEP meeting is part of a triennial re-evaluation (see "Annual and Triennial Assessments" on page 113), continuing eligibility will be considered.

In either case, a child may not be determined to be eligible if:

(1) The determinant factor for that eligibility determination is—

  (i) Lack of instruction in reading or math; or

  (ii) Limited English proficiency; and

(2) The child does not otherwise meet the eligibility criteria under Sec. 300.7(a). (34 C.F.R. § 300.534)

If a child is not determined to be eligible for special education, the next two steps in the IEP meeting process—development of goals and short-term objectives or benchmarks and determination of program, placement, and services—do not occur. The IEP team may instead do any of the following: (1) make some general recommendations to the classroom teacher for assisting student in the classroom, (2) refer the student back to the SST, or (3) refer the student to the 504 team for eligibility determination under SECTION 504 (see Chapter 8 "Section 504 and the Americans with Disabilities Act [ADA]"). In these situations, IEP teams should insure that some form of assistance is provided so that the child does not continue to struggle and fail in school.

If a child is determined to be eligible for special education, the next two steps in the IEP process do take place. The MDAT can determine that a student is eligible if the student has one or more disabilities that require special education and related services because of the disability(ies). The 13 eligibility categories identified under IDEA (1997) appear in the sidebar below. Notice that the terms *impairment* and *disability* occur. The World Health Organization (WHO) developed a helpful way to conceptualize the terms *impairment, disability,* and *handicap*.

Although these terms have been used interchangeably over the years, they do not mean the same thing. As you can see in Figure 4.1, developed by WHO in 1980 and embraced by ASHA in 1995, these terms have distinctly different meanings.

Impairment refers to the existence of an abnormality of the structure or function of the student's communication at an organic level (e.g., vocal nodules, a tongue thrust, a distorted /r/ phoneme, a hearing loss, repetition of the initial phoneme in words, or cognitive limitations). The presence of an impairment can be ascertained with the traditional instruments and STANDARDIZED TESTS that are common to the field. These tools will help determine if the person's communication deviates from the norms for age and ability. Traditional diagnostic measures can and should be used to determine impairment in any setting the student is seen for assessment. Impairment can be determined by comparing the child's standard score with age-appropriate norms (i.e., percentiles or similar measures, from a nondisabled population).

Federal Eligibility Categories for Special Education

Autism	Multiple Disabilities
Deaf-Blindness	Other Health Impairment
Developmental Delay (state option)	Orthopedic Impairment
Emotional Disturbance	Speech or Language Impairment
Hearing Impairment	Traumatic Brain Injury
Learning Disability	Visual Impairment
Mental Retardation	

States may also authorize school districts to include the condition of "developmental delay" for children aged 3 through 9, or a subset of this age group.

Source: 34 C.F.R. § 300.7 (a) (1)

Figure 4.1

World Health Organization (WHO) Categories
(Adapted for Communication Disabilities)

Impairment	Disability	Handicap
An abnormality in a person's structure or physical function	Actual effect an impairment has upon a person's life activities	Society's views of persons with disabilities
Examples: autism, dysarthria, hearing loss, voice disorder, stuttering, etc.	**Examples:** difficulty hearing conversation, reading problems, hard for others to understand, memory problems, etc.	**Examples:** limited social life and career options; less likely to make high income, attract desirable partner, become well educated
Measured by: Standardized, norm referenced tests in the discipline	**Measured by:** Functional outcomes in one's actual life activities; changes that occur due to interventions	**Measured by:** Quality of life indicators, society's beliefs and pre-conceptions, violation of laws
Use to decide eligibility if adverse effect on learning	Use for progress reports, year to year changes	Use to determine possible violations of civil rights

Source: WHO (1980)

Disability refers to the functional consequence of the known impairment. Speech-language pathologists must use functional status measures to determine what communication problems impede the student's daily life activities. In school, the broadest educational environment is used to determine functional status: class grades, class participation, self-esteem, oral and written work, school leadership, parents' concerns, peers' reactions, and so on. There are almost no functional status tests in common use for speech-language, so speech-language pathologists must rely on reports from teachers; parents; peers; the student; and a review of class performance, including grades. If functional status does not appear to be affected by the identified impairment, the student is not disabled and therefore not eligible for speech-language services under IDEA (1997). A preliminary set of functional status measures were made available by ASHA in 1998(e). See

"Functional Outcomes and the School-Based Speech-Language Pathologist" in Chapter 5 for samples of these statements.

Handicap refers to society's perception of what an individual can or cannot do based on what persons without disabilities believe is possible. There may be many genuine social consequences of a disability: joblessness, isolation, fewer friends, fewer educational opportunities, and other limitations on how one communicates with others. An impairment need not be handicapping in and of itself. Although an impairment causes a disability, it is the failure to ameliorate that disability that leads to a handicap. Because communication is such a vital activity of daily living, a communication impairment is usually disabling, but when remediated or modified to no longer limit a student's ability to learn or interact successfully, an impairment may not be a handicap. The term *handicap* is in the process

of being replaced by *participation,* a positive statement of what a student can do (Threats, 2000).

Special education once used only the term *handicap* to refer to all three conditions. Students found to have "handicapping conditions" were called "speech handicapped learners," and their education was defined in a federal law called the (1975) EDUCATION FOR ALL HANDICAPPED CHILDREN ACT (EAHCA). The use of this terminology has since been changed, specifically to highlight when and why services are provided in schools—not for impairments, but to reduce disabilities and their potentially handicapping effects.

In determining eligibility and placement, IDEA (1997) directs the IEP team to:

(1) Draw upon information from a variety of sources, including aptitude and achievement tests, parent input,

Avoiding Communication Handicapism

Students with communication disabilities may have artificial limitations placed on their lives when they are perceived by others as lacking in some way. For example, the attitude of other people made Nathan's stuttering become a handicap. Adults believed that his struggles with oral presentations were a problem, so they steered him away from a career in law, politics, teaching, or sales. Nathan even began to think his choices were limited by his stuttering. Keishia had a significant hearing loss, so the department chair in science talked her out of studying to be an audiologist. Jorge had strongly accented English, so his parents thought he should not bother with acting school. Kim had cerebral palsy and used a wheelchair, prompting her high school advisor to give her applications only for a two-year junior college. Each of these students was limited by others' ideas of what they could strive for as a person with disabilities. This pre-judgment is handicapism, just like racism or sexism. It is prejudicial and not founded on fact.

teacher recommendations, physical condition, social or cultural background, and adaptive behavior; and

(2) Ensure that information obtained from all of these sources is documented and carefully considered. (34 C.F.R. § 300.535)

There is a distinct and important difference between eligibility and placement. Eligibility refers specifically to considering the child's assessment results as they compare to the outlined eligibility criteria, to determine if the child has a disability and if that disability requires special education and related services.

Any of the 13 listed eligibility categories for special education can have speech-language issues involved with the presenting exceptionality. For example, when the IEP team determines that a student qualifies as a child with AUTISM or traumatic brain injury, such students likely present with speech or language disorders as well. The IEP team should identify speech and language as an area of need and subsequently discuss goals and services to address this need as part of the student's placement.

Speech-language services in schools are part of special education and must meet the requirements of IDEA (1997). Students are determined to be eligible for such services by following a two-step process. First, the student is assessed using traditional standardized tests and/or informal speech-language assessment tools, in addition to observational data. If the student scores significantly below expected levels, speech-language pathologists must go to the second step: determining if these identified communication deficits impede the student's educational performance. IDEA regulations state "Speech or language impairment means a communication disorder, such as stuttering, impaired articulation, a language impairment, or a voice impairment, that adversely affects a child's educational performance" (34 C.F.R. § 300.7 [c] [11]). The key to this definition is the requirement that the impairment "adversely affects a child's educational performance." When asked "Does a speech impairment always trigger eligibility under the IDEA or § 504?" Gorn (1997b) answered "No," pointing to the requirement for adverse affect. Speech-language pathologists may identify, for example, that a student has a myofunctional disorder resulting in a tongue thrust without a frontal lisp. Such a student is not considered eligible under IDEA (1997) because there is no adverse educational impact.

Under IDEA (1997), speech-language services (and all special education services) may be provided to students in school only if both conditions are satisfied: a disability exists and it adversely affects the child's educational performance. The adverse effect may be shown in one or more areas: academic, social, or vocational. This second step is a distinct departure from similar services in health care and private practice. An example of a form that speech-language pathologists in the Florida Department of Education use in determining the effect of the disability on educational performance is shown in Figure 4.2.

Figure 4.2

Educational Relevance of the Communication Disorder

_____ does/does not demonstrate a communication disorder
Name of Student that does/does not negatively impacts his/her ability to benefit from the educational process in one or more of the following areas:

Academic—ability to benefit from the curriculum
Social—ability to interact with peers and adults
Vocational—ability to participate in vocational activities

Academic Impact	Social Impact	Vocational Impact
List academic areas impacted by communication problems:	List social areas impacted by communication problems:	List job related skills/competencies student cannot demonstrate due to communication problems:
_____ Below average grades	_____ Peers tease student about communication problem	_____ Inability to understand/follow oral directions
_____ Inability to complete language-based activities vs. nonlanguage-based activities	_____ Student demonstrates embarrassment and/or frustration regarding communication problem	_____ Inappropriate response to coworker/supervisor/comments
_____ Inability to understand oral directions	_____ Student demonstrates difficulty interpreting communication intent	_____ Unable to answer/ask questions in a coherent/concise manner
_____ Grades below the students ability level	_____ Other: _____	_____ Other: _____
_____ Other: _____		

_____   _____
Speech-Language Pathologist   LEA (Designee)

_____   _____
Other Professional   Other Professional

_____   _____
Parent   Date

From *A Training and Resource Manual for the Implementation of State Eligibility Criteria for the Speech and Language Impaired* [Addendum] (p. 20), by the Florida Department of Education, Bureau of Instructional Support and Community Services, Division of Public Schools, 1997, Tallahassee, FL: Author.

This two-step process is frequently misunderstood. Nonschool agencies and parents may mistakenly conclude that school-based speech-language pathologists have poor skills in identifying some impairments, such as a mild articulation disorder, a tongue thrust, or even vocal hoarseness. In actuality, school-based speech-language pathologists are capable of making such diagnoses but are not allowed to conclude that services are necessary if there is not an adverse educational effect. In such cases, if the student is receiving passing grades and there is no evidence of constrained social interactions or other nonacademic disabling effects, speech-language intervention would not be considered a special education service that the student needs in order to receive educational benefit. The child may have an impairment, but not a disability. Although services may assist the student, it is not the responsibility of the education system to assume the cost of such services since there is no adverse educational effect. Federal regulations require that parents must receive a copy of the team's evaluation report and documentation of the eligibility determination (34 C.F.R. § 300.534).

Parents can make a decision to have speech-language services provided by an agency outside the school. Interestingly, approximately 3% of all speech-language services nationwide are provided by schools using their local funds to pay for non–special education intervention (ASHA, 1998d). Using local funds enables school districts to enroll students in speech-language services who do not meet state or federal criteria as children with disabilities. Therefore, it may appear to those outside the school system that some speech-language impairments are addressed with services, while others are not.

The fact is that only educational disabilities—and not impairments—are addressed in special education law. In contrast, health-care services do not address academic issues but do assess, treat, and pay for medical and functional issues. In private practice, any and all issues may be addressed if the client or family wishes to pay for the service, but not all families will have the resources to make such a decision.

State Eligibility Criteria for Speech-Language Services

IDEA (1997) regulations define a speech or language impairment as a "communication disorder such as stuttering, impaired articulation, a language impairment, or a voice impairment that adversely affects a child's educational performance" (34 C.F.R. § 300.7 [b] [11]). This definition is further interpreted by each of the states in their own special education laws. The combination of tests needed for a valid assessment, the number and types of tests, plus the "cut-off" points on standardized tests are determined by each state. Consequently, a student could have an educationally related communication disorder identified in one state, but not in another. This does not happen often, but it is possible.

Issues in determining eligibility for language intervention are complicated by several factors including what constitutes a significant level of language disability, as well as regulations imposed by government agencies and local school districts (ASHA, 1989a; Nelson, Cheng, Shulman, and Westby, 1994). Since IDEA's inception in the mid-1970s (then known as the EAHCA), *language disability* has been a confusing entity for states and regulatory agencies to define. Defining *language* and *language disorder* has been equally problematic for researchers, scholars, and speech-language pathologists in the field. Over the years, child language has grown from a simple notion of expressive and receptive vocabulary development to a sophisticated interplay of phonology, morphology, SYNTAX, SEMANTICS, and pragmatics. The three categories content, form, and use are used in some states. (See Chapter 6 for a discussion of how language now also encompasses reading and writing as the FUNCTIONAL OUTCOMES of language intervention that are related to academic success [ASHA, 2000d].)

According to ASHA (1989a), to determine a language disability, STATE EDUCATIONAL AGENCIES (SEAs) may adopt pre-existing eligibility criteria based on one or more of these four categories:

1. Approved lists of norm-referenced tests

2. Mandated use of a discrepancy formula

3. Predetermined age equivalent, standard deviation, or minimum percentile rank units

4. Exclusionary regulations for populations that are not considered

State-by-state variations in speech-language intervention eligibility criteria have been investigated for several decades with little change resulting (Apel, 1993; Nye and Montgomery, 1989). Apel compiled a unique profile of language impairment criteria by state into the categories of:

- General definition of communication disorders

- Five-aspect definition of language (semantic, syntactic, pragmatic, phono-

logical, morphological) or three-aspect definition (content, form, and use)

- Definitions of language that included oral, oral/written or no mention of either

- Descriptions of speech production errors for articulation, phonology, or both

- Qualifications for service based on units (standard deviation, severity, chronological age)

- How severity ratings for language of mild, moderate, severe were measured

An abbreviated list of states in each category from Apel's investigation are shown in the sidebar on page 98. The variance from state to state is notable.

States also determine which children with language impairments (and a corresponding adverse educational effect) are eligible for services. These eligibility criteria were collected by Apel (1993) and are summarized in the sidebar on page 99. Again, wide variability from state to state exists for service delivery to students with language disabilities. Appendix E provides examples.

Two of the more widely used approaches to determining eligibility are normative reference points and severity ratings. These approaches are discussed in the sections that follow.

Normative Reference Points

Several normative reference points for expected language development have been used by states to determine eligibility. Two are most common: MENTAL AGE (MA) and CHRONOLOGICAL AGE (CA). If language performance matches MA, some states declare the child ineligible for

---

Variation in Criteria Used by States to Determine Language Impairment

State Definitions of Impairment

1. General definition of communication disorders   **40%**

Maine	Illinois	Kansas	Louisiana
Alaska	Maryland	Massachusetts	Minnesota
Nebraska	New Hampshire	New Jersey	New Mexico
New York	Pennsylvania	Rhode Island	S. Carolina
Texas	Utah	D.C.	Wisconsin

2. Definition by 5 aspects (phonology, morphology, syntax, semantics, pragmatics) or 3 aspects (content, form, use)   **54%**

Alabama	Arkansas	California	Colorado
Connecticut	Delaware	Florida	Georgia
Hawaii	Idaho	Indiana	Iowa
Kentucky	Michigan	Mississippi	Missouri
Montana	Nevada	N. Carolina	N. Dakota
Ohio	Oklahoma	Vermont	Virginia
Washington	W. Virginia	Wyoming	

3. No definition   **6%**

Arizona	Oregon	S. Dakota

Source: Apel (1993)
Note: No data from Tennessee.

---

speech-language services. (This approach is referred to as cognitive referencing.) In other states, if language performance matches MA but still falls below CA expectations, the child may still be eligible for speech-language services. Researchers disagree on the relative value of these two methods and conclude that neither is clearly superior (Fey, 1996; Singer and Bashir, 1999). A speech-language pathologist needs to know the issues involved in MA referencing versus CA referencing (i.e., cognitive referencing)

and what his or her state requires (ASHA, 1989a; Butler, 1999; Cirrin, 1996; Issakson, 2000; Krassowski and Plante, 1997; Nelson, 1999).

The relationship of language to intellect is complex. Some educators try to separate the two; others believe there is a causal relationship between language and intelligence. Arguments in support of cognitive referencing contend that language skills can never exceed a student's intellectual capability; therefore, language intervention is not warranted if performance on language tests is equivalent to performance on

Variation in States' Criteria for Eligibility for Language Services

1. Two or more standard deviations below the mean on standardized tests

Minnesota	Montana	Nebraska	Vermont

2. One and one-half standard deviations (7th percentile) on two or more tests

California	Idaho	Missouri	Washington
Hawaii	Michigan	Montana	

3. One standard deviation below the mean with multiple sources of data

Oklahoma	W. Virginia	Florida
North Carolina	Missouri	

4. Determined by severity ratings

Alabama	Wyoming	Mississippi
North Dakota	Iowa	
Indiana		

5. General indications of delay

Alaska	Arkansas	Arizona
Colorado	Connecticut	Delaware
Georgia	Illinois	Kansas
Kentucky	Maryland	Massachusetts
Nevada	New Jersey	New Hampshire
New Mexico	Ohio	Oregon
Rhode Island	South Carolina	South Dakota
Texas	Utah	Virginia
District of Columbia	Wisconsin	

Source: Apel (1993)

intellectual measures. Determining intellectual capability is problematic, however, since most intelligence tests rely on students' verbal skills. Additionally, cognitive referencing emphasizes scores on static norm-referenced assessments and tends to overlook the potential of intervention to improve functional outcomes. Eligibility criteria for language disorders remain controversial (Secord, 1998) and the speech-language pathologist is advised to closely follow the dictates of his or her state department of education.

Severity Ratings

State severity ratings were reviewed by Nye and Montgomery (1989) and continue to be of interest to SEAs to manage the potentially large number of children who could qualify for services. There is considerable variation in the types of severity ratings used, and each year a few states will alter their eligibility criteria or coding process to some degree. This alteration can take several years to implement in large or heavily regulated states. Severity ratings are suggested by ASHA as useful tools for the school-based speech-language pathologist to manage CASELOAD and student needs (ASHA, 1999c; 2000b). Currently, 16 states refer to severity ratings for determining eligibility (Apel, 1993; ASHA, 1999c). These states may use scales with one to six levels and/or the terms *mild, moderate* and *severe*. Table 4.2 lists

Table 4.2

State Severity Ratings for Language Disorders

State	Terms Used	Measurements
Alabama	mild/moderate/severe	1.0 to 2.0 standard deviations
Florida	mild/moderate/severe	1.0 to 2.0 standard deviations
Georgia	mild/moderate/severe	calls attention; some disadvantage; not understood
Indiana	mild/moderate/severe	1–7 points based on SD of 1.0–2.0
Iowa	deviations to disorders	1–4
Kentucky	mild/moderate/severe	0 (normal) to 3
Maine	interferes/limits/prevents	
Maryland	Level 1 to Level 6	
Michigan	use the discrepancy model	
Missouri	determined by districts	
New Jersey	mild/moderate = instruction; severe = interferes with communication	
North Carolina	2–10 points	
North Dakota	mild/moderate/severe	1.0 to 2.0 standard deviations
Oregon	several models provided in state manual	
South Carolina	general characteristics of needs	
Virginia	1–6 scale	criteria for each disability

Source: ASHA (1999c)

the states that use a severity system to determine eligibility and their terminology.

Once a child is found to meet eligibility criteria, goals and short-term objectives or benchmarks are established in the identified area(s) of need. Following eligibility determination and establishment of goals in the area(s) of need, consideration is given to program placement and services (e.g., speech-language services). Placement may be thought of as the description of the program that meets the student's individual educational needs. After reviewing the student's present levels of performance and making an eligibility determination (if necessary), the next consideration is what skills and abilities the student needs to develop.

Development of Goals and Short-Term Objectives or Benchmarks

The second step in the IEP meeting process is to develop GOALS and SHORT-TERM OBJECTIVES or BENCHMARKS. At least one goal should be established for each identified area of need. Goals are written in only the identified area(s) of need and not for curricular or developmental areas that will be addressed in the scope of the CLASSROOM INSTRUCTION at the student's grade level or above. IDEA (1997) regulations require each IEP to include:

> A statement of measurable annual goals, including benchmarks or short-term objectives, related to—
>
> > (i) Meeting the child's needs that result from the child's disability to enable the child to be involved

---

Practical Application of Goal Setting

During the IEP process, goals and short-term objectives or benchmarks are developed based on the student's present levels of educational performance.

Sequence	Application for Kara, a 4th Grader
1. The IEP team identifies the area of need by examining present levels of performance.	1. Kara uses less than 100 words in free-write activities.
2. The IEP team identifies a goal area.	2. Kara will use second-grade vocabulary in spoken and written language.
3. The IEP team develops either short-term objectives or benchmarks or both to contribute to attainment of the goal.	3. Short-Term Objective: Use 10 new vocabulary words each week in reading and writing. Benchmark: During second semester, read and use vocabulary from a book written at the 2.5 level.

in and progress in the general curriculum (i.e., the same curriculum as for nondisabled children), or for preschool children, as appropriate, to participate in appropriate activities; and

(ii) Meeting each of the child's other educational needs that result from the child's disability. (34 C.F.R. § 300.347 [a] [2])

The regulations also require that the public agency "make a good faith effort to assist the child to achieve the goals and OBJECTIVES or benchmarks listed in the IEP" (34 C.F.R. § 300.350).

Short-term objectives for students are defined as "measurable intermediate steps" as opposed to benchmarks which are "major milestones" (34 C.F.R. Part 300, Appendix A, Question 1)

Short-term objectives are described as discrete components of the annual goal, and benchmarks describe the amount of progress the student is expected to make within specified segments of the year. An IEP team may use either short-term objectives or benchmarks or a combination of the two depending on the nature of the annual goal and the needs of the child. (34 C.F.R. Part 300, Appendix A, Question 1)

Reading/Language Arts Content Standards

Reading

Word Analysis, Fluency, and Systematic Vocabulary Development (Grade 1)

Concepts About Print

- Match oral words to printed words

Phonemic Awareness

- Distinguish initial, medial, and final sounds in single-syllable words

Comprehension and Analysis of Grade Level Appropriate Text

- Respond to who, what, when, where, and how questions
- Retell the central ideas of a simple expository or narrative passage

Source: California Department of Education (1998)

Language Arts

Demonstrates competence in general skills and strategies of the reading process (Grades 6–8)

- Generates interesting questions to be answered while reading
- Represents abstract information (e.g., concepts, generalizations) as explicit mental pictures
- Understands stories and expository texts from the perspective of the attitudes and values of the time period in which they were written

Source: Kendall and Marzano (1996)

Since school districts across the country have adopted standards that students are expected to master, there should be no doubt what students are expected to learn. Standards-based reform, of course, is not without its own controversy. As discussed in Chapter 1, standards-based systems include accountability components of high-stakes testing and consequences to systems that

What Is a Benchmark?

Benchmark Definitions

- In general education, benchmarks "are checkpoints that may be tied to designated grade levels at which student's progress toward mastery of a standard is measured" (Council of Administrators of Special Education [CASE], 1999a, p. 9).

- Benchmarks "translates standards into what the student should understand and be able to do at developmentally appropriate levels" (Contra Costa Special Education Local Plan Area [SELPA], 1998, p. 2).

- "Benchmarks are grade-level expectations for student achievement, using age appropriate materials. They mark progress toward achievement (of identified standards.) Indicators may accompany each benchmark. Indicators are specific learning behaviors that can be taught and that demonstrate student achievement of a benchmark. Benchmarks and indicators describe what students should be able to do without teacher assistance. Benchmarks are performance goals for all students. It is anticipated that some students will progress beyond the grade level benchmarks while other students may need specialized support to reach their goals. Teachers provide appropriate challenges for these students while directing and assisting all students in activities that stretch their learning capabilities" (CASE, 1999a, p. 9).

- The state of Wisconsin (O'Donnell, 1999) clarifies "The purpose of the short-term objectives or benchmarks is to specify which path meets the needs of our student. The short-term objectives or benchmarks must state specific, measurable behaviors that will be observed as the student makes progress from the present level of performance to the goal. These objectives or benchmarks may be sequential (crawl, then walk) or they may be parallel (comb hair and brush teeth)" (p. 54).

Council of Administrators in Special Education (CASE) Benchmark Considerations for Using Benchmarks in the IEP Process

- Benchmarks establish expected performance levels at different points during the IEP year.

- Benchmarks allow for regular checks of progress that coincide with the reporting periods for informing parents of their child's progress toward achieving annual goals.

- Benchmarks reflect the direction of student progress toward meeting IEP goals. (CASE, 1999a, p. 9) do not show improvements in student performance. When examining the requirement for accessing the general education curriculum, the U.S. Department of Education (1999) expressed the following concern to Congress regarding standards:

> Virtually every State has developed standards in at least one academic content area; however, there is no "standard" for the State standards (McDonnell et al., 1997). They differ in what they are called (e.g., goals, benchmarks, expectations, frameworks) as well as in subject areas and levels of specificity. While there are variations in levels of expectation for student demonstration of proficiency, there is an increasing trend to assess the student's ability to apply or demonstrate the use of skills in higher order thinking or problem-solving activities. As noted earlier, academic standards are typically included in large-scale assessments, while nonacademic standards are rarely included. (p. I–24)

While there are limitations and concerns about standards, this should not impede speech-language pathologists and other special educators from looking to their district-adopted standards for guidance when establishing goals and short-term objectives or benchmarks for students. The documents guide general education. Recall the dissertation study mentioned in Chapter 1 (Moore-Brown, 1998), which demonstrated that goals and short-term objectives were set for lower-level skill development, and not challenging to students in special education programs. A change toward using the standards to guide IEP goal development should help bridge the gap and meet the congressional

intent of raising expectations for students receiving special education (see Chapter 2).

The academic orientation of the standards might be limiting for students whose goals must include functional or social-emotional skills. However, for the majority of students on the speech-language pathologist's caseload, using standards as a guide for IEP goal development should be an everyday practice.

Benchmarks can be derived from standards by identifying intermediate accomplishments that lead to reaching the standards. The advantage of using benchmarks in the IEP process is that they:

- Help link IEPs to the general education curriculum

- Facilitate increased communication with general educators through the use of a common language

- Promote collaboration among all educators

- Provide for adjustment during the year without reconvening the IEP team

- Correlate with the IEP reporting periods for the purpose of sharing progress

- Establish a more user-friendly process for team members and parents than the short term objectives IEP teams have historically used (CASE, 1999, p. 2)

Speech-language pathologists in public schools have expertise in speech and language acquisition, development, and disorders. Curriculum and standards are constructed based on the developmental levels (e.g., cognitive, linguistic, and social-emotional) that children are expected to have reached at any given grade level. When writing a goal and developing a short-term objective or benchmark, the speech-language pathologist will need to examine the learning expectations and classroom instructional environment to determine how the student's identified disability or delay will impact his or her achieving such expectations. From this information, goals and short-term objectives or benchmarks can be developed.

One rule of thumb that might help speech-language pathologists and others who need to develop goals and short-term objectives or benchmarks will be to consider the type of curriculum the student is mastering. If the curriculum is functional or if the areas of identified need are social, behavioral, or pragmatic, then the use of objectives (i.e., short-term, measurable, intermediate steps) might be the appropriate approach. If the student is participating in the academic curriculum, then benchmarks might be a preferred approach, thereby connecting the student to the curriculum. In examining assessment information, the speech-language pathologist might note that the student's language abilities are two or more years behind his or her grade-level peers. When examining the requirements of the classroom, then, the speech-language pathologist may wish to look at the benchmarks in the year or two prior to the current grade to find a skill that can serve as the baseline from which to build.

Consider an example taken from California's content standards (California Department of Education, 1999d):

Reading Comprehension: Students will identify the basic facts and ideas in

what they have read, heard, or viewed, drawing on such strategies as generating essential questions and comparing information from several sources.

Comprehension and Analysis

Grade 1: respond to who, what, where, when, and how questions (p. 62)

Grade 2: ask clarifying questions concerning essential textual elements of stories (why, what-if, how). (p. 78)

Speech-language pathologists have written goals for *wh-* questions for many years. Here is evidence of when such a skill is needed not only for oral language communication, but also to facilitate reading comprehension. The speech-language pathologist might consider writing the following goals and benchmarks for a second-grade student who has difficulty answering and asking *wh-* questions.

Goal: Manuel will answer and ask *wh-* questions about narrative stories and about stories read in class from the grade-level text.

Benchmarks:

- By the first reporting period, Manuel will answer *who, what,* and *where* questions about narrative stories told to him by his teacher or speech-language pathologist.

- By the second reporting period, Manuel will answer *who, what, where, when,* and *how* questions about stories read aloud to him from the first-grade text.

- By the third reporting period, Manuel will ask clarifying questions about narrative stories told to him by his teacher or speech-language pathologist.

- By the fourth reporting period, Manuel will ask clarifying questions concerning essential textual elements of stories read to him from his grade-level text.

Consider another example in which the identified area of need is vocabulary with the goal for vocabulary development to enhance spoken and written comprehension. What would short-term objectives and benchmarks look like for Sarah, a fourth grader?

Short-term objective: Sarah will identify 10 members of identified categories with 80% accuracy.

Benchmarks: Sarah will:

- Understand and explain common antonyms and synonyms

- Use knowledge of individual words in unknown compound words to predict their meaning

- Know the meaning of simple prefixes and suffixes

- Identify simple multiple-meaning words at the second- and third-grade level

These benchmarks were taken directly from the reading/language arts content standards found in the California framework (1999d, p. 77) for second graders. If the speech-language pathologist and classroom teacher, as well as Sarah's parents, begin to systematically address these areas, Sarah will not only develop her vocabulary, but also will be mastering skills identified as necessary to be successful in the curriculum. As Sarah develops these skills, the members of the IEP team can look to the next benchmarks for third and fourth graders, so that Sarah can develop skills identified for her same-age peers. See sidebar for examples of goals and benchmarks for two more students.

When writing goals and short-term objectives or benchmarks to the general education curriculum, remember the concept of universal design, which organizes curriculum into tasks that can be performed by students with a wide range of skills using a variety of modalities:

> Ideally, effective universal design does not result in lowered expectations or watered-down instruction. Rather, it calls for multiple ways of expressing competency in regards to a given standard. Universal design also results in blending of different types of standards. (U.S. Department of Education, 1999, pp. 1–25)

Universal design helps speech-language pathologists and educators understand that demonstration of knowledge attainment may vary. Universal design will help support the alternatives for achieving and measuring goal attainment.

Since passage of the EAHCA in 1975, goals were written as broad statements, such as "to improve reading comprehension." Under IDEA (1997), such a statement is considered too vague to be measurable. IEP goals should always describe in measurable terms what the team determines the student is expected to achieve one year from the date of the IEP meeting. Goals and short-term objectives or benchmarks should never identify what adults (i.e., teachers, instructional assistants, or parents) do; they should always have the "who" identified as the student. Additionally, they should always be written in positive language, not in a way that reflects a decrease in negative behavior. If the desired behavior is identified, then the competing negative behavior will correspondingly decrease or disappear. According to Contra Costa SELPA (1998), a good format for writing

IEP objectives or benchmarks is something like the following:

  How:

  Who: (the student)

Does What:

Criteria:

Evaluation Method:

By When:

How Speech-Language Services Can Be Integrated within the Curriculum Using Annual Goals and Benchmarks

A. Measurable Annual Goal: Theresa will produce her target phonemes correctly in initial and final position in words when practicing the passages selected for her third-grade oral-reading rate exercises.

Benchmarks:

- She will recognize her target phonemes in the words that contain them in a third grade reading passage. (first report card)

- She will produce her target phonemes correctly in single words selected from the books used in class. (second report card)

- She will self correct when reading for the weekly check of Words Read Correctly Per Minute (WRCPM) in class and in therapy. (third report card)

- She will correctly produce target phonemes in initial and final positions in words in third-grade oral-reading rate exercises. (fourth report card)

Note:

The fourth report card report should show Theresa reaching the goal in one school year. A percentage correct at each stage is not required as long as she continues to make progress toward the goal, and this is reported meaningfully to parents at each reporting period. While oral-reading rate is a general education benchmark, age-appropriate articulation skill is a speech and language standard. One supports the other. Progress in speech links to academic performance. Average oral-reading rate is the child's age × 10. Reading passages aloud will be the next step toward complete carryover to conversation which the speech-language pathologist may write as the next goal. With continual practice on the classroom material, students frequently generalize on their own. Concurrently, they become better readers because they are reading more.

Continued on next page

Continued

B. Measurable Annual Goal: Tuan will demonstrate phonological awareness skills needed to succeed in the second-grade reading program in his classroom.

Benchmarks:

- He will recognize spoken word boundaries by stating correctly the number of words in an utterance. (first report card)

- He will correctly count the number of syllables in multisyllabic words read to him from his textbooks. (second report card)

- He will say aloud at least 3 words that rhyme with a given word presented orally. (third report card)

- He will accurately match a spoken word with its corresponding graphemes selected from his reading workbook. (fourth report card)

- He will be able to decode 5 unfamiliar words presented in therapy and in class as well as any three other students in his grade. (last report card)

Note:

Tuan's IEP benchmarks represent the developmental sequence for phonological awareness skills for reading, plus they are typical auditory processing skills presented in therapy. Combined, they enable Tuan to acquire both emergent reading skills and language and communication skills in his speech and language program. The speech-language pathologist would likely use many therapeutic strategies to help Tuan develop these auditory processing skills, however the IEP goals and objectives would reflect the functional use or generalization of those skills into the school curriculum.

Local guidelines or forms will give the speech-language pathologist direction in how each LEA requires measurement to be reflected for the goals and objectives or benchmarks.

IDEA (1997) has a reporting requirement that aligns reporting on IEP goal progress to the reporting periods of general education. This requirement mandates that IEPs include a statement of:

i. How the child's progress toward the annual goals will be measured; and

ii. How the parents will be regularly informed (by such means as periodic report cards), at least as often as parents are informed of their nondisabled children's progress, of—

(A) their child's progress toward the annual goals; and

(B) the extent to which that progress is sufficient to enable the child to achieve the goals by the end of the year. (34 C.F.R. § 300.347 [a] [7])

Including some measurement component in the short-term objectives or benchmarks may more easily identify "the extent to which progress is sufficient," meeting the intent of point B of the reporting requirement. Most states have interpreted this new reporting requirement as "report cards" for IEPs. Forms have been developed in many school districts to accommodate this requirement. What is important is that written communication exists between the service provider and the parent, regarding the progress that the student makes toward IEP goals.

Determination of Program, Placement, and Services

Determination of program, placement, and services is the third step in the IEP meeting process. The IEP team uses the information obtained in the first two steps to decide in what setting the goals and objectives or benchmarks can be implemented. Discussing placement or services before identifying present levels or goals can lead to unintended difficulties. Further, according to Gorn (1997a), "Each IEP goal should have corresponding items of instruction or services identified. Having goals without related programming indicates that the school district is not providing FAPE" (p. 2:14).

Students qualify for special education by meeting eligibility criteria; they do not qualify for any particular program. Common vernacular periodically refers to "qualifying for a special class" or some such phrase. Speech-language

> Students qualify for special education by meeting eligibility criteria; they do not qualify for any particular program.

pathologists and other professionals must be careful not to make this error. A student may qualify as having a disability in any of the eligibility categories (see page 91). Placement and services are decided later, as the last step of the IEP meeting process.

At times, the determination of program, placement, and services can be contentious. It is not unusual for parents and teachers to have experienced a great deal of frustration prior to finally arriving at the point of an IEP meeting. Failure in school has been the experience of the family and the student, and in many cases, this has been a tough road. Teachers may believe that the identification process has taken too long. Teachers and family members may feel that they know what program the student needs, and so they come to the IEP meeting with a specific intention in mind.

Once a student has been identified as being eligible for special education by meeting eligibility criteria, that student is entitled to receive any service that the IEP team determines is needed. The IEP team must follow the requirements and philosophy of LEAST RESTRICTIVE ENVIRONMENT (LRE) when determining placement and services, that is:

(1) That to the maximum extent appropriate, children with disabilities...are educated with children who are nondisabled; and

(2) That special classes, separate schooling or other removal of children with disabilities from the regular educational

environment occurs only if the nature or severity of the disability is such that the education in regular classes with the use of supplementary aids and services cannot be achieved satisfactorily. (34 C.F.R. § 300.550 [b])

One of the most important considerations for IEP teams in making determinations of placement is to keep children in the neighborhood school, or as close to home as possible, and attending the school that they would attend if they did not have a disability, unless their IEP requires some other arrangement. IDEA (1997) regulations specifically direct that "A child with a disability is not removed from education in age-appropriate regular classrooms solely because of needed modifications in the general curriculum" (34 C.F.R. § 300.552 [c]).

For children with "speech only" disorders (e.g., articulation, fluency, or voice disorder), speech services may be the only special education provided to the student. For children with language impairments that have an academic impact, support from the RESOURCE TEACHER or learning disabilities specialist may be provided. As the nature of the student's disability becomes more complex, it is more likely that the student will receive additional services. Sometimes the speech-language pathologist will be the only provider of special education services. Other times, the speech-language pathologist will be a member of a larger team. The service provider who is with the student the most usually assumes case management responsibility. Service delivery and how to make these decisions is discussed in Chapter 5.

Speech-language is identified as a related service (i.e., a service necessary for the student to benefit from special education) under federal law. Speech-language services can be also be identified as special education if they are considered so under state guidelines (34 C.F.R. § 300.26 [a] [2] [i]). Speech-language services are defined as:

i. Identification of children with speech or language impairments;

ii. Diagnosis and appraisal of specific speech or language impairments;

iii. Referral for medical or other professional attention necessary for the habilitation of speech or language impairments;

iv. Provision of speech and language services for the habilitation or prevention of communicative impairments; and

v. Counseling and guidance of parents, children, and teachers regarding speech and language impairments. (34 C.F.R § 300.24 [14])

The determination of what services a student requires to meet his or her identified goals and receive educational benefit is a most important function of IEP teams. Issues such as caseload management and service delivery options are also tied to placement determination but should only be discussed at the IEP meeting if the issues pertain to the student. In other words, caseload size is an issue for the speech-language pathologist, but is not an IEP issue. Figure 4.3 recaps the IEP meeting process.

Figure 4.3

IEP Meeting Process

Determination of Present Levels of Educational Performance

- Review evaluation data
- Review classroom performance
- Review other related information
- Consider input from parents, teachers, and specialists

↓

Development of Goals and Short-Term Objectives or Benchmarks

- Based on identified areas of need
- Designed to enable the child to progress in the general education curriculum
- Are measurable

↓

Determination of Program, Placement, and Services

- Includes services needed in order for goals to be achieved
- Designed to confer meaningful educational benefit

Record Keeping and Documentation

In keeping with accountability requirements and to clearly explain the course of intervention to parents, teachers, the student, and others, documentation is critical to the work of public school speech-language pathologists. To verify what activities were completed with the student and how these activities were designed to meet IEP goals, it is recommended that speech-language pathologists maintain records for each student. The following are suggestions of what might be recorded in this documentation:

1. A schedule of when students were seen for service and for how long

2. A log of intervention activities and outcomes

3. A portfolio of student performance/student work

4. Records of communication with parents, teachers, and others regarding the student

5. A student file with all IEP and assessment information, as well as IEP procedure documentation and progress report cards

Speech-language pathologists should be aware that if parents request their child's records, copies of all documentation, such as that mentioned above, in addition to the typical school records, must be provided to them. For this reason, all professionals must be cautious and prudent about the notes they include in files. Speech-language pathologists should also have records of the intervention strategies being used, the success they are having with them, the modifications being made, and the conditions in which the intervention is taking place. Not only must goals be measurable, but the speech-language pathologist must also document when and how those measurements are taken. Data sheets and logs need to be readable and complete. Using tried-and-true documentation forms such as those found in *The Survival Guide for School-Based Speech-Language Pathologists* (Pritchard Dodge, 2000) and *Social Skill Strategies* (Book A and Book B) (Gajewski, Hirn, and Mayo, 1998) can be useful for speech-language pathologists.

Langdon (2000) provided excellent suggestions for enhancing interactions with families of English-language learners. Langdon's suggestions are generally GOOD PRACTICES:

- Avoid using professional jargon and provide examples instead.

- Ensure that the parents understand the assessment procedures and reason(s) why the student may have a language-learning difficulty.

- Invite the parent to offer their perspective about their child.

- Respect the parents' comments about their child's problem. Also, understand how various handicapping [sic] conditions can be viewed by various cultures and individuals within a culture.

- Offer suggestions that are realistic.

- Provide as many examples as possible from the school setting.

- Avoid insisting that the parents use English.

- Invite the parents to attend and participate in the intervention process. (pp. 382–383)

Participating as a member of the IEP team, writing and developing an IEP, and conducting intervention based on the plan outlined in the document is a complex process. Speech-language pathologists who are new to the field or new to a school system should seek a mentor to learn the specifics of the IEP process for the system in which he or she works. If a speech-language pathologist is a Clinical Fellow (CF), then his or her CF supervisor may be able to serve in this capacity. Other non–speech-language pathology professionals in the school district may also be able to assist a new speech-language pathologist learning the way.

All educators must be aware of the confidentiality requirements under the FAMILY EDUCATIONAL RIGHTS AND PRIVACY ACT (FERPA, 1974, § 513 of Public Law 93-380 [The Education Amendments of 1974]), which applies to IDEA (1997) and all school records. Under FERPA, students' and parents' rights to privacy are protected with regard to personally identifiable information in education records. An IEP is an education record; therefore, to disclose improperly the contents of an IEP would be a violation of FERPA (Gorn, 1997a).

In practical terms, this means that all educators must be extremely careful when they discuss cases. Revealing the names of children and parents would be considered a violation of their rights, if the receiver of the information is not involved in the case by virtue of their position with the LEA. Make it a personal rule not to reveal the names of children or families to anyone who does not have direct involvement in the case and never to use the names of children on your caseloads in public, even when discussing a case with a team member. If speech-language pathologists make this their personal habit, they will not have to worry about being overheard by a child's relative or family friend.

> Make it a personal rule not to reveal the names of children or families to anyone who does not have direct involvement in the case.

Speech-language pathologists and other special education personnel often complain about paperwork demands, which can be overwhelming. All requirements, however, are procedurally driven. In order to comply with the law, documentation must be completed. In addition to completing forms correctly and following appropriate procedures, timelines must be kept. Teams that work closely together find the process moves along smoothly, assuring compliance and quality.

Annual and Triennial Assessments

IDEA (1997) requires that students who are eligible for special education services have their progress reviewed at least annually by the IEP team. This is called the annual review, and the intended date is written on a child's current IEP. Every three years, the IEP team needs to decide if further testing is needed and determine if the student should remain in special education. Because "comprehensive evaluation is the critical foundation for developing an educationally relevant IEP" (Brannen et al., 2000, p. 20), each type of evaluation will be discussed below.

An ANNUAL REVIEW of the student's IEP is conducted each year for a student to measure and record the amount of change that occurred for each of that student's written annual goals. In addition, specific short-term objectives, benchmarks, or both are reviewed to determine if they are needed and remain relevant to the general education curriculum. Although a speech-language pathologist may choose to reassess a student using some standardized tests, these tests are not required and, in fact, may be less effective. The results of standardized testing are useful for qualifying students for services, since these tests compare the abilities of a student with the expected abilities of other students his or her age, usually nationwide. However, these tests do not offer results in functional terms. When used to measure change, test scores offer a numerical value of how a student responded to a testing probe, but not his or her actual performance in the classroom, with peers, or in other true-life situations. The FUNCTIONAL COMMUNICATION MEASURES (FCMs) described at the end of Chapter 5 are more useful. Speech-language pathologists use nonstandardized tests, observations, checklists, portfolios, and other formal and informal measures to determine progress toward the goals in a year. State- or districtwide administered assessments, which are grade level specific, may be used if the student took the tests (either with or without appropriate accommodations) as directed on the IEP. If the student is not to take the state- or districtwide assessments, the IEP must contain such a statement, and the reason must be based on why it is not appropriate for that student. Report-card-type grades, or periodic narratives, though required by IDEA (1997), do not always describe progress sufficiently to meet the state standards or the student's individual objectives. Therefore, all student evaluations should be conducted and interpreted using multiple means of assessment.

Every three years, an IEP team must determine if a student continues to have a disability. In some cases, standardized testing may be used. The same evaluation measures used for annual assessments may be used at the triennial assessment with the same cautions. IDEA (1997) allows the IEP team to determine if additional data are actually necessary to make the determination of the student's continued disability. If it is judged not necessary,

the district must notify the parents and the parents have the right to request an assessment. The district is required to assess all students whose parents request these services. Since parents are a part of all decision making for their child's program, they are involved in the discussion of which, if any, triennial reassessments are needed. At times, student needs are clear without formal testing. For example, a child making year-to-year progress on speech-language goals for communication disabilities related to cognitive impairment would not need to have a triennial assessment to determine if he or she still has a cognitive impairment. The disability would not have to be reaffirmed unless parents specifically request that to be done. This clarification of IDEA in the 1997 reauthorization was designed to better utilize a child's instructional time and not repeat comprehensive testing cycles every year or every three years.

The school district must administer the tests and other evaluation materials needed to produce the data identified by the IEP team. Parents are asked to help define the data needed for their child. The IEP is the vehicle that links this vital evaluation information to the desired outcomes for each child. These outcomes become the basis for determining the particular services that the student needs, which professionals can best provide them, and in what setting they should be offered. Annual reviews and triennial re-evaluations, when determined to be needed, serve this purpose for students and families. Local policy directs procedures for assessments.

Exit or Dismissal Criteria

Although this chapter emphasizes how to place children with communication disorders into intervention programs, of equal importance is to describe the criteria for successfully completing that intervention. It is good practice to think about exit criteria at the beginning of the intervention cycle, because the criteria should serve as the "beacon" that guides the intervention process.

Reassessment of a student is required by IDEA to make a dismissal decision. The student should be dismissed when his or her communication no longer has an adverse effect on education. This can be difficult to ascertain unless functional outcomes have been collected throughout the intervention. If the speech-language pathologist or the team focused on impairment, then retesting to see if there is still an impairment (standardized testing) will not provide the information needed to determine dismissal. Focusing on reducing the effect of the impairment (i.e., the disability) will provide the information needed to decide on dismissal. The data that have been gathered while the student was receiving speech-language services can be used for the dismissal decision.

Intervention should not continue until a student is "perfect" or "100%." This is often not realistic. Dismissal may occur before a student demonstrates complete mastery of all targeted skills. Reassessment for dismissal requires the speech-language pathologist to revisit the options of standardized, performance-based, and DYNAMIC ASSESSMENT (as discussed in Chapter 3) to determine which will provide the most useful information. Dismissal criteria should be functionally based, not test-based, as shown in the samples that follow.

States have been slower to design exit criteria than eligibility criteria. Some have more exacting statements than others. Some school districts have developed their own dismissal criteria to help support their statements to parents and teachers that a student has made sufficient progress, or may benefit more from a different service. In a few instances, a decision to terminate speech-language services may be based on mutually agreed on circumstances such as the student's interest, motivation, or available time.

Each of the methods described in the next section on exit criteria gives the school-based speech-language pathologist a basis for making dismissal decisions with some degree of confidence and connection to school academic expectancies and IDEA (1997) accountability.

California

The following exit criteria for four types of communication disorders were developed by a large county-based school system—Merced County—with a culturally diverse population and comprehensive urban and rural service delivery plans. This list (from the Merced County Office of Special Education, 1998) begins with general considerations for exiting intervention and continues into specific disorders.

Articulation Therapy
General Considerations

There are several factors for the IEP team to consider when making decisions regarding exit from articulation therapy:

1. Correct production of the target phoneme is reached with the speech sample reflecting criteria as designed on the IEP.

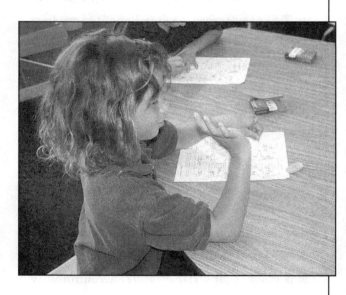

2. Articulation skills are determined to be commensurate with chronological and developmental age.

3. After one year of direct therapy, there is a lack of significant progress in articulation skills as evidenced by probes, therapy data, and teacher/parent observation.

4. The student consistently demonstrates behaviors that are not conducive to therapy such as a lack of cooperation, motivation, or

chronic absenteeism. In these circumstances the IEP Team should consider the initial eligibility decision since these behaviors may reflect social maladjustment, environmental, cultural, or economic factors rather than an actual disability. The IEP team may also explore alternative services or strategies to remedy interfering behaviors or conditions.

5. Other associated and/or disabling conditions prevent the student from benefiting from further therapy. Examples are dental abnormalities, velopharyngeal insufficiency, or inadequate physiological support for speech. (p. I-2)

Articulation Exit Criteria

A student no longer qualifies for articulation therapy when the IEP team determines that any one or more of the following general conditions exist:

1. The student's disability no longer negatively affects his/her educational performance in the regular education or special education program.

2. The student no longer meets the qualification criteria for a speech and language disorder under which he or she is receiving articulation therapy as a primary special education service OR the student no longer requires articulation

therapy as a related/DIS service in order to benefit from his/her special education program.

3. The student's needs will be better served by an alternative program and/or service.

4. He/she reaches the age of 22 years (or the end of the school year in which he/she turns 22 years of age).

5. He/she graduates from high school.

6. Parent (or student over 18 years of age) refuses to allow the continuance of special education services. (p. I-3)

Voice Therapy General Considerations

There are several factors for the IEP team to consider when making decisions regarding exit from voice therapy:

1. The SLP's professional judgement indicates that the student's voice is within normal limits as related to age, gender, and culture.

2. Other associated and/or disabling conditions prevent the student from benefiting from further therapy. Examples are dental abnormalities, velopharyngeal insufficiency, or inadequate physiological support for speech.

3. Persistent inappropriate vocal behaviors prevent the student from benefiting from therapy.

4. The student consistently demonstrates behaviors that are not conducive to therapy such as a lack of cooperation, motivation, or chronic absenteeism. In these circumstances the IEP Team should consider the initial eligibility decision since these behaviors may reflect social maladjustment, environmental, cultural, or economic factors rather than an actual disability. The IEP team may also explore alternative services or strategies to remedy interfering behaviors or conditions. (p. II-2)

Voice Exit Criteria

The student no longer qualifies for voice therapy when the IEP team determines that any one or more of the following general conditions exist:

1. The student's disability no longer negatively affects his/her educational performance in the regular education or special education program.

2. The student no longer meets the qualification criteria for a speech and language disorder under which he or she is receiving voice therapy as a primary special education service OR the student no longer requires voice therapy as a related/DIS service in order to benefit from his/her special education program.

3. The student's needs will be better served by an alternative program and/or service.

4. He/she reaches the age of 22 years (or the end of the school year in which he/she turns 22 years of age).

5. He/she graduates from high school.

6. Parent (or student over 18 years of age) refuses to allow the continuance of special education services. (p. II-2)

Fluency Therapy Exit Criteria

1. He/she achieves the fluency goal as designed on the IEP, and/or the student perceives him/herself to a normal speaker.

2. Student has failed to respond to intensive intervention over a 1- to 2-year period of remediation, following exposure to a variety of therapeutic techniques.

3. The student consistently demonstrates behaviors that are not conducive to therapy such as a lack of cooperation, motivation, or chronic absenteeism. In these circumstances the IEP Team should consider the initial eligibility decision since these behaviors may reflect social maladjustment, environmental, cultural, or economic factors rather than an actual disability. The IEP team may also explore alternative services or strategies to remedy interfering behaviors or conditions.

4. Other associated and/or handicapping conditions such as neurological impairments prevent the student from benefiting from further therapy. (p. III-2)

The exit criteria listed for fluency are the same as for articulation and voice.

Language Therapy General Considerations

There are several factors for the IEP team to consider when making decisions about exiting from language therapy:

1. The student demonstrates receptive and expressive language skills within the range expected for his/her developmental level.

2. The student is performing at a predetermined level as designated on the IEP.

3. The student uses augmentative communication aids appropriately, effectively, and independently.

4. The student uses compensatory communication skills appropriately, effectively, and independently.

5. There is a lack of progress in language skills within 2 years time as evidenced by formal tests, therapy records, observations, teacher, parent, consultation, or other documentation.

6. The student consistently demonstrates behaviors that are not conducive to therapy such as a lack of cooperation, motivation, or chronic absenteeism. In these circumstances the IEP Team should consider the initial eligibility decision since these behaviors may reflect social maladjustment, environmental, cultural, or economic factors rather than an actual disability. The IEP team may also explore alternative services or strategies to remedy interfering behaviors or conditions.

7. The student's communication skills are best reinforced and monitored in a classroom setting. (p. IV-2)

The exit criteria listed for language are the same as for articulation, voice, and fluency.

Illinois

Exit criteria can also be stated for speech-language services directly from IDEA (1997). There are basically three statements that the Illinois State Board of Education (1993) has used as their criteria:

1. The need for specialized services to address the adverse effects on educational performance is no longer present.

2. The disability no longer has an adverse effect on the student's educational performance.

3. The disability no longer exists. (p. 21)

Florida

State guidelines may provide an outline against which the speech-language pathologist can measure a student's satisfactory performance. Florida Department of Education's manual (1995) lists some of the following measures for speech and language dismissal criteria:

A student will be dismissed when evidence has been documented that the student has satisfactorily achieved the program goals resulting in acceptable language, articulation, fluency and/or voice based on re-evaluation.

Satisfactory achievement of program goals is defined as:

(a) At least 85% correct and acceptable use of language articulation, fluency and voice in a conversational sample, and/or

(b) Communication skills at or above (1) standard deviation from the mean based on chronological age or expected level of functioning, and/or

(c) Communication skills at or above the 16th percentile, and/or

(d) Communication skills at or above the 3rd stanine.

Dismissal may be appropriate when the following criteria are documented:

1. The student's achievement of program goals has resulted in maximum expected improvement (but not at a level of satisfactory achievement as defined above), or

2. The communication disorder no longer adversely interferes with the student's pre-academic, academic, social, emotional, or vocational adjustment. (pp. 18–19)

CHAPTER 5

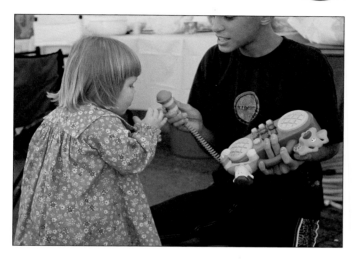

Service Delivery Options

IN THIS CHAPTER

Service delivery in speech-language and special education has traditionally been conceptualized as discrete programs organized by disability, location, and degree of contact between the professional and the client (Neidecker and Blosser, 1993). However, when viewed in the broadest sense, every activity on behalf of, or in contact with, a client—screening, consultation, assessment, identification, goal setting with functional outcomes and links to the curriculum, intervention, collaboration, re-evaluation, parent contacts, and dismissal—is service delivery. This chapter scans the larger picture of special education, of which speech-language services are a part. The role of school-based speech-language pathologists in inclusive education, models of speech-language intervention, good practice issues, working with a school team, functional outcomes, linking services to consumer satisfaction, and functional communication measures are also described.

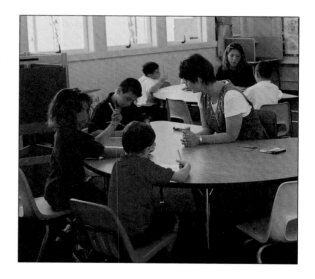

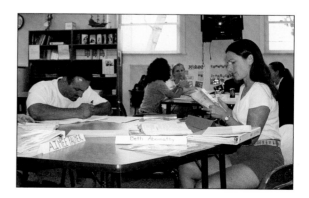

1. What are the components of service delivery in speech-language programs in schools today? How have they changed in the last decade? Why?

2. What are the essential features of the ASHA inclusive practices paper (see page 131)? How do you think the position statement will shape the design of service delivery systems in schools?

3. How did speech-language pathologists attempt to answer the four basic questions that center on functional outcomes (see Figure 5.5) before considering a functional approach? What resources can you use to respond to the four questions today?

4. Review the section on functional outcomes, and write three outcome statements for each of the students described in the case studies (see page 154). What elements do you need to address to make the outcomes functional?

5. Use Figure 5.4 to make up a school schedule for a speech-language pathologist who does any nine of the activities in the bulleted list.

6. What program characteristics may be used to show consumers that a student will receive appropriate benefit from an IEP? Give examples of measures that would demonstrate student benefit.

7. Use the sample functional communication measures (FCMs) in the sidebar on page 153 to project a one-year goal for a student performing at Level 3 for language comprehension. Design assessments or probes to use in gathering data for quarterly progress reports to parents.

Concept of Service Delivery

Traditionally, speech-language pathologists scheduled students for intervention based on physical factors, such as what type of disorder a student presented, the age of the student, the size of the speech room, the school's academic schedule, and the number of days per week the speech-language pathologist was at that site. While these are all factors in a school-based program, they are not critical to obtaining the best FUNCTIONAL OUTCOMES for the student. (See "What Are the Steps in the IEP Meeting Process?" in Chapter 4 for a discussion of the importance of functional outcomes related to disability instead of impairment.) Increasing emphasis will be placed on using research-based strategies in the future, with the intent to increase the efficiency and functionality of all SPECIAL EDUCATION intervention programs. SERVICE DELIVERY will need to be based on what approach provides the most appropriate treatment for the student, requiring speech-language pathologists to adjust models and time constraints to fit. Blosser and Kratcoski (1997) stated that the current "concept of unique and discreet options has in effect limited, instead of expanded, clinician's [sic] thinking about how to develop appropriate treatment programs" (p. 101).

New ways to think about and plan for school-based speech-language service delivery, including direct and indirect intervention, have been posed. Early texts urged "speech correctionists" to use "forms of practice" such as "singing, perceptual reorganization, naming, oral reading, radio speaking, choral speaking, catharsis" and other "adjustive techniques." Public school interventions were described with four models for service delivery: "1.) schools for exceptional children, 2.) itinerant remedial speech correction, 3.) speech improvement, and 4.) classroom teachers who felt the need to know something about speech handicaps, and in the process of professional preparation for teaching, have taken one or more courses dealing with speech disorders" (Johnson, Brown, Curtis, Edney, and Keaster, 1956, p. 413).

An Overview of Special Education Services

Perhaps the best way to understand how speech-language services fit into the fabric of special education services begins with a review of the interventions common to that part of public education. The INDIVIDUALS WITH DISABILITIES EDUCATION ACT (IDEA) AMENDMENTS OF 1997 were discussed in detail in the first three chapters of this book; however, the actual delivery of school-based services requires further description. With the possible exception of assessment, service delivery is the most visible part of IDEA. While there are state-to-state differences, the general practice of assisting struggling learners identified with exceptional needs in the public education system is applied in all 50 states.

Prevalence of Speech-Language Disorders

The prevalence of speech-language disorders in public school populations has consistently been reported to be 3 to 4% of students enrolled in general education (Neidecker, 1987). This number is misleading, however, as it does not take into account all the students who have medical or educational disabilities that include COMMUNICATION DISORDERS. Students identified as having special education needs represent approximately 10% of the school population, with a range from 8 to 18% across states. Within this special education population, about 22% are students with speech-language impairments (not those with hearing disorders or students in other groups who commonly also have communication disorders, such as traumatic brain injury, developmental disabilities, and LEARNING DISABILITIES), the second highest percentage after learning disabilities at 51% (U.S. Department of Education, 1999).

The largest proportions of special education students served primarily in general education classrooms are those students with communication disorders (see Table 5.1). Of the students with speech-language impairments, 95.1% are served primarily in the general education classroom (U.S. Department of Education, 1998). This meets the letter and the spirit of the federal law and assists states in meeting federal guidelines for least restrictive settings.

The breadth of service delivery expected of speech-language pathologists in school programs is evident from states' plans for educational relevancy written to meet federal guidelines (Brannen et al., 2000). These usually include all services delivered, not simply intervention services. One state can be used as an example. Beginning at the top of Figure 5.1 (see page 126), it is obvious that service delivery is greater than the small "Implementation" box in the center. This box may be thought of as the "hub" of the schematic since intervention to assist the learner is also the reason we engage in all the other activities. Figure 5.1 includes the dimensions addressed in the next three chapters of this book.

Levels of Special Education Services

A classic diagram of seven levels of service delivery in special education, presented in Figure 5.2 (see page 127), was introduced in 1976 after the passage of the EDUCATION FOR ALL HANDICAPPED CHILDREN ACT (EAHCA) and credited to Deno (1970). It shows that the greatest number of students are in the LEAST RESTRICTIVE ENVIRONMENT (LRE) of level one (general education classroom) cascading down to the most restrictive level seven (nonpublic school). Most students with speech-language disabilities, even those with multiple needs, are served in levels 1–4. They spend most, if not all, of their school day in the general education classroom with their peers. The general education curriculum, taught by classroom teachers, is the most prevalent form of education for students that speech-language pathologists serve. This is the single most important factor in the creation of speech-language service delivery models in schools today. The identification, focus, frequency,

Table 5.1

Disability Categories and Proportion of Students Currently Served Primarily in General Education Classrooms for Students Ages 6–21

(Full-Time Regular Class Placement, or Regular Class Placement with Resource Room Service)

Disability Category	Proportion of Students Served Primarily in Regular Classrooms
Speech/Language impairments	95.1%
Learning disabilities	81.7%
Other health impaired	73.4%
Visual impairments	68.3%
Orthopedic impairments	61.5%
Hearing impairments	55.0%
Emotional/Behavioral disorders	47.1%
Mental retardation	38.8%
Multiple disabilities	24.2%
Traumatic brain injury	53.4%
Deaf-blindness	20.7%
Autism	22.7%
All categories	74.0%

From *Twentieth Annual Report to Congress on the Implementation of the Individuals with Disabilities Education Act* (p. 14), by the U.S. Department of Education, 1998, Washington, DC: Author.

intensity, purpose, and progress assessment of students with speech-language disabilities is predicated on their general education program.

Levels 5, 6, and 7 in the cascade refer to self-contained classrooms in which MAINSTREAMING (i.e., including a student with his or her peers developing typically) is the only way a student has access to same-age peers. In these settings, students are typically grouped by disability with an age span of 4 to 6 years due to the low incidence of such conditions. This is even more likely to be the case in rural or low population areas. Educational time with peers needs to be arranged for most of these students and can be difficult logistically. Students might even be at segregated sites, where only students with special needs are educated. These sites make peer contacts even more awkward to manage. In some cases, speech-language sessions might provide the only contact with age-appropriate peers. Students identified with speech-language needs could receive services in a PULLOUT program with same-age peers and a grade-appropriate

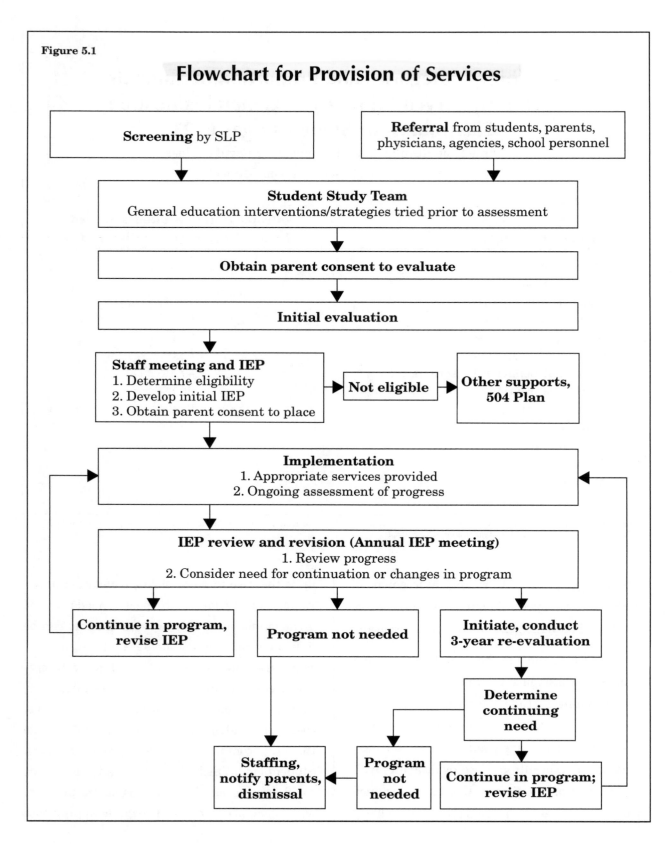

Figure 5.1

Flowchart for Provision of Services

Screening by SLP

Referral from students, parents, physicians, agencies, school personnel

Student Study Team
General education interventions/strategies tried prior to assessment

Obtain parent consent to evaluate

Initial evaluation

Staff meeting and IEP
1. Determine eligibility
2. Develop initial IEP
3. Obtain parent consent to place

Not eligible

Other supports, 504 Plan

Implementation
1. Appropriate services provided
2. Ongoing assessment of progress

IEP review and revision (Annual IEP meeting)
1. Review progress
2. Consider need for continuation or changes in program

Continue in program, revise IEP

Program not needed

Initiate, conduct 3-year re-evaluation

Determine continuing need

Staffing, notify parents, dismissal

Program not needed

Continue in program; revise IEP

Figure 5.2

Application of the Seven Levels of Service in Special Education to Communication Disabilities

Level One
General education classroom—the greatest number of
options are available here, especially in inclusive settings nationwide.

Level Two
General education classroom with consultation—
students are supported by speech-language pathologist/teacher
teams in collaborative ways.

Level Three
General education classroom with designated instruction
and services—pullout types of sessions are typical here.

Level Four
General education classroom with resource
assistance—speech-language pathologists and resource
teachers work together to offer greater support.

Level Five
Full-time special education classroom—
classes may be taught by speech-language
pathologists or other qualified teachers.

Level Six
Special school—larger numbers
of students with communication
disabilities are grouped together.

Level Seven
Nonpublic school—a
clinical or educational
setting in the community.

From "The Casccade of Special Education Services," by E. Deno, 1970, *Exceptional Children, 39,* p. 495. © 1994 by the Council for Exceptional Children. Adapted with permission.

curriculum. (Highly innovative speech-language pathologists do make a difference for the student!) Speech-language services for students in these service levels often lack the range of options available on other levels. Careful planning and implementation are needed to assure that all students' services are not lessened by the restrictions of the setting.

Types of Special Education Services

Related Services

Students may be eligible to receive FREE APPRO- PRIATE PUBLIC EDUCATION (FAPE) through special education alone or with corresponding RELATED SERVICES that support the special education services for the primary disability area and enable a child to benefit from his or her special education program. According to 34 CODE OF FEDERAL REGULATIONS (C.F.R.) § 300.24 (a):

> [T]he term *related services* means transportation and such developmental, corrective, and other supportive services as are required to assist a child with a disability to benefit from special education, and includes speech-language pathology and audiology services, psychological services, physical and occupational therapy, recreation, including therapeutic recreation, early identification and assessment of disabilities in children, counseling services, including rehabilitation counseling, orientation and mobility services, and medical services

for diagnostic or evaluation purposes. The term also includes school health services, social work services in schools, and parent counseling and training.

Students with speech-language disabilities may also have other cognitive, educational, behavioral, emotional, or health challenges. In fact, speech-language disabilities may be manifestations of other congenital or acquired conditions, such as developmental delays, Down syndrome, head trauma, AUTISM SPECTRUM DIS- ORDERS, and cerebral palsy. Speech-language development plays an integral part in the educational success of children with such conditions, so speech-language services may be recommended as a related service when a student meets the criteria for one of the other 12 special education eligibility categories (see Chapter 4, page 91). Speech-language pathologists would then provide services that would allow a student to benefit from a special education program. For example, developing an AUGMENTATIVE AND ALTERNATIVE COMMUNICATION (AAC) system may be a related service that would allow a student with cerebral palsy to participate more effectively in his or her special education instruction. The most frequently requested and provided related service is speech-language assessment and intervention (U.S. Department of Education, 1999).

Mainstreaming and Inclusion

The realization that education in this country must be valid for *all* children began with mainstreaming. Mainstreaming was later referred to as the REGULAR EDUCATION INITIATIVE (REI) (Will,

1986), which evolved into the INCLUSION MOVEMENT and eventually had a far-reaching effect on the delivery of all instructional services in schools (Biklin, 1992; Hoskins, 1990; Stainback and Stainback, 1996). Speech-language pathologists have described the profound differences that inclusion brought to service delivery in schools (Creaghead, 1999; Hoskins, 1995; Power-deFur and Orelove, 1997). "The movement toward inclusionary education for children with special needs has dramatically changed the professional roles of special educators working in schools. A remedial framework, previously the cornerstone of intervention for special education services, has been challenged" (Merritt and Culatta, 1998, p. ix). All school and community-based services for children with disabilities have been influenced by the Inclusion Movement.

Educators have used the term *mainstreaming* to refer to students with exceptional needs who are served in self-contained special education classrooms but join their same-age peers in recess, lunch, art, music, and classroom academics for perhaps 10–40 percent of their day (Biklin, 1992; Mastropieri and Scruggs, 2000). This part-time program has been gradually replaced in many schools with *inclusion*. In the inclusive environment, students are with same-age peers for the majority of the school day, but may leave from time to time for services outside the classroom. Speech-language intervention is one of those services. The Inclusion Movement "has also challenged the manner in which speech language pathologists (SLPs) plan and deliver services to children with communication impairments" (Merritt and Culatta, 1998, p. ix). Power-deFur and Orelove (1997) believe that

the inclusion trend will increase steadily. All service providers have already altered, or will soon be altering, their programs to include children with and without disabilities (Hoskins, 1995; Mastropieri and Scruggs, 2000; Montgomery, 1997a, 1997b). Many national organizations—including the AMERICAN SPEECH-LANGUAGE-HEARING ASSOCIATION (ASHA) and others with large numbers of members who are speech-language pathologists in schools—have issued brief policy and position statements on inclusion (see sidebar on page 130 for a list of examples on the Web). These organizations' statements range from strongly worded opposition (like those of the American Federation of Teachers or the Learning Disabilities Association of America [LDA]) to cautious support (like those of the National Association of Elementary School Principals or the National Association of School Psychologists) to enthusiastic endorsement (like those of the National Association of State Boards of Education or The Association for Persons with Severe Handicaps [TASH]). State departments of education often have official statements on inclusive schooling, so it is wise for speech-language pathologists to know the philosophy of the various organizations, educators, and parents involved in the school.

Parents and educators have had strong feelings on both sides of the theory and practice of inclusion. Some felt that students needed to be with same-age peers as much as possible to make friends and to help all students learn social roles (Stainback and Stainback, 1996). Others have stated that the amount of modification necessary for some children is disruptive to the students with disabilities and their peers without disabilities (Kauffman and Hallahan,

---

Position Statements on Inclusion

Many organizations took positions on inclusion during the mid-1990s. A sampling of viewpoints are available online.

American Federation of Teachers — *www.aft.org/about/resolutions/1994/inclusion.html*

The Association for Persons with Severe Handicaps — *www.tash.org/resolutions/R33INCED.html*

Learning Disabilities Association of America — *www.ldanatl.org/positions/inclusion.shtml*

National Association of Elementary School Principals — *www.naesp.org/misc/platform2000.htm*

National Association of School Psychologists — *www.schoolhousedoor.com/media/teacher/haggart-inclusiveprog.txt*

National Education Association — *www.nea.org/publiced/idea/neainclu.html*

National Joint Committee on Learning Disabilities — *http://ldonline.org/njeld/react_inclu.html*

1995; National Joint Committee on Learning Disabilities [NJCLD], 2001). Many parents and professionals, especially those in the field of hearing loss and deafness, believe each student is so highly individualistic that the exact same set of learner characteristics could indicate inclusion in one case, but not in another (Seal, 1997).

Speech-language pathologists have relied on ASHA's (1996b) "Inclusive Practices for Children and Youths with Communication Disorders" to help clarify service delivery for students with disabilities who receive their support in general education classrooms. This position paper supports an array of settings for students but recognizes the powerful effect that peer interactions have on the development of communication skills. (See sidebar for the full text of ASHA's position statement, which falls in the range of cautious support with a strong focus on individual needs.)

As mentioned in the prevalence section of this chapter (see "Prevalence of Speech-Language Disorders," page 124), a large percentage of students with communication disorders are educated in inclusive settings. Those students with communication disorders in addition to another special education condition are likely to be in more restrictive environments using the mainstreaming concept of "visiting their peers' classrooms" (Mastropieri and Scruggs, 2000, p. 23). This practice will continue to change as well. If successful, students with more significant disabilities may gradually spend a larger portion of their day with same-age peers. However, greater amounts of time in inclusive environments require more targeted modifications for students, especially as they reach the secondary level (Montgomery, 1997a; Seal, 1997). Seal suggests that differentiated classes for DEAF students, or those with severe hearing loss, might include deaf culture, ASSISTIVE

ASHA's Position Statement on Inclusion

It is the position of the American Speech-Language-Hearing Association (ASHA) that an array of speech, language, and hearing services should be available in educational settings to support children and youths with communication disorders. The term "inclusive practices" best represents this philosophy. The inclusive-practices philosophy emphasizes serving children and youths in the least restrictive environment that meets their needs optimally. Inclusive practices consist of a range of service-delivery options that need not be mutually exclusive. They can include direct, classroom-based, community-based, and consultative intervention programming. Inclusive practices are based on a commitment to selecting and designing interventions that meet the need of each child and family. Factors contributing to the determination of individual need include the child's age, type of disability, communication competence, language and cultural background, academic performance, social skills, family and teacher concerns, and the student's own attitudes about speech, language, and hearing services.

ASHA recognizes that the provision of speech, language, and hearing services in educational settings is moving toward service-delivery models that integrate intervention with general educational programs, often termed *inclusion* [italics added]. Inclusion has numerous strengths, including natural opportunities for peer interaction, and available research suggests cautious optimism regarding its effectiveness in promoting communication abilities and skills in related developmental domains. ASHA believes that the shift toward inclusion will not be optimal when implemented in absolute terms. Rather, the unique and specific needs of each child and family must always be considered.

The broad goal of inclusive service delivery should be compatible with continued recognition of the individual's unique needs and concerns. Inclusive practices are recommended as a guide in the development of intervention programming for children and youths with communication disorders.

After SPED placement – should…

TECHNOLOGY, self advocacy, and others. Montgomery (2000b) listed three guidelines for successfully beginning the inclusion process. An INDIVIDUALIZED EDUCATION PROGRAM (IEP) team should ensure that students re-entering an inclusive classroom after special class PLACE-MENTS should initially be supported to:

- Make one or more friends
- Have a job or responsibility in the classroom
- Have a schedule based on what the class is learning

Each of these guidelines relies heavily on a student's functional communication and, if warranted, becomes a GOAL on the child's IEP. These supports have been found to be valid for elementary- and secondary-level students (Montgomery, 1997a).

Choosing a Service Delivery System

Speech-language service delivery in schools is a synthesis of the inclusive education philosophy and IDEA's (1997) mandate for universal access to the general education curriculum. Models of service delivery presented here were selected from a review of the current literature in school-based practice, surveys of school-based speech-language pathologists (Peters-Johnson, 1998), and experiences of both authors as school-based speech-language pathologists. Service delivery models are described using ASHA's *Preferred Practice Patterns for the Profession of Speech-Language Pathology* (1997c), school realities, and the most appropriate student outcomes.

Speech-language pathologists perform many activities on behalf of students from birth to age 22 nationwide, and age 25 in Michigan. The diversity of these activities is illustrated in Figure 5.3. Some of these activities have already been discussed in preceding chapters and others will be addressed later in this book (see Chapters 6 and 7). To do their jobs successfully, speech-language pathologists need to carefully schedule their time and duties, especially if they are working at multiple sites. These services are all used in school-based programs, though speech-language pathologists will not necessarily conduct them all.

Components of Service Delivery

Blosser and Kratcoski (1997) posed a framework for designing service delivery models that would take into account all the conventional criteria and allow speech-language pathologists to embrace new models as they became necessary. They felt that a speech-language pathologist's role was continually evolving with an increased understanding of individuals with communication disorders and the effects on learning and daily living tasks. Throughout the field, consumers of speech-language services have become more involved in their own treatment. In schools, partnerships are formed with parents and community agencies, technology has made the improbable likely, and documentation of student outcomes drives education and rehabilitation. Speech-language pathologists need a framework that encompasses all service delivery models, not a proliferation of more and more models. Blosser and Kratcoski's framework (see Table 5.2 on page 134) appears to conclude at the year 2000, but the three foci of treatment will dominate decision-making for the foreseeable future.

Every service model should address four ideas: overall effectiveness, coordination with other programs and services, commitment of all parties, and resources available. A student should receive services that are matched to his or her needs at that point in time and are flexible to changing conditions. According to Blosser and Kratcoski (1997), this requires flexing the provider, the activities, and the context. In the following descriptions, the provider arrangement changes, the range of activities is broad but primarily curriculum-centered, and the

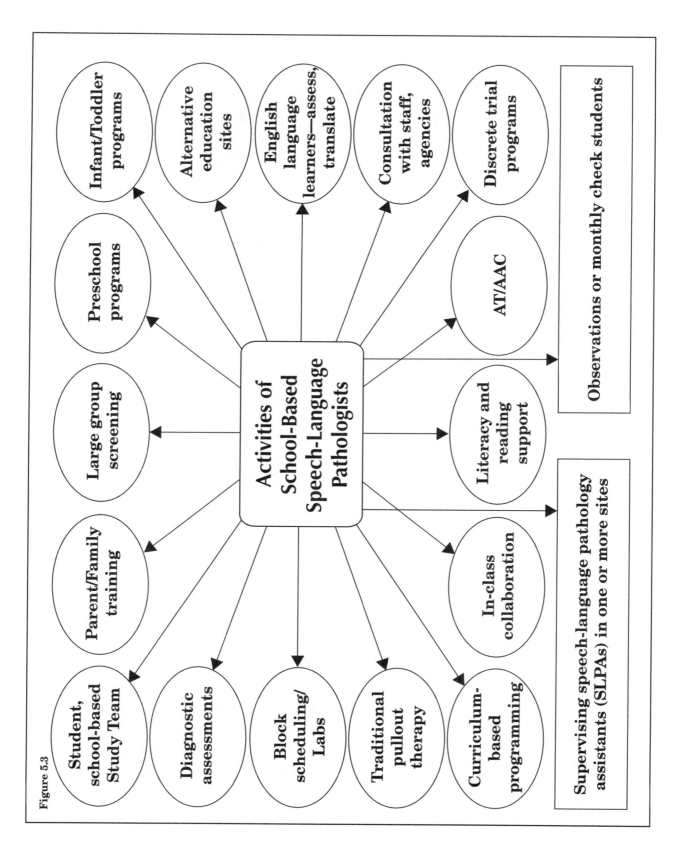

Figure 5.3

Infant/Toddler programs

Alternative education sites

English language learners—assess, translate

Consultation with staff, agencies

Discrete trial programs

Preschool programs

AT/AAC

Observations or monthly check students

Large group screening

Activities of School-Based Speech-Language Pathologists

Literacy and reading support

Parent/Family training

In-class collaboration

Supervising speech-language pathology assistants (SLPAs) in one or more sites

Student, school-based Study Team

Diagnostic assessments

Block scheduling/ Labs

Traditional pullout therapy

Curriculum-based programming

Table 5.2

The Evolution of Speech-Language Pathologist Service Delivery Models

	1970s	1980s	1990s	2000
Focus for treatment	Mechanistic view of language	Pragmatics	Functional, interactive communication Preparation for learning, living, and working	Outcomes
Speech-language pathologist's role	Specialist model	Expert model	Collaborative-consultative model	Facilitator of the service delivery
Emerging issues	Language use is important	Language and learning are linked	Inclusion, transition, efficacy, account-ability, outcomes	To be decided
	syntax / semantics / phonology	content / form / use	communication / learning / collaboration	context / providers / activities

From "PACs: A Framework for Determining Appropriate Service Delivery Options," by J.L. Blosser and A. Kratcoski, 1997, *Language, Speech, and Hearing Services in Schools, 28,* p. 100. © 1997 by the American Speech-Language-Hearing Association. Reprinted with permission.

contexts are school-related. Flexibility among provider, activities, and context is important in the following models, as in the curriculum models in Chapter 6 and the expanded and specialized service delivery models presented in Chapter 7.

The Concept of Good Practice

The term GOOD PRACTICE is used in school-based programs (and other settings) to denote the use of research-based, effective, and measurable techniques to provide intervention or instruction for students who experience communication disorders and disabilities. In contrast to BEST PRACTICE, which establishes one intervention as better than all others, good practice can be defended successfully in legal proceedings and mediations. What is best for one student's circumstances may not be best for another. Professionals in speech and language, and other educational pursuits, are ethically bound to apply good practice principles to all their responsibilities, with a vigilance for new information and research. "To use only one [approach]…is not malpractice. To use more than one is merely enriched practice" (Rosenbek, 1984, p. 361).

Some speech-language pathologists teach classrooms of students with communication disorders; some may co-teach with RESOURCE TEACHERS; and others use multiple approaches of pullout therapy (i.e., removing children from a classroom for speech-language services), co-teaching, and classroom support. There are many models based on the needs of students, the culture of school districts, and the innovative ideas and skills of speech-language pathologists everywhere.

Good practice in schools requires speech-language pathologists to recognize the commonalties and differences among three macrodelivery systems—CLASSROOM INSTRUCTION, CONVENTIONAL THERAPY, and COLLABORATIVE INTERVENTION—and to choose the system or combination of systems most likely to result in progress for a student. Progress in speech-language skills was initially the goal of school-based speech-language pathologists, but since the advent of IDEA (1997), this progress must also be linked to academic achievement at a student's appropriate level (Brannen et al., 2000).

Speech-language pathologists choose one or more of the macrodelivery systems, or alternates from one to another, over the period of time a student receives speech-language services. "Service delivery is a dynamic concept and should change as the needs of the students change. No one service delivery model should be used exclusively during treatment" (ASHA,

1999c, p. 58). STATE EDUCATIONAL AGENCIES (SEAs), through their consultant staff and committees of speech-language pathologists from the field who volunteer their time, publish guidelines for assessment, ELIGIBILITY, and service delivery for speech-language and hearing services in their states (see "Who to Ask When You Have a Question on the Job" in Chapter 9). These comprehensive manuals specify the school service delivery models encouraged in a particular state. They help speech-language pathologists select an appropriate assessment procedure, followed by one or more intervention programs. Figure 5.4, the schematic from the Indiana Speech-Language-Hearing Association (ISHA, 1997), has been included for the reader to appreciate the breadth of information available for the school-based speech-language pathologist. The model from a school service area in Illinois (see sidebar on page 137) and the generic model for schools (see Table 5.3, page 138) provide further examples of the guidance available regarding service delivery.

Classroom instruction is typically delivered by a classroom teacher, a supervised instructional aide, or a SUBJECT AREA SPECIALIST (e.g., music, art, or biology).

- In self-contained classrooms for students with special needs, this person can be a special education teacher or a speech-language pathologist.

- The intent in this setting is to teach students the grade- or age-level curriculum.

- Speech-language skills are directly or indirectly taught by a teacher as part of the subject area (e.g., auditory attention skills, opposites, descriptive labels, public speaking, oral book reports, noun-verb

135

Indiana's Overview of Good Practice in Schools

Figure 5.4

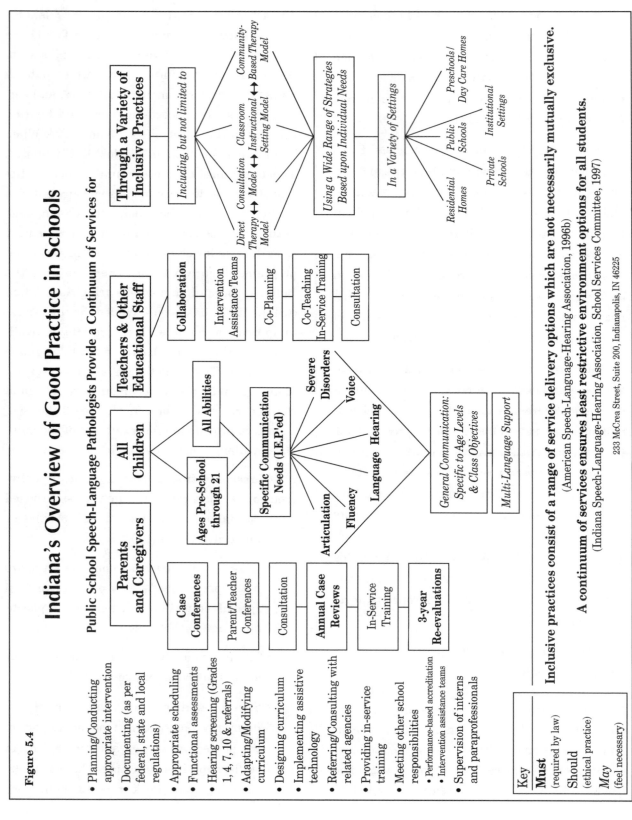

Inclusive practices consist of a range of service delivery options which are not necessarily mutually exclusive.
(American Speech-Language-Hearing Association, 1996b)

A continuum of services ensures least restrictive environment options for all students.
(Indiana Speech-Language-Hearing Association, School Services Committee, 1997)

233 McCrea Street, Suite 200, Indianapolis, IN 46225

From *Indiana's Overview of Good Practice in Schools*, by the Indiana Speech-Language-Hearing Association (ISHA), 1997, Indianapolis, IN: Author. © 1997 by ISHA. Adapted with permission.

136

Service Delivery Provision Options

Service options may include: direct intervention, consultation, monitoring, biweekly or monthly sessions to reinforce carryover, and so on.

A. Factors that may influence intervention time or may contraindicate intervention events though an identified problem exists:

1. Identified speech deviation does not interfere with the child's educational or social or emotional progress and, therefore, cannot be considered a handicap.

2. Physiological factors interfere with speech-language intervention.

3. Other areas of service need to precede speech-language services if speech-language intervention is to be beneficial.

4. Immaturity may prohibit progress in speech-language intervention.

5. When viewing the child's needs as a whole, other educational needs have priority.

A child may be dismissed from speech-language intervention services through an IEP conference when the goals and objectives have been met and no new ones are needed or when one of the above factors has priority.

B. Considerations in implementing options for individual children:

1. When a factor that would contraindicate therapy is present, the problem should still be identified. Note the reason why intervention is not indicated at this time on the IEP.

2. The factors that may influence the amount and type of speech-language service should be considered for each child at the multidisciplinary conference (MDC) when the IEP is written. The LRE mandate requires justification for the amount of time the child is missing in his or her general education program to participate in speech-language intervention.

3. This requirement to justify speech-language intervention time in view of the child's total needs can be a consideration when dismissal may be indicated although a problem still exists.

4. The rating scales were designed for use with children whose primary language is English. Bilingual children and those with regional dialects, cultural dialects, or both may require different service options.

Source: Illinois State Board of Education, Black Hawk Area Special Education District (1993)

Table 5.3

Service Delivery Model for Speech-Language Pathologists

	Itinerant Program (Direct Service)	Resource Room Program (Direct Service)	Self-Contained Program (Direct Service)	Consultation Program (Indirect Service)
Cases Served	• All communicative disorders. • All ranges (mild to severe).	• All communicative disorders (moderate to severe).	• Severe and/or multiple communicative disorders. • Primary handicapping condition is communication regardless of etiology.	• All communicative disorders. • All ranges (mild to severe).
Services Provided	• Program development, management, coordination and evaluation. • Direct services. • Provision of speech-language services in coordination with classroom teacher and/or other special educators.	• Program development, management, coordination and evaluation. • Direct service and/or self study. • Provision of speech-language services in coordination with classroom teacher and/or other special educators. • Primary responsibility for academic instruction rests with classroom teacher.	• Program development, management, coordination and evaluation. • Direct speech-language services plus academic instruction provided by speech-language pathologist with SEA Guidelines.	• Program development, management, coordination and evaluation. • Indirect services: Develops clinical program to be carried out by others.
Group Size	• Individual or small group. • Up to 3 students per session.	• Individual or small group. • Up to 5 students per session.	• Up to 10 students per speech-language pathologist. • Up to 15 students per speech-language pathologist and aide.	• Individual or group (through indirect service).
Time Per Day	• Variable: ½ hr. (mild) to 2 hr. per day for (severe).	• 1 to 3 hrs. per day.	• Full school day.	• Variable: Possible range ½ hr. (mild) to 3 to 4 hrs. per day.
Time Per Week	• 2 to 5 times per week.	• 4 to 5 times per week.	• Full-time placement.	• 1 to 5 times per week.
Rationale for Caseload Size	• Moderate-severe cases require more service. • Increased clinical time required to produce change. • Amount and type of service needed is considered in determining caseload numbers.	• Moderate-severe cases may require more intensive services. • Consistent with some state regulations for classes of special education.	• Consistent with some state regulations for classes of special education. • Provides for intensive services.	• Amount of time necessitated by organizational and structural variety of personnel/agencies involved. • Variability of student needs and of the needs of those being trained.
Caseload Maximums	• Up to 25 severe. • Up to 25–55 maximum.	• Up to 15–25 students.	• Up to 15 students with aide. • Up to 10 students without aide.	• 10–15 severe. • 15–55 mild moderate. • As needed.

Sources: ASHA (1998d); Peters-Johnson (1998)

agreement in written discourse, vocabulary, or narrative scripts).

- The instruction is directed to the ability level of the middle of the class, and although students earn individual grades on report cards, whole class improvement is sought.

Conventional therapy is typically delivered in individual or small-group pullout sessions in a small room or area designated for intervention.

- A speech-language pathologist or a supervised SPEECH-LANGUAGE PATHOLOGY ASSISTANT (SLPA) presents a task, introduces the directions, and often interacts directly with a student during the session.

- The intent in this setting is to modify a student's specific deficient communication skill. Some groups are composed of students who all have the same type of deficiency while others may have different areas of need.

- The skills are selected from developmental hierarchies, standardized testing levels, and expectancies for children at various ages. Speech-language skills are directly modeled, encouraged, and reinforced using a wide range of materials and interest areas (e.g., toys, games, books, cards, practice workbooks, and kits).

- The therapy is designed for a particular student, and only that individual's improvement is measured and recorded.

Collaborative intervention is typically delivered in a classroom in a co-teaching arrangement with a teacher or in a less distracting environment or pullout session using materials from the classroom.

- A speech-language pathologist or SLPA uses tasks from the classroom, and modifies the presentation, scaffolds a students' responses, or both to assure success.

- The intent is to increase the amount of interaction a student has with the curriculum and thereby address deficient speech-language skills in a way that will rapidly impact grade-level work. New skills are taught using the student's areas of strength.

- Speech-language skills are directly modeled by a speech-language pathologist and peers, encouraged, facilitated, and reinforced by a student's successful completion of some or all of the assigned curriculum. Examples are:

  Class plays

  COOPERATIVE LEARNING group assignments

  Question-and-answer sessions

  Journal writing

  Recalling facts from a textbook

- The intervention is directed at the juncture of a student's deficient communication skills and the requirements of the curriculum.

- Although advancement of the whole class is the focus, an individual student's progress on predetermined communication goals is also monitored and recorded.

The Role of a Case Manager in Service Delivery

Decisions regarding the nature (direct or indirect), type (individual, group, or class), and location (resource room, classroom, home, or community) of service delivery are based on the need to provide FAPE for each student in the LRE and consistent with a student's individual needs as documented on an IEP. The role of a speech-language pathologist is to assist an educational team in selecting, planning, and coordinating appropriate service delivery using various scheduling options throughout the duration of services. This begins with the initial placement decisions, extends through all re-evaluations and special circumstances, and culminates when the student is dismissed from the speech-language program.

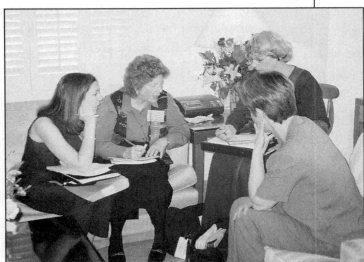

Speech-language pathologists serve as CASE MANAGERS for students whose primary need is communication or whose program is constructed around speech-language goals. They may also serve as case managers for students who are included in a general education program and monitored by one or more special educators. As a case manager, a speech-language pathologist may:

- Serve as the point of contact for a student's special education services

- Schedule and coordinate both school-based and community-based assessments

- Assume a leadership role in developing an IEP or INDIVIDUALIZED FAMILY SERVICE PLAN (IFSP)

- Assist families in identifying available service providers and advocacy organizations within a community

- Coordinate, monitor, and ensure timely delivery of special education services, related services, or both

  - Schedule and coordinate any requested re-evaluation processes

  - Facilitate the development of IDEA-required TRANSITION plans at any level

  - Coordinate services or provide CONSULTATION for students in charter schools, private schools, or other educational agencies off a school campus (ASHA, 1989a)

If a speech-language pathologist is not a case manager, he or she remains an active team member, providing appropriate services to identified students and following through on all joint responsibilities coordinated by the case manager. The speech-language pathologist is the most knowledgeable person to select the service delivery model for speech-language services; however, input from parents and other team members is always considered. According to ASHA (1999c), when choosing the most promising service delivery model, the speech-language pathologist acting as case manager must give consideration to a student's:

1. Strengths, needs, and emerging abilities

2. Need for peer modeling

3. Communication needs as they relate to the general education curriculum

4. Need for intensive intervention

5. Effort, attitude, motivation, and social skills

6. Disorder(s) severity

7. Disorder(s) nature

8. Age and developmental level

Case managers must weight these factors when assisting the team to select appropriate service delivery models.

In the *Twenty-first Annual Report to Congress on the Implementation of the Individuals with Disabilities Education Act* (U.S. Department of Education, 1999), the continuing need for a full continuum of services for students with disabilities was stressed. Because there is no single special education setting that benefits all students, a large number of options should be available, with different levels of support and opportunities for independence. The review of special education models in this text, plus ASHA's (1996b) position state-

ment on INCLUSIVE PRACTICES, enables speech-language pathologists to conclude that "an array of speech language and hearing services should be available in educational settings to support children and youth with communication disorders" (ASHA, 1996b, p. 35). This further underscores the need for a variety of possible settings, so that the best match can be made and changes are systematic and encouraged within the natural environments of school, home, and community. During the course of his or her intervention, a student might participate in many different service delivery models. Three important concepts that drive all service delivery model decisions are:

1. Service delivery is a dynamic concept, and it changes as the needs of the student change.

2. No one service delivery model is to be used exclusively during intervention.

3. For all service delivery models, it is essential that time be made available in the weekly schedule for collaboration/consultation with parents, general educators, special educators, and other service providers. (ASHA, 1996b)

Preferred Practice Patterns for Intervention

PREFERRED PRACTICE PATTERNS are generic and universally applicable for all service delivery models. They are based on the "Classification of Speech-Language Pathology and Audiology Procedures and Communication Disorders" (ASHA, 1987). The practice patterns were developed as a guide to enhance the quality of professional services, as an educational tool for persons outside the profession, and as a method to help ensure uniformity of service delivery across settings. Therapeutic practices provided in schools, for example, will be essentially the same in a nonschool agency. Each practice pattern describes the same elements (e.g., see how they were listed in the sidebar on page 75 in Chapter 3).

The principles of ASHA's (1997c) preferred practice patterns for SCREENING, assessment, and intervention services have been used to describe the models chosen throughout this book. Refer to Appendix B to review the preferred practice patterns for intervention, or visit ASHA's Web site (*www.asha.org*) for a complete list.

Functional Outcomes and the School-Based Speech-Language Pathologist

FUNCTIONAL OUTCOMES are defined as "the results of care" in health-care circles (Rao as cited in Crawford, 1998) and the "results of intervention" in educational settings (Amiot, 1998; Montgomery, 1999b). They can be considered evidence of progress. The bottom line for all service delivery programs is contained in this question: When you provide services for a student with communication disorders, how do you determine that the intervention has made a meaningful difference in that student's life?

This may seem like a straightforward question, but in determining what tools and procedures speech-language pathologists need to find the answer, several other questions are raised:

- Can speech-language pathologists rely on standardized test scores to capture the improvement?

- Is it more authentic if persons other than speech-language pathologists report the changes they observe?

- Does only the student know if the intervention was helpful?

- Do speech-language pathologists know if most students with similar diagnoses make similar improvements? How can this be found out? If students do not, why not?

- Does the student's rate of improvement change with different speech-language pathologists?

- Does one service provider see results more quickly or more slowly than another? How can speech-language pathologists alter that rate?

All of these questions and more arose after the speech-language pathology and audiology professions began to focus on functional outcomes in the 1990s (Ferguson, 1994–1995; Spahr, 1996). Meanwhile, speech-language pathologists had conducted their professional responsibilities successfully for more than 60 years without directly confronting these questions. Of course, the field of speech-language pathology is not without accountability. For years, speech-language pathologists have responded to questions about individual effectiveness (Enderby and Emerson, 1995). For example, researchers and speech-language pathologists have investigated if one clinical approach is more effective than another (Bain and Dollaghan, 1991; Kamhi, 1991). Speech-language pathologists have asked if clients receiving a certain type of intervention scored higher on the same battery of tests at the end of a cycle of treatment (ASHA, 1999a; Enderby and Emerson, 1995). The profession has queried itself about whether clients actually had less communication difficulty at the conclusion of therapy, if clients regressed or maintained their skills, or if clients received direct assistance from a speech-language pathologist a second time (Crawford, 1998; Enderby and Emerson, 1995). These were closely related and interesting questions, but they did not adequately address an underlying concern in health care and education posed in the 1990s: Is there a research base to show that speech-language pathology services are valuable and necessary for persons with communication disorders? According to Enderby and Emerson, the answer is a strong yes. Measuring and reporting that value, and then linking it directly to a speech-language pathologist's intervention process is the purpose of functional outcomes (Campbell, 1999a; ASHA, 1998e). Moore-Brown, Montgomery, Biehl, Karr, and Stein (1998) emphasized how critical it was for school speech-language pathologists to "make sure the goals are well written and truly reflect the outcomes desired for this child.... We need to be able to provide this information and answer questions as to what it is we're doing, what difference it makes, how long it takes, and what it costs" (p. 11).

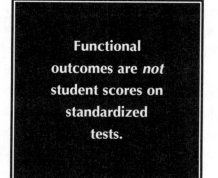

Functional outcomes are *not* student scores on standardized tests.

Functional Outcomes Defined as Results of Intervention

The employers, agencies, insurance companies, school boards, legislators, and clients who pay for speech-language services want to know what meaningful change occurs because speech-language pathologists are members of health-care or education teams. These payers want to know consumers' functional outcomes. Because speech-language pathologists are most often employees of a school district or a regional system (ASHA, 1997b; ASHA, 1998d), the idea of these agencies as service payers may seem out of place at first glance. Speech-language pathologists and all professionals who work in school systems must remember that taxpayers support all educational services. Criticism of the costs of special education can be meaningfully addressed by functional outcome measures.

"Documentation of accountability in schools is important to assist in developing reasonable cost/benefit ratios for program planning purposes. Effective utilization of this documentation can be a highly persuasive tool" (Ferguson, 1994–1995, p. 8). Cost/Benefit ratios and similar methods of accountability make a difference in whether school-based speech-language pathologists are hired, the opinions and respect of fellow professionals, and how responsibilities are assigned.

Functional outcomes are *not* student scores on STANDARDIZED TESTS. Nor are they a list of the OBJECTIVES an individual has mastered.

Instead, they are an accounting of the cost, time, and resulting restoration (or newly acquired performance) of the client (Rao as cited in Crawford, 1998; Wolf, 1997) and a treatment tool that shows close relationship to reimbursement in all work settings. While the use of functional outcomes is a relatively new concept for some speech-language pathologists, it has been noted in the professional literature since 1993 (Montgomery, 1997b).

Functional outcomes for adults are measured in terms that reflect a life context beyond therapy. An adult may return to work or previous social activities, interact with family and friends, and be independent at selected tasks again after treatment for a communication disorder. These changes are called RESTORATIVE. For children and youth, functional outcomes are framed in broader educational standards—progress in academics or a life-skills curriculum, friendship development, and age-appropriate interdependence and interaction with family members and care providers. Functional outcomes for children are HABILITATIVE, or newly acquired performances. An exception to this might be a traumatic brain injury, where the focus of therapy would be to restore previous functioning and learn new academic information at the student's grade level. See Table 5.4 for a list of ASHA functional status measures for students.

Functional Outcomes' Relationship to Health Care

Schools were able to watch the evolution of functional outcome measures in health care during the early 1990s. Speech-language pathologists providing services through health care were jarred by the sudden restrictions on reimbursement imposed by HEALTH MAINTENANCE ORGANIZATIONS (HMOs) and fee capitation (Wolf, 1997). In an even tighter managed care system introduced in 1998, speech-language pathologists were expected to share the risk of habilitation or rehabilitation of a client with parties paying for the intervention services. Significant change in patient-functioning level was required in a prescribed amount of time to receive a maximum payment. If it took longer to reach the expected level of function, in most cases, there were no additional payments (Crawford, 1998).

The restrictions required health-care administrators to accurately estimate the time it would take for speech-language pathologists to meet patients' goals; otherwise speech-language pathologists or health-care facilities found it was not cost-effective to offer services. Insurance companies did not deny services, but they did deny payment. Speech-language pathologists were expected to know how many sessions would be needed for a client to reach a certain performance level. Conversely, they had to decide how much patient progress was reasonable in the amount of intervention time that was covered by insurance. Speech-language pathologists also needed to recognize clients who could not be expected to make meaningful change and judiciously not schedule them for therapy reimbursed by a particular payer. New MEDICARE fee schedules, PROSPECTIVE PAYMENT, and a SHARED CAP on rehabilitation services intensified the treatment/reimbursement issues for the profession (ASHA, 1998a). While many speech-language pathologists decried this

Table 5.4

ASHA Functional Status Measures

For each statement, indicate on a scale of 0–7 how much assistance is needed for a student to function in each area within the educational environment.

0 = No basis for rating
1 = Does not do
2 = Does with maximal assistance
3 = Does with moderate to maximal assistance
4 = Does with moderate assistance
5 = Does with minimal to moderate assistance
6 = Does with minimal assistance
7 = Does independently

a. The student's speech is understood.

b. The student responds to questions regarding everyday and classroom activities.

c. The student produces appropriate phrases and sentences in response to classroom activities.

d. The student communicates wants, needs, ideas, and concepts to others either verbally or by use of an augmentative communication system.

e. The student uses appropriate vocabulary to function within the classroom.

f. The student describes familiar objects and events.

g. The student knows and uses age-appropriate interactions with peers and staff.

h. The student initiates, maintains, and concludes conversations with peers and staff within classroom settings.

i. The student initiates, maintains, and concludes conversations with peers and staff in non-classroom settings.

j. The student indicates when messages are not understood.

k. The student completes oral presentations.

l. The student demonstrates the ability to give directions.

Continued on next page

Table 5.4—*Continued*

m. The student demonstrates the ability to follow directions.

n. The student demonstrates the ability to recall written information presented in the educational environment.

o. The student demonstrates the ability to recall auditory information presented in the educational environment.

p. The student demonstrates the ability to use verbal language to solve problems.

q. The student demonstrates appropriate listening skills within the educational environment.

r. The student recognizes and demonstrates comprehension of nonverbal communication.

Definitions for Evaluating the Functional
Status Measures on the Scale of Independence

0	No basis for rating	Includes circumstances in which a behavior is not observed, directly tested, and/or the information is not available from other sources.
1	Does not do	Child does not perform the communication behavior, even with maximal assistance or prompting.
2	Does with maximal assistance	Child performs the communication behavior with constant assistance and prompting only.
3	Does with moderate to maximal assistance	Child performs the communication behavior but frequently needs assistance and prompting.
4	Does with moderate assistance	Child performs the communication behavior, often needing assistance and prompting.
5	Does with minimal to moderate assistance	Child performs the communication behavior, occasionally needing assistance and/or prompting.
6	Does with minimal assistance	Child performs the communication behavior, rarely needing assistance and/or prompting.
7	Does independently	Child performs the communication behavior, needing no assistance and/or prompting.

From *User's Guide Phase I—Group II, National Treatment Outcome Data Collection Project,* (pp. 41–44), by the American Speech-Language-Hearing Association (ASHA), 1995, Rockville, MD: Author. © 1995 by ASHA. Adapted with permission.

health-care environment as fiscally driven, it was apparent that this fiscal pressure fueled the need for accurate outcome data in speech-language pathology and audiology (Baum, 1998; Grimes, 1997; S. Karr, personal communication, November 19, 1999).

Functional outcomes have been measured therapeutically, fiscally, and emotionally in adult health care before the terms reached the schools. Slightly tongue in cheek, Rao (as cited in Crawford, 1998) noted that success in adult rehabilitation in speech-language services was formerly measured with the six Ds: death, disease, dollars, disability, discomfort, and dissatisfaction. School-based speech-language pathologists, pressed to demonstrate success in their programs, might also have selected five Ds: dollars, departure, dissatisfaction, diploma, and dismissal!

Functional Outcomes as Reflected in IDEA (1997) Amendments

According to IDEA (1997), all special educators are mandated to link intervention with a student's core curriculum and overall academic goals (Campbell, 1999b). Further, special educators must report student progress to parents on the same schedule as general educators as well as address curriculum BENCHMARKS on an IEP.

Speech-language pathologists may write SHORT-TERM OBJECTIVES for increasing a child's AUDITORY PROCESSING skills to build a foundation for other skills, or they may write benchmarks and goals to show the level of spelling

and LITERACY skills that comprise the educational standards the child needs to reach. Benchmarks, objectives, or both that relate to academic or school behaviors identify functional outcomes while those that relate to processing deficits usually do not. Benchmarks and short-term objectives are points along a path to a goal. If the early parts of intervention are focused on changing underlying skills only, a speech-language IEP may not appear to be connected with the student's *use* of these new skills. Speech-language pathologists need to link skills with daily functional activities from the beginning (Moore-Brown et al., 1998). Examples of functional outcomes written as measurable annual goals and benchmarks can be found in Chapter 4.

Four Basic Questions for Functional Outcomes

The systematic search for practical intervention benchmarks has pushed speech-language pathologists in all settings to begin to explore and use functional outcomes. Four basic questions, like the borders of a picture frame illustrated in Figure 5.5, characterize these functional outcomes. Side one asks "How many sessions does it take to show meaningful change?" Side two queries "How will each assessment streamline the costs of serving this student?" Side three asks "Is this the most cost-effective way to provide this service?" Side four asks "Can you prove that the services you provide make a difference for the student?" (Montgomery, 1997b).

When an individual speech-language pathologist answers one or more of these questions

Figure 5.5

Four Essential Questions for Functional Outcomes in School-Based Service

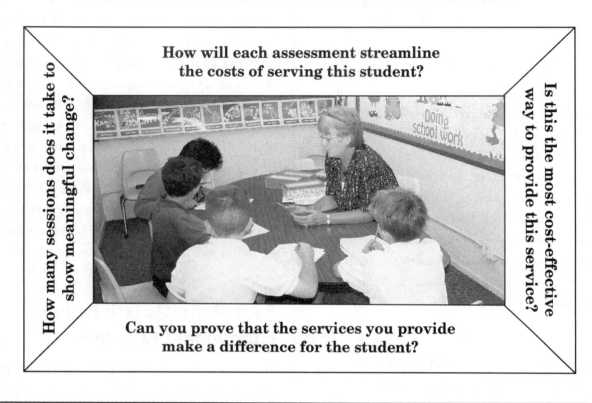

How will each assessment streamline the costs of serving this student?

How many sessions does it take to show meaningful change?

Is this the most cost-effective way to provide this service?

Can you prove that the services you provide make a difference for the student?

From "Using Functional Outcomes in the Schools," by J.K. Montgomery, 1997b, *CSHA Magazine, 26*(2), pp. 7–8. © 1997 by the California Speech-Language-Hearing Association. Adapted with permission.

with confidence, he or she has ventured that much closer to restructuring services around a student's and payer's expectancies, which leads to greater customer satisfaction and more consistent remuneration for speech-language pathologists. While tying speech-language services so closely to the payment system has been considered crude or commercial in some circles, or lacking in professionalism by others, it is precisely this results-based approach that demonstrated the speech-language pathologist's value in the health workplace (Spahr, 1996). Keeping track of the client's functional outcomes, instead of reporting more trivial changes in discrete communication skills or comparing scaled scores on a pre-and posttest, demonstrates that the speech-language pathologist is applying resources wisely (Larson and McKinley, 1995a; Mullen, 2000).

School-based speech-language pathologists learned quickly that changes in reporting student progress were necessary for accountability within educational reforms (Moore-Brown, 1998) (see Chapter 1 for a discussion of educational reforms). Speech-language pathologists need to align their intervention with students' academic or developmental progress. Results must document increased functional performance levels of students who receive speech-language services.

Clinically Significant Change

Functional outcomes must be the paramount product of speech-language pathologists' planned intervention for students. Speech-language pathologists must design measurable goals and select meaningful benchmarks that truly matter to students, families, and systems educating students. Speech-language pathologists want to be sure that their work results in clinically significant change for individuals with communication disorders. The criteria for clinically significant change from Bain and Dollaghan (1991) is perhaps the most widely cited in the field. They suggest that clinically significant change must be:

1. Due to intervention, not maturation

2. Real, not random

3. Important, not trivial

The Bain and Dollaghan (1991) guidelines assist speech-language pathologists in selecting consumer-driven goals. "The documentation of clinical significance is useful in prospective, on-line, and retrospective decision-making" in service delivery in schools (Ferguson, 1994–1995, p. 8), and IEPs must be designed to confer educational benefit. What better way to do this than to use functional outcomes?

Unlike the fiscally based decisions of cost and length of speech-language services, functional outcomes (also called PERFORMANCE OUTCOMES) evolve directly from a speech-language pathologist's assessment of a student's functioning level. Functional or performance outcomes are the best estimate of the student's anticipated communicative status. Functional outcomes for students actually vary little by practice setting since all the statements focus on how individuals

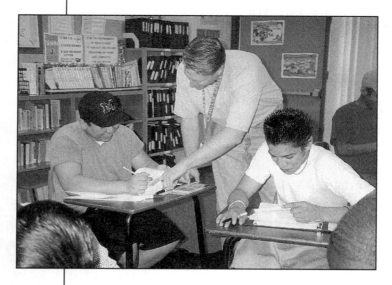

will have more effective and satisfying lives. In education, curricular goals are the focus; in health care, life or workplace expectancies are emphasized. Eventually the use of functional outcomes may actually draw together education and health care, private- and public-sector speech-language pathologists, in common benchmarks and even common agreement of termination points for therapy. The benchmarks, or points along the path to a goal, will be recognizable to health-care, education, and family stakeholders. Speech-language pathologists may differ dramatically on the process they use to reach these benchmarks, but they can all agree that they are seeking the same client (student) performance. Functional outcomes have a universal appeal to multidisciplinary teams, families, and payers (i.e., insurance agencies and state taxpayers). When students' IEPs are designed to confer educational benefit, functional outcomes are easier for speech-language pathologists to document.

Direct Versus Indirect Outcomes

Outcomes can be viewed as either direct or indirect (Montgomery, 1997b). DIRECT OUTCOMES are behavioral changes that are planned. For example, if Felicia learns to convey accurate information to another person during a telephone call by practicing telephone dialogues, it would be a direct outcome. INDIRECT OUTCOMES may occur if a new and appropriate behavior emerges that was not anticipated (Blackstone and Pressman, 1996). Likewise, if Jason learns to take turns and to follow the rules in a playground game with his peers, the indirect outcome is Jason using appropriate social language and pragmatics. Taking turns and following rules should be documented as functional outcomes even if they were not specifically planned in the IEP. Speech-language pathologists need to be alert to the manifestations of improved communication skills.

Outcomes may also be categorized as intended versus unintended. When Connie learns to write statements about a character's feelings, using adjectives and adverbs, in her collaborative speech and language sessions, writing such statements about a novel read in class is an intended outcome. Another time, if Connie uses her writing skills to write notes to a friend in her class about an argument with her boyfriend, her text is an unintended outcome. The unintended outcome, though a personally valuable activity, demonstrates the skill even if she did not write the class assignment correctly (Montgomery, 1999b). Though learning the playground game and writing notes to friends may not have been these students' predicted outcomes, their emergence may be credited to intervention. Although we plan for direct, intended skill development, speech-language pathologists need to identify the indirect, unintended outcomes that signal progress as well!

An example of this phenomenon is the incidental learning of sight words by students during articulation therapy (Stewart, Gonzalez, and Page, 1997). Changes in academic behavior occurred that no one expected when students were found able to read the words they used in each speech session to practice their target phonemes. Students increased their reading skills because the words were printed on the picture cards and students read the print repeatedly during their speech-language sessions.

When communication events are related to the anticipated new or restored skills, they should be recorded as outcomes. Speech-language pathologists may need to look beyond traditional intervention sessions for unexpected outcomes

> When communication events are related to the anticipated new or restored skills, they should be recorded as outcomes.

with children. In writing about augmentative and alternative communication (AAC), Blackstone and Pressman (1996) have challenged speech-language pathologists to know their intervention techniques thoroughly to assure that outcome measures are matched to consumers. They cautioned about the distinct differences and expectancies for AAC users in schools versus those with acquired conditions and those with severe physical disabilities. The outcomes in these three groups were not interchangeable. In schools, academic expectancies were set noticeably higher, resulting in few intended outcomes. Social or interpersonal goals were set more conservatively, resulting in more unintentional outcomes. This occurred without regard to the student's etiology (congenital or acquired disabilities) or other medical conditions. Thus, school-based speech-language pathologists should anticipate recording both intended and unintended outcomes when measuring student progress. Both types of outcomes are examples of clinically significant change as defined by Bain and Dollaghan (1991).

Linking Services to Consumer Satisfaction

Consumer satisfaction is a fitting conclusion to a discussion of functional outcomes. Speech-language pathologists may be unaware of how their services appear to consumers. In infant and preschool services provided by schools, children and families are primary consumers. For schools-age consumers, we add their teachers, peers, and state legislatures. They are all seeking satisfaction, often for diverse outcomes.

When a speech-language assessment indicates the need for an intervention program, a consumer wants to know the best program for him or her or, as a parent, for his or her child. Finding what is best for each client means focusing on consumer satisfaction. "Best" is a thoughtful combination of what functional outcomes are desired, when and where services are provided, and the amount of time and resources needed. IDEA (1997) requires schools to provide intervention that is of educational benefit for a student. It does not require that the best or maximum intervention be sought. IDEA and SEAs require the highest qualified personnel to use research-based practices and adequate resources to ensure that all students have access to the curriculum and can benefit from their education. Speech-language pathologists recognize that this may translate into good practice instead of best practice (see "Appropriate Benefit" in Chapter 7 for a discussion of appropriate versus best practice).

Selecting more effective interventions, with some individual variance, will become easier if we use the academic outcome data being gathered on elementary and secondary level students (Gillon, 2000; Larson and McKinley, 1995a). What is best for one student may not be best for another. For speech-language pathologists "there is a continuing problem of specifying which treatment is likely to work with which child" (Enderby and Emerson, 1995, p. 126). All students in special education should receive appropriate services resulting in clinically significant change and educationally functional outcomes. A parent/guardian observation of student change subsequent to services showed 97% satisfaction with speech-language services in schools, and 92% believed there was improvement (Whitmire, Karr, and Mullen, 2000).

Even though more data are needed to reach any conclusions (Whitmire, Karr, and Mullen, 2000), speech-language pathologists who respond to the four basic questions in the picture frame of Figure 5.5 for students on their CASELOAD or in their classroom will be able to address consumer satisfaction. There is a great need for outcome data for school-age children that is collected nationwide from school-based speech-language pathologists serving individuals with communication disorders (Mullen, 2000). This is an immense undertaking and efforts will continue into the future.

Functional Communication Measures (FCMs)

Pilot studies or comprehensive data collection based on functional outcomes have been conducted yearly in schools since 1995 (ASHA, 1999a). A seven-point rating scale of FUNCTIONAL COMMUNICATION MEASURES (FCMs) was designed and field-tested in K–12 settings by school-based speech-language pathologists (ASHA, 1999a). ASHA's FCMs are the most comprehensive set of functional outcomes for school-based speech-language pathologists available. There are statements of student abilities in 15 areas: articulation/phonology, AAC comprehension, AAC production, cognitive communication, dysphagia, fluency, language comprehension, language production, central auditory processing,

hearing sensitivity, hearing loss, hearing gain from amplification, hearing aid use, hearing aids, and ASSISTIVE LISTENING DEVICE (ALD) operation and management. The sidebar includes a description of the seven levels for language comprehension.

FCMs enable speech-language pathologists to rely less on standardized test scores to determine present levels of performance by defining performance at a particular number level (1–7) as a base line. Speech-language pathologists can probe many times during the intervention sessions to record improvements and speech-language pathologists, teachers, and families can observe changes. FCMs resemble the process of DYNAMIC ASSESSMENT discussed in Chapter 3. They keep the intervention process linked to the functional activities of students at any developmental level. Students who were judged to be performing at a Level 1 or 2 on the FCM might have short-term objectives (or benchmarks) written to reach a Level 3 while students at initial Level 4 or 5 could be expected to reach Level 6 or 7 in one year or less. Students who perform at Level 6 should not be enrolled in speech-language intervention unless there are extenuating circumstances (e.g., recurrent otitis media or adverse educational impact) since they are most likely to improve without it (ASHA, 1998e).

According to IDEA (1997), all special education service providers, including speech-language pathologists, must measure student progress in a functional and educationally relevant way (Brannen et al., 2000). Functional measurement is a critical part of the reforms in general and special education that require increased accountability of

Functional Communication Measures for Language Comprehension

CNT/DNT	An aspect of communication that one could not test (CNT) due to the level of functioning or should have tested but did not test (DNT) due to time or other factors.
Level 1	Profound impairment: No understanding of verbal language.
Level 2	Severe impairment: 10–20% comprehension of single words in restricted contexts, Cannot participate in conversations.
Level 3	Moderate to severe impairment: 30–40% comprehension of words and phrases in restricted contexts. Minimal response as a conversational participant.
Level 4	Moderate impairment: 50% comprehension of phrases and sentences in typical contexts. Moderate response as a conversational participant to one or two topics.
Level 5	Moderate to mild impairment: 60–70% comprehension of sentences and conversation in familiar contexts. Good participation in conversations for a limited number of topics.
Level 6	Mild impairment: 80–90% comprehension of conversation in broad contexts. Full participant in most conversations.
Level 7	Normal comprehension of language.

From *User's Guide Phase I—Group II, National Treatment Outcome Data Collection Project,* (p. 54), by the American Speech-Language-Hearing Association (ASHA), 1995, Rockville, MD: Author. © 1995 by ASHA. Adapted with permission.

all educators and related services professionals. Using the FCM levels discussed in this chapter, preliminary data from a three-year study have shown that 87% of speech-language students on caseloads of 40 or less made progress in a year while only 64% of those on caseloads of 60 or more did so (Whitmire, Karr, and Mullen, 2000). This has far-reaching implications for all school-based speech-language pathologists. Stating how the child's disability limits educational performance, and then how the student has responded to the instructional adaptations and supports put in place, must be functionally described and measured. FCMs make this possible in the schools of the twenty-first century (Brannen et al., 2000).

Once a student is identified with an impairment that results in a disability and is found eligible for services in school, a speech-language pathologist can use the FCMs to ascertain the student's functional level and plan the expected outcome in one year of services. The FCMs can also help an IEP team decide if particular communication goals are reasonable for the student. If the student has a FCM of Level 2, the team could examine the likelihood that the

---

Clinically Significant Change: Two Cases

Sara, a 6-year-old, had dysarthric, mostly unintelligible speech due to cerebral palsy. Although she was able to learn in her inclusive classroom, few of her peers or teachers knew her abilities until she began to use a powerful augmentative communication system with voice and print output. Finally, she could demonstrate what she knew, participate in class, and become a reader and writer. The speech-language pathologist taught Sara the AAC methods she needed, and the educational successes followed.

Matthew, a 9-year-old, experienced severe stuttering behavior in the classroom and in most social situations. He was thought to be—and even considered himself—a slow learner with poor organizational skills, low self-esteem, and a limited grasp of new concepts in the curriculum. He rarely participated in a noisy, highly interactive fourth-grade classroom. After successful speech intervention reduced his disfluencies and gave him new strategies to compete in the classroom, he took greater responsibility for learning, began to feel successful, participated more often, and lifted his grades from mostly Ds to mostly Bs.

In both cases, change was clinically significant.

---

student will achieve an FCM of Level 3 by the end of the year. An IEP team should not recommend an intervention plan for a change in level if progress is not anticipated within a year. Some students with physical or cognitive limitations may not be able to advance past a certain communication level. Stability at one FCM level could be one of the indicators for dismissal as discussed in Chapter 4.

It is possible for a student to make progress toward more functional communication in a form that cannot be recorded with available FCMs. These behaviors may fall in the unintended outcomes discussed in this chapter under "Direct Versus Indirect Outcomes" (see page 150). More work on FCMs in the next decade will help to close this gap.

CHAPTER 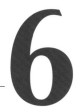6

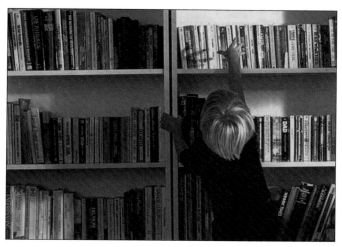

Meeting School Standards and Providing Access to the Curriculum

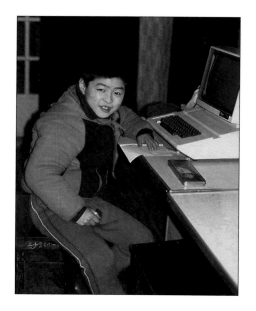

IN THIS CHAPTER

This chapter introduces issues surrounding service delivery. One section focuses on managing caseloads. Service delivery is discussed in the form of specific intervention models that are based on ASHA guidelines, incorporate both direct and indirect forms of contact with students, and link to the curriculum. Helpful grouping strategies and specific models for consultation and collaboration are described. Examples of literacy and preschool programs and a focus on secondary students are included.

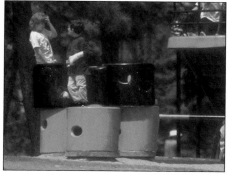

1. Discuss the ASHA position statement on reading and writing in light of what you know about the important role of reading in being a successful student. Find the list in this chapter of roles and responsibilities in promoting reading and writing (see page 185), and compare yourself to the expectancies for speech-language pathologists. Where can you get more information to be prepared?

2. Why is there is feeling of urgency when working with preschoolers? How does that urgency affect the delivery of services? Plan a series of questions to ask a parent to help you understand how the child communicates at home.

3. Should high school students receive speech-language services if they have had more than three years of service in the elementary grades? Defend your answer.

4. From your viewpoint, discuss the effect of Year-Round Education (YRE) on all students, students with disabilities, and the professionals who work with them, especially speech-language pathologists. Would YRE affect functional outcomes? In what way?

5. What factors would you consider when deciding how to group students for intervention?

6. Collaborative consultation assumes cooperativeness among professionals. Project what might be done when resistance to the process exists.

7. Practice writing a behavioral objective that is linked to a child's general education curriculum versus one that is not. If you do not know how, what resources might you tap?

Caseloads and Service Delivery

Speech-language pathologists in schools have the same responsibilities as all employees in a school district. They must enforce the academic standards of STATE EDUCATIONAL AGENCIES (SEAs) and LOCAL EDUCATIONAL AGENCIES (LEAs) while they support students with communication disabilities to be successful in school. Fortunately, the AMERICAN SPEECH-LANGUAGE-HEARING ASSOCIATION (ASHA), researchers, and speech-language pathologists have developed many effective SERVICE DELIVERY methods for speech-language pathologists to use with confidence.

Service delivery takes on many forms in the school environment. Speech-language pathologists should not only use a variety of methods and delivery models, but they should be able to categorize or describe them to fellow professionals to build administrative support at the school or district level. Using and advocating for a range of service delivery models promotes new ideas and gains support for speech-language pathologists as school team members (Montgomery, 1990). These models also guide speech-language pathologists in becoming an integral part of a school team, able to apply their expertise to the goals of the school and the curriculum.

ASHA Service Delivery Options

ASHA has issued guidelines for seven service delivery options that help speech-language pathologists become more effective members of a total school team. Note that they revolve around the good practice options summarized in Chapter 5: CLASSROOM INSTRUCTION, conventional intervention, and COLLABORATION. ASHA's *Guidelines for the Roles and Responsibilities of the School-Based Speech-Language Pathologist* (1999c) represented in the sidebar (see page 158) offers a valuable list of service delivery models for use in schools. These options provide speech-language pathologists with great flexibility to address the needs of students on their CASELOAD.

These options are simply frameworks within which students of any age, disability, or learning situation can receive services. After an assessment and identification process is completed and an INDIVIDUALIZED EDUCATION PROGRAM (IEP) meeting is held, the team, the parents, and many times the student determine what arrangement of time, resources, and location will serve that individual best. Voice, articulation, fluency, language, and other communication disabilities can be served in any of these configurations. The authors encourage "thinking outside the box" when designing intervention services and schedules. A list of models is helpful to speech-language pathologists and school teams in the same way a menu encourages one to consider new choices. Although models may be helpful in this way, it is important to remember that intervention can be provided in any form that speech-language pathologists create for students.

Caseload Size

Examining school-based speech-language pathologists' typical caseloads by day and by week has

Service Delivery Options

Monitor: The speech-language pathologist sees the student for a specified amount of time per grading period to monitor or "check" on the student's speech and language skills. Often this model immediately precedes dismissal.

Collaborative Consultation: The speech-language pathologist, regular and/or special education teacher(s), and parents/families work together to facilitate a student's communication and learning in educational environments. This is an indirect model in which the speech-language pathologist does not provide direct service to the student.

Classroom Based: This model is also known as integrated services, curriculum-based, transdisciplinary, interdisciplinary, or inclusive programming. There is an emphasis on the speech-language pathologist providing direct services to students within the classroom and other natural environments. Team teaching by the speech-language pathologist and the regular and/or special education teacher(s) is frequent with this model.

Pullout: Services are provided to students individually and/or in small groups within the speech-language resource room setting. Some speech-language pathologists may prefer to provide individual or small group services within the physical space of the classroom.

Self-Contained Program: The speech-language pathologist is the classroom teacher responsible for providing both academic/curriculum instruction and speech-language remediation.

Community Based: Communication services are provided to students within the home or community setting. Goals and objectives focus primarily on functional communication skills.

Combination: The speech-language pathologist provides two or more service delivery options (e.g., provides individual or small group treatment on a pull-out basis twice a week to develop skills or preteach concepts and also works with the student within the classroom).

From *Guidelines for the Roles and Responsibilities of the School-Based Speech-Language Pathologist* (p. 37), by the American Speech-Language-Hearing Association (ASHA), 1999c, Rockville, MD: Author. © 1999 by ASHA. Reprinted with permission.

long been considered a factor in choosing models of service delivery. The authors believe that this factor should not be the focus. Caseload size will vary greatly across the country with lows of 35 to 40 students per speech-language pathologist (e.g., Nebraska and Iowa) and reported highs of 90 or more students per speech-language pathologist (e.g., Illinois, New York, and California). In 1999, a nationwide survey found even greater ranges of 3 to 145 students per speech-language pathologist (Council for Exceptional Children [CEC], 1999). States determine their caseload minimums and maximums, thus the incredible variations. Caseload size and management was the number one issue for speech-language pathologists in schools on an ASHA (1998d) survey and was selected as the first priority issue for the ASHA Legislative Council in 2000 (Whitmire, 2000a). Advocating for a reduction in the size of caseloads for public school speech-language programs is a politically and economically volatile issue because of competing needs and limited resources.

GOOD PRACTICE and good service delivery, however, are not based on political and economic issues. Regardless of caseload size, consumers expect speech-language pathologists to make professional decisions that must include choosing interventions wisely, matching students' performance levels with available services, and measuring progress with FUNCTIONAL OUTCOMES (see "Functional Outcomes and the School-Based Speech-Language Pathologist" in Chapter 5). Nevertheless, speech-language pathologists do need to advocate for reasonable caseloads, so that they can perform their duties. As will be discussed in "Professional Organizations" in Chapter 9, maintaining a political voice through membership in professional organizations and

being on alert for proposed legislation is a responsibility of speech-language pathologists. Vigilance and tenacity in reshaping state caseload maximums does reap benefits for students and their families.

Although maintaining a lower caseload may allow speech-language pathologists to schedule more frequent or intensive services for some children, data on improved outcomes in these circumstances have not been collected in a standardized manner (Mullen, 2000). Such data have not yet been used to convince lawmakers to reduce caseload size (Moore-Brown, Montgomery, Biehl, Karr, and Stein, 1998; Whitmire, Karr, and Mullen, 2000).

Scheduling the Caseload

Caseload size can significantly influence the service delivery choices that speech-language pathologists make; however, individual student needs must be the overriding factor. This can cause anxiety and require great flexibility from everyone involved. It is important to remember that no single method of delivering services is appropriate for the entire intervention period. Model changes are inherent in the scheduling process and should be based on students' needs, not on the time of year, space, or other external factors. Practically, of course, all these factors must be worked into a schedule. For example, a student may need one-to-one service for a phonological disorder for six weeks, then an in-class model to begin the generalization process with meaningful classroom-based cues for eight weeks, and finally a once a month "drop-in group" (i.e., checkup) for reinforcement for the remainder of the school year.

Speech-language pathologists need to be able to make adjustments whenever necessary. As long as a student is making steady progress toward IEP GOALS, the existing service model may be maintained. Lack of progress indicates a need for change in service delivery. One of the great advantages of a school-based model is the many options available that are not in hospital programs, day clinics, or private-practice settings. In these other settings, the pool of typical peers is simply not there, and the learning environment provides limited opportunities for naturalistic practice.

Table 6.1 offers ideas for how to schedule programs in elementary and secondary schools as well as for speech-language pathologists who serve multiple school sites. Schedules must allow for some assessment and meeting time and use every available minute of the school day to serve students. Most school days allow about 6 to 6½ hours of student contact time, so time is at a premium. Almost 60 percent of speech-language pathologists' days are spent in direct intervention (ASHA, 1998d). Despite the pressure to use every available minute for intervention, speech-language pathologists must wisely allocate time for lunch, breaks, and required assigned duties that are expected of all school personnel.

Year-Round Education (YRE)

Traditional school calendars were established to meet the needs of an agrarian society in which entire families needed to devote uninterrupted time to harvest crops each year. Year-round education (YRE) is an alternative to the traditional 180-day, September through June schedule.

Year-round education centers on reorganizing the school year to provide more continuous learning by breaking up the long summer vacation into shorter, more frequent vacations throughout the year. It does not eliminate the summer vacation, but reduces it and redistributes it as vacation or intersession time during the school year. Students attending a year-round school go to the same classes and receive the same instruction as students on a traditional calendar. The year-round calendar is organized into instructional periods and vacation weeks that are more evenly balanced across 12 months than the traditional school calendar. The balanced calendar minimizes the learning loss that occurs during a typical three-month summer vacation. (National Association of Year-Round Education [NAYRE], 2001, ¶ 2).

The *Encyclopedia of American Education* (Unger, 1996) defines *year-round school* as:

A school that operates a 12-month-a-year academic program to ensure maximum utilization of school facilities and accommodate a larger number of students without investing in plant expansion. (p. 1095)

During the 1999–2000 school year, 561 school districts in 43 states used a YRE schedule. This equated to 2,880 public schools serving over 2 million children through this type of alternative scheduling. YRE schools use several calendar variations that typically schedule three quarters of the students to attend "on-track," while one quarter of the students are "off-track." Although YRE was begun to maximize

Table 6.1

Creating Schedules for Service Delivery

There are several different types of schedules that must be created by speech-language pathologists each year. They serve as the evidence of delivery of services as specified in student IEPs. Each schedule has a distinct purpose, a different audience, and a corresponding format. Some features will be found in every schedule while others are unique to a specific format. Schedules with student names on them are considered a part of confidential records and are not shown to unauthorized persons. Types of schedules used in school programs are outlined below.

Type of Schedule	Purpose	Audience(s)	Format
Daily	Used to record daily activities at a specific location	Education team, site administrator	By time and names
Daily with assistant	Used to record daily activities of speech-language pathologist and assistant(s) at a specific location	Education team, site administrator, assistant(s), supervisor(s)	By time and names
Weekly	Used to track weekly locations for services if more than one location, week at a glance if one location. Important for block scheduling and monitoring students	SLP, education team, district administrator(s), parents	By time and activity
Weekly with assistant	Same as above with assistant(s) added where appropriate	Same as above, classified staff administrators(s), assistant(s)	By time and activity
Monthly	Kept for documenting monthly responsibilities, such as school staff meetings, out-of-district or agency meetings, district meetings, professional growth conferences, CEUs, and so on. Important if using block scheduling, curriculum-based instruction (off-campus), or monthly monitoring and checking	Same as above	By month and activity; usually includes contact information such as names or phone numbers
Yearlong	Primarily used for documenting long-range planning, evidence of contacts with agencies, out-of-district commitments, and so on. May have screening dates, IEPs, triannual re-evaluations, school-based teams for prereferral, and special education interventions	Administrators, hearing officers, court orders, subpoenaed records	By activity and contact time expended; may include names of others at meetings

facility usage in crowded buildings, academic benefits may be realized for students, especially those in need of SPECIAL EDUCATION, due to shorter nonschool breaks.

Teachers generally follow the same track or schedule as their students, but scheduling becomes more difficult for support services providers (e.g., speech-language pathologists). Special education services must be provided across all tracks throughout the entire 246 or 247 days that school is in session in YRE. Speech-language pathologists need a work calendar that provides service to students throughout the school year. Some solutions include:

- Speech-language pathologists' contracts and salaries are extended, covering between 200 and 230 days of the school year.

- Certain days of the year are identified as "no speech" days and are nonwork days for speech-language pathologists, such as the first week of school, the three days before the Thanksgiving holiday, the week before the winter holiday break, or the last week or two of school.

- Speech-language pathologists coordinate schedules to provide coverage for each other during others' off-track time.

- Speech-language pathologists work a four-day workweek.

Once a work calendar is established for speech-language pathologists, the challenge of how to serve students must be tackled. The most significant difference for speech-language pathologists in a YRE school is the fact that the groupings of students can change every month (if on a multi-track YRE schedule). Although this may sound like a daunting task (and it is at first), skilled scheduling may allow speech-language pathologists to realize greater variation and effectiveness in service delivery. The changing mix of students on the caseload will allow for greater intensity at times with certain groups and will also allow children greater opportunities to work with different peers.

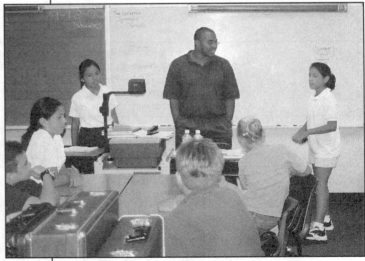

Speech-language pathologists working in YRE schools must learn how to calculate special education procedural timelines according to the various tracking systems in the schools. Mandated timelines are on hold when students are off-track, but not when speech-language pathologists are. Most YRE school districts publish a timeline calendar in order to make this calculation easier for staff.

Other members of a team may not have the same vacation schedule as a speech-language pathologist, so planning forward and backward is a good idea when working in a YRE school. Scheduling meeting dates when everyone will be available should be done at the beginning of the year. Some assessments may need to have plans signed early to accommodate vacation schedules. Moving a timeline up is always acceptable practice, but being late on completing an assessment or IEP, especially due to vacation schedules, is never acceptable and would be considered noncompliant with the INDIVIDUALS WITH DISABILITIES EDUCATION ACT (IDEA) AMENDMENTS OF 1997. Team coordination takes exceptional planning in a YRE school, but it is possible.

Tables 6.2 and 6.3 (see pages 164–165) show schedules for a speech-language pathologist who serves a multitrack YRE school. There are four tracks: A, B, C, and D. One track is always "off," and three are always "on." Table 6.2 shows A, B, and D on and Table 6.3 shows B, C, and D on. When A track students are on vacation, C track students replace them on the schedule. For example, in the 11:00 to 11:30 a.m. slot on Monday, four children are seen for intervention. Two children, Matt and Chris, continue in the second schedule. Jason and Gabriel go on vacation and are replaced by Tabitha and Adam.

There is great potential in YRE for positive effects for students and greater flexibility in service delivery models. Remember that although the YRE schedule may seem like a different amount of time, it is really the same amount, spread over a 12-month period.

There are two keys to ensuring successful implementation of alternative scheduling. The first is to remain open and creative. School speech-language pathologists have met numerous challenges with patience, understanding, and creativity... The second key is to stay involved and be proactive (Bland, 1998, pp. 34–35).

Should You Organize by Disability?

Organizing service models by communication disability has been reported in several sources (ASHA, 1998d; Neidecker, 1987). The authors believe this approach restricts creativity in service delivery for speech-language pathologists and students. PREFERRED PRACTICE PATTERNS do not indicate that particular service models are reserved for certain disabilities (ASHA, 1997c). In fact, the IDEA (1997) requirements for IEPs preclude the use of a one-size-fits-all program.

The ASHA (1998d) schools survey used a disability-based model to organize questions about service delivery. Survey data reflected the numbers of students served in each "disorder," instead of numbers served with various service delivery models. The use of disability categories awarded some implied validity to this organizational framework. In the future, analysis of functional outcomes for each service delivery model might reveal more interesting and useful data on effective service delivery for America's school children.

Table 6.2

YRE Schedule for Speech-Language Services—Part 1
Calle Lakeview School

Tracks A, B, D

	Monday	Tuesday	Wed	Thursday	Friday
9:00–9:40 Primary class	Jose Casey Travis	Andrew Nadia	Christie Daniel Devon	Sofia Kennisha	Assessments
9:45–10:15 Upper-level class	Artesia Andrea Denise Rebecca	Steven Mattie	Chrissy Missy	Andrew	
10:30–11:00 Pull-out	Special ed class Denise	Daniel Andrew	Chrissy Mikla Ennis	Daniel Nikki Alex	
11:00–11:30 Kgn	Matt Chris Jason Gabriel	Travis	Matt Chris Jason Gabriel	Travis	
11:00–12:00 Pull-out/Class	Darren Brian	Special ed class	Darren Chris		
1:00–1:30 Primary-level class	Andrew Kevin Bura	Bernice Joanna Nick Kristine	Andrew Kevin Brian	Lonnie Joanna Kevin Nick Kristine	
1:30–2:00 Upper-level class	Nick Bryan Dereck Robert Jimmie	Justin Tearah Christine	Nick Bryan Dereck Robert Jimmie	Justin Tearah Christine	
2:00–2:30 Pull-out	Courtney Heather Darryl	Gabriel	Courtney Heather Darryl	Jill Toya	
2:30–3:00 Pull-out	Kristin Matt Ashlee	Kevin Andrea Marlie Cody	Kristen Matt Ashlee	Andrea Marlie Cody Kevin	

Table 6.3					
YRE Schedule for Speech-Language Services—Part 2					
Calle Lakeview School				Tracks B, C, D	
	Monday	**Tuesday**	**Wed**	**Thursday**	**Friday**
9:00–9:40 Primary class	Jose Casey Travis	Andrew Nadia	Christie Daniel Devon	Sofia Kennisha	Assessments
9:45–10:15 Upper-level class	Artesia Andrea Denise Rebecca	Steven Mattie Kennisha	Andrew	Chrissy Missy	
10:30–11:00 Pull-out		Daniel Mikla Ennis Kelly		Daniel Mikla Ennis Kelly	
11:00–11:30 Kgn	Matt Chris Tabitha Adam	Travis	Off Campus Head Start Collaborative Program	Home Visits Curriculum Team Meetings	
11:00–12:00 Pull-out/Class	Brian Chris	Special ed class			
1:00–1:30 Primary-level class	Andrew Kevin Bura	Bonnie Kyle Zachary			
1:30–2:00 Upper-level class	Nick Bryan Dereck	Justin Eric Taylor			
2:00–2:30 Pull-out	Courtney Tony Nate Barstow	Adolfo Sarah Darryl			
2:30–3:00 Pull-out	Kristin Matt Ken	Kristin Matt Ken			

Support Personnel Model

Using support personnel in a school speech-language program is a recent innovation. Although support personnel have been routinely used in other special education settings since the early 1970s, they have had little involvement with speech-language services. Some states (e.g., Kansas and Nebraska) established special training and employment categories for speech-language support personnel early, but many states were hesitant to start until the field formally embraced the idea of trained and registered support personnel in 1995 through its national professional organization, ASHA (see "Speech-Language Pathology Assistants (SLPAs) and Aides in Schools" in Chapter 9).

The SPEECH-LANGUAGE PATHOLOGY ASSISTANT (SLPA) is typically regulated in a school program through at least two levels: the state LICENSING or CERTIFICATION of training level and the local school district employment level. States were concerned with meeting IDEA (1997) requirements to use qualified providers and trained and supervised SLPAs. Local districts were concerned with hiring practices, salary, benefits, seniority issues, and a new category of instructional staff that was more highly trained and costly than previous ones. Trained and supervised SLPAs can be very helpful to speech-language pathologists, especially if caseload numbers are high, and SLPAs allow greater numbers of children to be seen for more intensive services.

Using SLPAs dramatically changes the way speech-language pathologists manage the intervention schedule and organize service delivery. A short list of the roles and responsibilities of SLPAs shows the potential parameters of this expanded model:

- Conduct speech-language SCREENINGS

- Provide direct intervention to students

- Follow documented intervention plans and IEPs

- Document student progress

- Assist during student assessments

- Assist with informal documentation, prepare materials, perform clerical duties

- Schedule activities; prepare charts, records, graphs, or otherwise display data

- Perform checks and maintenance of equipment

- Participate in research projects, in-service training, and public relations programs (ASHA, 1996a)

The SUPPORT PERSONNEL MODEL enables speech-language pathologists to provide a greater range of services to students on the caseload, but SLPAs cannot maintain their own caseload. They must serve students who are identified by a speech-language pathologist and an IEP team only. They must be directly supervised 10–30 percent of the time they are working with students. Initially, SLPAs will require greater amounts of supervision to assure that intervention and other activities are conducted accurately and uniformly. However, SLPAs can provide services to students using all available models and may work simultaneously with speech-language pathologists. This allows daily intensive therapy for some students, in-class support for some students, and discrete trial sessions for others. Carryover and generalization sessions can be set up on a routine basis for students about to be dismissed.

The support personnel model is actually a cluster of models that can be managed by a communication team (i.e., the speech-language pathologist and one, two, or three SLPAs). Speech-language pathologists are responsible for the complete program but delegate tasks to SLPAs. SLPAs are the trained eyes and ears of speech-language pathologists when they are in the classroom and are equally effective at using the therapy room for small groups when speech-language pathologists are team-teaching in the classroom. SLPAs are also able to monitor students who need to be checked each week for hearing aid batteries, oral motor exercises, and written journal entries.

> **SLPAs are the trained eyes and ears of speech-language pathologists when they are in the classroom and are equally effective at using the therapy room for small groups.**

Schedules remain flexible throughout the year. One method that facilitates flexibility is to use cards in a pocket chart, so that assignments can be moved around as conditions change. A master schedule of all students seen for speech-language intervention may be necessary to share with other team members who may have difficulty coordinating with an ever-changing schedule that involves several speech-language service providers on the communication team.

Grouping Strategies

Scheduling and professional collaboration can be enhanced by using thoughtful grouping strategies. A body of research on the effectiveness of grouping strategies exists, linking cooperative learning groups to academic success (Johnson and Johnson, 1989; Kagan, 1994; Slavin, 1990). Children learn in groups throughout their school years. Recognizing that groups are the natural context of the classroom can help speech-language pathologists build collaborative working relationships with teachers and other education professionals. Students learning in groups should be a communication goal.

Grouping students for intervention can occur in traditional PULLOUT models, classrooms, and collaborative teams. Three types of groups are used in schools— SKILL GROUPS, FRIENDSHIP GROUPS, and RANDOM/PURPOSE GROUPS. Speech-language pathologists can use all three.

Skill Groups

Skill groups are composed of children who cannot independently do an assigned task or lack an underlying skill necessary to complete a task. Educators and speech-language pathologists commonly group children with similar skill levels together. These professionals need to work intensively with skill groups because there are no models in these groups who can do the task. If a whole class is divided into skill groups, as is often done for reading, instructors must move rapidly from group to group to provide teaching.

Speech-language pathologists frequently use skill groups, assigning children with peers who have the same perceived or tested deficits. Perhaps a student does not demonstrate a skill, such as conversational turn-taking or consistent production of a phoneme. All students near that student's age who have the same difficulty would be place together in a skill group. Skill grouping is labor-intensive for speech-language pathologists who do all the modeling, facilitating, and reinforcing. Students must wait, not always patiently, for professionals to provide cues and evaluation. Skill grouping often results in teaching isolated communication skills in an unnatural communication context, which can limit generalization.

Skill groups are easy to assemble and plan. Progress can be easily measured using only one probe for the group. Once a student shows improved skills, he or she is likely to be moved to another skill group. Students will be reassigned to join a new group of students who also need assistance with the next task that they need to learn. As frustrating as this might seem, students have been known to seek out ways to stay in their skill group if they like it. If improvement in the target skill means leaving the comfort and routine of a group of friends, students choose to not demonstrate that they can do the task. Progress dissipates when some students conclude that they like to attend speech sessions just to be with their group, even though they can already perform the expected task successfully. Speech-language pathologists need to observe

their skill groups conscientiously to assure that students are moving ahead at a steady pace.

Friendship Groups

Friendship groups are comprised of students who choose to be together or who adults assign together because they are friends. In these groups, students may be highly motivated and often quite social. They enjoy each other's company and will often work much harder just to keep all their friends together. Educators find these groupings to be full of energy and surprisingly productive. Much work can be accomplished quickly in a friendship group.

Speech-language pathologists rarely group this way since they are less aware of the social groupings of their students or may not be able to place classmates, let alone friends, together. However, when social groups are possible, speech-language pathologists remark on how exciting the activities are and how supportive the students are of each other, especially considering the variety of target goals a group may have. Friendship groups often get an extra boost in their effectiveness because students genuinely like each other, enjoy the opportunity to practice together, and are powerful models for each other. The targeted need of one student is a strength of one or more of the other students, providing peer facilitation, social rewards, and motivation. Natural contexts provide many opportunities for practice and generalization of communication skills. These groups can be exuberant and noisy or require the speech-language pathologist to monitor the social conversation that occurs.

Random/Purpose Groups

Random/purpose groups are the most time consuming to assemble but result in the most facilitative learning environment for children. They appear random, but speech-language pathologists have a purpose for putting them together. Educators group children by selecting students who can do various aspects of a task, so that they must join together to get it done. In the classroom, this usually means a group composed of some students who read easily and some who struggle, some students who write well and some who avoid it, some students who have artistic talent, and some students who can organize others. This group of 5 to 6 students can pull together and accomplish something that none of them can do alone. They may or may not be friends, but they recognize that together they can accomplish the task. The term COOPERATIVE LEARNING is often used for this type of group in variations known as jigsaw learning, pinwheels, or share pairs.

In speech-language intervention, a group of students with various phonological disabilities can operate like a random/purpose group. Children with multiple articulation errors, sometimes unintelligible, are grouped together and cycled through many phoneme productions. Different phonemes are targets for different children. This enables some students to be models for others in the group rather than depending on an adult model, who is often less motivating than peers. In random/purpose groups, speech-language pathologists structure services to accommodate strengths and needs of all children. Random/purpose groups of four to nine unintelligible children were found very successful in phonological remediation programs, with 85 percent of the students demonstrating significant change in 17 weeks or less of therapy (Montgomery and Bonderman, 1989). Groups of this type take considerable time and effort to organize. Changes in the group can upset instructional goals and activities.

Methods for Enhancing the Grouping Process

Educators often assign students who are to be in a random/purpose group (also referred to as "flexible grouping" or "heterogeneous grouping") through some type of matching task. Speech-language pathologists might enhance this grouping process by using language-oriented sorting methods, such as passing out cards with words, phrases, or pictures printed on them. Speech-language pathologists might ask students with picture cards to move around the room and talk to other students to determine what "scene" they belong in, such as a rain forest, a desert, a grassy plain, or a mountain. The picture card belongs to one of the scenes. Content from the classroom can be used, such as recent books read, science words, or adjectives that go with nouns. The process of finding one's group is an authentic language and communication experience. Speech-language pathologists may want to assure that caseload students receive cards that will place them in the appropriate group. Speech-language pathologists who work in collaborative classrooms use these types of activities often.

Educators have reported to the authors that they often keep effective random/purpose groups together for several subject areas as students become more and more productive and eventually learn to blend their skills. Speech-language pathologists can use this strategy also, moving previously unsuccessful students into already functioning groups without the limitations of matching a child's specific area of need as is done in skill groups.

Successful grouping of students on school caseloads is an important and easily overlooked responsibility of speech-language pathologists. The effectiveness of group therapy lies in the thought behind the grouping, which can result in greater effectiveness and motivation in students.

Using wise grouping strategies is an important component of COLLABORATIVE CONSULTATION. Flexible grouping of children provides services for vastly different communication needs. Purpose grouping can be a great assistance to teachers and can bring speech-language pathologists into classes for a wide variety of communication intervention activities.

Consultation and Collaboration

CONSULTATION and collaboration, distinctly different approaches, evolved as models for all aspects of service delivery nationwide in the 1990s as a consequence of the REGULAR EDUCATION INITIATIVE (REI) and a focus on the general education curriculum (Montgomery, 1992). After 20 years of special education legis-lation, school districts wanted to know if the programs were effective and if students receiving special education were learning.

Districts attempted to integrate their special education services into the mainstream of education and combine some of the specialized intervention with grade-level academic activities. This integration promoted the idea of professionals working with each other to support students, rather than each professional always working directly with each student. New speech-language school services have been enthusiastically described in the literature (e.g., Creaghead, 1999; Ehren, 2000; Ferguson, 1991; Miller, 1989; Montgomery, 1992; Moore-Brown, 2000; Nelson and Hoskins, 1997; Prelock, 2000; Secord, 1999; Secord and Damico, 1998).

Broadly speaking, speech-language intervention services may be provided in three forms— direct, indirect, or collaborative/consultative.

- A student can be served directly by a speech-language pathologist individually or in a group of students, either separately from the classroom or in the classroom.

- A student can be served indirectly by a speech-language pathologist individually, in a small group, or with the whole class in the student's classroom.

- A student can be served by a trained person, who is directed by a speech-language pathologist, in any relevant setting. This collaborative/consultative arrangement can be with an SLPA, a classroom teacher, another special educator, a peer, a parent, a bus driver, and so on (Montgomery, 1992).

IDEA (1997) requires that service delivery be directed by qualified professionals (e.g., speech-language pathologists), but it does not have to be administered directly by these professionals. In some cases, intervention is much more effective if it is not directly administered. The support personnel model reviewed earlier in this chapter (see page 166), for example, can be an effective consultative model. It is another way to structure meaningful intervention services for students and release speech-language pathologists for assessment, consultation, or work with families. For another example of indirect services through consultation (see "Infants and Toddlers" in Chapter 7). Service delivery can happen wherever it is arranged to happen. The essential component is that services are planned, supervised, measured, and evaluated for their effectiveness by speech-language pathologists.

Delivery models can be differentiated between consultation, collaboration, and collaborative/consultation approaches:

Consultation is **a voluntary process** in which one professional assists another to address a problem of a third party. It is a process rather than a style. It is voluntary and entails an indirect relationship. It involves shared participation, effective communication, teamwork, sharing, and problem solving.

Collaboration is **a style** in which two co-equal parties engage voluntarily in shared decision making as they work toward a common goal. It involves shared participation, resources ownership, accountability, and rewards. (Secord, 1999, p. 7)

Collaborative-consultation is **an interactive process** that enables teams of people with diverse expertise to generate creative solutions to mutually defined problems. The outcome is enhanced and altered, and produces solutions that are different from those that the individual team members would have produced independently. (Idol-Maestas, Paolucci-Whitcomb, and Levin, 1986, p. 1)

All of these service delivery approaches constitute the way speech-language pathologists function as support professionals in an educational setting. Speech-language pathologists in medical settings are often referred to as allied-health professionals. In the same way, speech-language pathologists in schools are allied-education professionals. They provide services in an array of direct and indirect ways to meet student needs.

It's no longer appropriate for speech-language pathologists to provide their services independently. The classroom teacher is the expert on curriculum. The SLP is the expert on language acquisition. Putting those two together will facilitate the most efficacious treatment for the student. (Shulman, as quoted in Campbell, 1999a, p. 7)

> The essential component is that services are planned, supervised, measured, and evaluated for their effectiveness by speech-language pathologists.

ASHA's 1995 nationwide survey on school services revealed that direct (i.e., traditional pull-out services) were used 24% of the time in infant and toddler programs, 50% with preschoolers, 78% with elementary-aged students, and 65% in secondary schools. Thirty-one percent of the preschool services, and 13% of the elementary-level services were classroom-based (i.e., indirect). Collaboration and consultation techniques were used 5% of the time with elementary students but 52% with infants and toddlers (ASHA, 1998d). In one of few studies comparing the three service delivery models, the collaborative model was the most effective in teaching curricular vocabulary for students who qualified for speech-language services (Throneburg, Calvert, Sturm, Paramboukas, and Paul, 2000).

Using any of these consultative constructs with deliberative planning allows speech-language pathologists to work in conjunction with classroom teachers, resource specialists, occupational therapists, social workers, and others. The curriculum is incorporated into therapy and therapy into the curriculum. Solutions to taxing service delivery issues present themselves when more than one individual assumes ownership for services. This assures more functional interventions, reduces the fragmentation of students' days, and enables speech-language pathologists to take a more active part in the schools. Collaboration begets more collaboration as team members begin to rely on each other, meet more often, and get pleasure from each others' successes.

Types of Teams

IDEA requires the use of a group of qualified professionals representing different disciplines and parents, often called a MULTIDISCIPLINARY TEAM (MDT), to plan and implement a student's IEP (see "Team Approach" and Figure 3.4 in Chapter 3 for a description of this team's activities). Appropriate service delivery (i.e., planning and implementing the IEP) for the student with communication disabilities is directly linked to how well the MDT functions. The MDT differs from an INTERDISCIPLINARY TEAM (IDT) and a TRANSDISCIPLINARY TEAM (TDT) in important ways (Donahue-Kilburg, 1992; Secord, 1999). The limited degree of cross-disciplinary work found in the MDT gives rise to the need for consultation and collaboration in schools to create effective ways to support students throughout their school days and their school career. This collaborative work can be accomplished by using the interdisciplinary and transdisciplinary methods described in Table 6.4. Both these teams extend the effectiveness of service delivery for children and families and enhance generalization to other contexts (Montgomery, 1992).

It is obvious that although an MDT is identified in IDEA (1997), it is the least collaborative of the three types. Effective service delivery rests on a TDT model that functions well. Therefore, the collaboration and consultation concepts inherent in TDT need to be formally taught to members of school MDT teams. Speech-language pathologists who are aware of this mismatch can promote and participate in cross-discipline training that makes service delivery models outside of traditional pullout

Table 6.4

Team Methods

	Multidisciplinary Team (MDT)	Interdisciplinary Team (IDT)	Transdisciplinary Team (TDT)
Definition	This is either a generic term for coordinated services or a specific term for a group of professionals who play their traditional roles with little coordination of services (Donahue-Kilburg, 1992; Wilcox, 1989).	Members work together on the evaluation and treatment team but evaluate and treat the student and family separately. They often have formal channels for communication and a functioning case manager (Donahue-Kilburg, 1992).	Members divide their work into direct and indirect student services. Not everyone works with every student, but all members consult with each other to carry out the service delivery plans the group, including parents and care-givers, designs together (Donahue-Kilburg, 1992).
Typical Activities	Work independently and make decisions regarding their areas of expertise; review findings at a team meeting with all the other disciplines in attendance; conduct assessments, establish objectives independently, and then share assessments and objectives	Have members with an area of expertise who are aware of the other team members' expertise; designate a team leader to coordinate all activities; develop two-way communication channels to exchange ideas often; conduct assessments, establish objectives independently, and then share assessments and objectives	Engage in role release and move across discipline boundaries, teaching, learning, and sharing with each other; design goals based on what a student and family believe is important, add their ideas, agree to carry out the plan that evolves; conduct assessments together, observe students functioning while another team member works with them, work closely with and rely on reports from families

therapy feasible in schools. Some long-standing school teams have evolved into IDT or TDT models, and collaborative service delivery is less stressful for them. Speech-language pathologists need to appraise their teams' methods of interaction and expand their comfort levels in sharing expertise to encourage collaborative models.

Writing Goals Together

An effective way for speech-language pathologists and other educators to begin collaborative/consultative service delivery is to write and implement shared goals for students with disabilities. Teams in a suburban school district have used the following methods to write shared goals by using transdisciplinary planning even though their IEP process was still basically multidisciplinary.

- The speech-language pathologist and two special educators met and planned their actions together, resulting in three joint goals rather than a series of goals from each specialist.

- For some children, only one common goal was most effective. All the team members responsible for the child's program contributed to the writing of this statement and rotated the responsibility for monitoring it throughout the year.

- Educators wrote goals and objectives in their own areas of expertise (speech and language; resource; adaptive physical education), however, other adults or peers were assigned to carry them out.

- Speech-language goals were written for a child which required that one objective be carried out at home (parent responsible) and another objective carried out at school (speech-language pathologist responsible). Both objectives needed to be met to reach the goal. The parent had agreed to do this at the meeting.

- Parents and educators wrote goals and objectives together, with a single monitoring system carried back and forth by the child, each night in his backpack. A separate monitoring system in each setting could be used and routinely compared to measure progress in different settings.

- Teams wrote embedded skill goals, where all objectives lead to a single goal such as functional communication. For example: Theresa will use her communication board to meaningfully respond to an adult greeting once a day. Occupational therapy and physical therapy had embedded motor goals, while the teacher had embedded cause and effect cognition goals, and the vision therapist had embedded left to right sequencing goals.

- The student's school day was viewed through life domains (homeroom, hallways, bus stop, scouts, cafeteria, etc.) and service plans and objectives written by the team were taught to the non-special education personnel in each setting or domain. Data was [sic] kept on a large chart by eight adults and one peer. (Montgomery, 1993b, p. 23)

Record Keeping Is Critical

Record keeping is important with all service delivery models and often serves useful functions for many team members involved with indirect service models. When speech-language pathologists act as consultants, a form helps to structure the discussion and keep it focussed on positive problem solving. The form can also guide a team in setting expectations for each member's activities and examining results. The Collaborative Consultation Form (see Figure 6.1 on page 176) is one example of a record-keeping form (Merritt and Culatta, 1998; Secord, 1999).

Records of a consultative meeting should include identification information regarding a student, family, and team participants. A clear description of the problem should be stated in terms that are observable and measurable along with a statement of the desired behavior or outcome. A review of past attempts to resolve the problem can be helpful. A range of options to address the problem may be listed, and the action that is agreed on should be clearly identified. The consultative meeting should never adjourn without first setting a date to check on progress or results.

Consultative forms should be used to clearly identify action plans, including persons responsible, what they will do, and timelines for implementation. These actions should be clearly tied to the functional outcomes desired for a student. See "Functional Outcomes and the School-Based Speech-Language Pathologist" in Chapter 5 for a discussion of functional outcomes.

Consultants need to display empathy and support for staff members, but that is not the purpose of the meeting. When acting as consultants, speech-language pathologists will guide team members to focus on problems, identify successes as well as concerns, and clearly identify the desired functional outcomes for a student. A well-designed form helps draw the discussion away from frustrations and toward a vision of what is desired for the student.

Action plans should clearly identify responsibilities, deadlines, and expected outcomes. This format helps reinforce the concept of teamwork and avoids the assumption that consultants have taken on the responsibility of solving problems independently. Consultants may use consultation forms to check back with team members to monitor their progress toward deadlines. When teams meet at their assigned follow-ups, they will have the information needed to determine the success of intervention and any adjustments that need to be made.

Peer Tutors as Part of Service Delivery

Once planning is focused on the environment of a student, peers take on greater significance in

> When speech-language pathologists act as consultants, a form helps to structure the discussion and keep it focussed on positive problem solving.

Figure 6.1

Collaborative Consultation Form

Student _____ DOB _____ Grade _____

School _____ Parent(s) _____

Speech-Language Pathologist _____ Date of Meeting _____

Team Members _____

_____

How was student involved in consultation? _____

DESCRIBE PROBLEM IN BEHAVIORAL TERMS:

DESCRIBE OUTCOME AND HOW IT WILL BE MEASURED:

BRAINSTORM STRATEGIES TO ASSIST STUDENT IN REACHING OUTCOME:

DEVELOP ACTION PLAN:

Date of Follow-up Meeting:_____

WHO	ACTION	TIMELINE	DESIRED STUDENT OUTCOME

Sources: Merritt and Culatta (1998); Secord (1999)

the delivery of services. Some students respond much more favorably to peers than adults and can demonstrate faster progress if the work is connected to peer interactions. This is a distinct advantage of school-based intervention that many speech-language pathologists may overlook. Speech-language pathologists can gradually shift responsibilities for monitoring to peer tutors or cooperative learning groups using the collaborative/consultative approach. This is also effective with adolescents (Larson and McKinley, 1987). Speech-language pathologists need to make the shift gradually, select peer models carefully, orient and train peers, have supports readily available for peers, and monitor and follow up with students and peers conscientiously. The advantages to peer tutoring are numerous and match many overall communication and academic goals designed for target students by speech-language pathologists. Some of these advantages include:

- Increases time for support and assistance for target students

- Increases the number of contexts in which target students can be supported

- Provides more natural intervention as most students learn with peers not with adults

- Supports a give and take between target students and peer tutors

- Models collaboration without directly involving other professionals, which can serve as a first step in a resistive school environment

- Provides opportunities for incidental learning and social and academic scripts that serve target students well in school and beyond (German, 1992; Larson and McKinley, 1987)

Building Relationships with General Educators

General educators are good resources to help identify and serve children who may need services since children with language disabilities often exhibit concomitant problems with grammar, vocabulary, or effective conversation skills (Secord, 1999). Speech-language pathologists should team with teachers to jointly observe a student's interactions in class and other school settings. Teaming facilitates all types of service delivery, especially collaboration. Successful collaboration means all professionals involved with the child's services will attend referral and IEP meetings together. "Teachers can augment the speech-language pathologist's observations with their own anecdotes or test results" (Campbell, 1999a, p. 8).

Statement from IDEA (1997)

The IDEA (1997) amendments added a requirement that each child's IEP team must include "at least one regular education teacher of the child (if the child is, or may be, participating in the regular education environment)" (34 CODE OF FEDERAL REGULATIONS [C.F.R.] § 300.344 [a] [2]). This should be someone who teaches or would have taught the student in a general education class. This person may be a grade-level teacher, a subject-area teacher, or a teacher at the home school of a student placed in a specialized school. The intent of this section of IDEA is to have a person at the meeting who keeps the conversation grounded in general education instruction, curriculum, and expectancies. If the student has significant educational needs, it may be difficult for specialists to recall what students at that age and grade are doing in the classroom. This context had been previously overlooked, and the amendments assured there would be a realistic and thoughtful appraisal of the student in the natural environment.

General Educators at the IEP Meeting

General educators can make great contributions to the development of a student's IEP. Speech-language pathologists will find that "language of the classroom" issues are indeed relevant to educators, and therapy is more successful when the whole team is aware of and working on the student's communication goals (Throneburg et al., 2000, p. 13).

There are specific actions that general educators can take prior to or during meetings to be helpful members of teams. Speech-language pathologists can share ideas with general

---

What General Educators Can Do as Required Members of IEP Teams

- Listen carefully to the discussion of a student's strengths and needs without undue concern about the label or diagnosis the student may carry.

- Bring a copy of the age-appropriate curriculum to the meeting. Be sure it is the one actually used to create that class.

- Describe a project or product students produce at your grade level.

- Bring or name a few books that are read to students at this grade.

- Describe how supplies and materials are acquired and stored by students in your classroom.

- Bring a list of what you believe are the five most important concepts your students will learn that year.

- Be prepared to answer questions about instructional methods that you use frequently.

- Give examples of the type of instructional support that is provided to students in your class.

- Describe the technology used by you and students in your class.

- Discuss the teaming activities of teachers at your grade level.

- Think about and share experiences you have had with paraprofessionals or other support person.

From *Inclusive Practices in the Middle School* [Handout], by J.K. Montgomery, 2000b, presentation at Hewes Middle School, Tustin Unified School District, Tustin, CA. © 2000 by J.K. Montgomery. Adapted with permission.

education peers that seem appropriate for the age and grade of a student (see sidebar for a list of ideas). General educators have a unique perspective on education that is often unfamiliar to special education teams. Appropriate decisions for a student's level of INCLUSION or support can be made at subsequent meetings if facts and opinions are shared early in the process. Again, it is important to have a classroom teacher be aware of the speech-language goals for a student by joining this discussion, rather than being given a completed IEP several weeks later "so you know what services he's receiving this year."

Speech-language pathologists can and should take a leadership role in this area of communication with and about students on their caseloads. General educators make important contributions when accommodations and modifications are discussed (Bateman and Linden, 1998). It is the responsibility of classroom teachers to assure that all students in their classrooms learn. Special education teams support general educators to meet that expectancy based on each student's present level of performance.

Linking Services to the Curriculum

During the 1990s, speech-language intervention services gradually evolved from clinically based therapy to broader-based educationally and developmentally related intervention services. Individual or small group sessions with speech-language pathologists were once the norm. Collaborative therapy using the core curriculum was reported as the new model by every state and the District of Columbia association presidents (Moore-Brown and Montgomery, 1999). Larger student groupings with technology-assisted, curriculum-related sessions conducted in classrooms are used in many districts. Descriptions of these exciting models are available in the literature (see "Literacy, Reading, and Writing," page 181), and several will be discussed in this chapter.

Several models have been developed to compare purposes and characteristics of therapy versus instruction. One such model (see Table 6.5 on page 180) has been observed by the authors in numerous schools and follows the spirit and letter of IDEA (1997). It links all the communication services to a student's educational goals and includes roles for speech-language pathologists to provide CONVENTIONAL THERAPY and classroom instruction. This approach has been used by many speech-language pathologists who use the student's curriculum as the vehicle for practicing targeted communication skills.

Some states tap the expertise of speech-language pathologists to work as communication teachers in self-contained classrooms. These professionals teach the content of the curriculum, guided by a strong language component, to children who have pervasive communication disabilities. This reduces the fragmentation that occurs with pullout services. A thorough description of service delivery in schools must include speech-language pathologists who apply all the therapeutic practice directly to the teaching of a content area. This position may require additional coursework or another

Table 6.5

Blended Therapeutic/Educational Role
for Collaboration in the Curriculum

Factors to Consider	Classroom Instruction	Conventional Therapy	Collaborative Intervention
Learning	Deals with learning new information and skills in the normal course of development	Deals with remediating or compensating for deficient skills that have not developed or that have been lost	Focuses on a combination of learning new information plus research-based intensive strategies using individualized instructional accommodations with a sensitivity for different learning styles and varying levels of student support
Student Engagement	Involves a captive audience with varying degrees of active engagement at different times	Depends on a student's ongoing, active participation in a self-help process	Combines the advantages of students working in multiskilled groups of same-age peers with individual empowerment possible with effective scaffolds
Planning	Uses a teaching sequence based on external criteria, curriculum standards, and progression	Uses a sequence of activities based on individual needs and progress	Uses a sequence based on individual needs and progress within the larger framework of curricular expectations for students at a particular grade level
Needs of Learners	Is oriented to group goals and uses a standard approach	Incorporates selection of individual goals and uses a diagnostic approach	Incorporates a selection of individual, measurable annual goals but encourages use of state or local standards as benchmarks under those goals
Pace	Is determined by the majority of group and average ability	Is determined by a student's mastery and the speech-language pathologist's judgements	Demands more intense efforts and adjusted pace to promote mastery; actions of all members of the team, including the general education teacher, are contingent on the actions of the student
Interaction	Has teachers teach the planned lesson and students provide feedback after specific tasks	Incorporates the speech-language pathologist's actions contingent on a student's reactions; informative and corrective feedback are essential and ongoing	Uses informative and corrective feedback provided in both formal and informal ways from educators, speech-language pathologists, peers, and support personnel

From *Inclusive Practices in the Middle School* [Handout], by J.K. Montgomery, 2000b, presentation at Hewes Middle School, Tustin Unified School District, Tustin, CA. © 2000 by J.K. Montgomery. Adapted with permission.

credential in some states (California Department of Education, 1999d).

In the environments of classroom instruction, conventional therapy, and COLLABORATIVE INTERVENTION, speech-language pathologists blend therapeutic goals and methods with educational standards, so that generalization of common skills is enhanced. Compatible with IDEA (1997), this model shows how educators and parents can be made aware of the impact of students' evolving communication skills.

The three macrosystems presented in Table 6.5 may use many broad-based instructional strategies. A service delivery model is similar to the outside walls of a house or the fence around a yard. Each occupant can furnish or plant it to fit his or her tastes, interests, and resources. Once the parameters of service are established, numerous therapeutic strategies will fit.

Literacy, Reading, and Writing

ASHA Position Statement

It is the position of the American Speech-Language-Hearing Association (ASHA) that speech-language pathologists (SLPs) play a critical and direct role in the development of literacy for children and adolescents with communication disorders, including those with severe or multiple disabilities. SLPs also make a contribution to the literacy

efforts of a school district or community on behalf of other children and adolescents. (ASHA, 2000d, p. 1)

This forthright statement acknowledged the strong connection between spoken and written language, asserting that speech-language pathologists would play a major role in supporting students with reading and language difficulties. It was motivated by the national interest in promoting LITERACY for all individuals, the acknowledgement that speech-language pathologists serve students whose language difficulties involve reading and writing, the role of speech-language pathologists as advocates for these students, the benefits of collaborative partnerships between educators, and the questions that speech-language pathologists had regarding their role in literacy (ASHA, 2000d). There is a considerable body of research that confirms the connection between language and reading from the COMMUNICATION DISORDERS, linguistics, and education fields (Catts and Kamhi, 1999; Sanders, 2001). Reading, language arts, and communication skills are linked interdependently in the educational process.

Reading and Reading Disabilities

Literacy is defined by Section 3 of the National Literacy Act of 1991 as "an individual's ability to read, write, and speak in English and compute and solve problems at levels of proficiency necessary to function on the job and in society, to achieve one's goals and to develop one's knowledge and potential." Literacy encompasses reading, writing, speaking, listening, and thinking. Literacy is the purpose of schooling in this country (Goldsworthy, 1996). "Of all school learning, nothing compares in importance with reading; it is of unparalleled significance" (Bettleheim and Zelan, 1982, p. 5).

Some descriptions of reading explain the reading event but are not helpful to explain why some students struggle to learn to read. Each definition seeks to include the two basic elements of reading: comprehension and decoding. Catts and Kamhi (1999) call reading "thinking guided by print" (p. 3). Snow, Burns, and Griffin (1998) combined the ideas of a national panel of 17 reading experts into a definition of reading:

> Reading as a cognitive and psycholinguistic activity requires the use of form (the written code) to obtain meaning (the message to be understood), within the context of the reader's purpose (for learning, for enjoyment, for insight). (p. 33)

Goldsworthy (1996), in one of the early texts on intervention for reading disabilities for speech-language pathologists, felt some simple definitions were misleading if reading was defined as an event rather than a process:

> During the reading process, information extracted from the printed page, whether at the level of decoding and word recognition or comprehension of text, is analyzed and compared with previously stored information. If it were a simple matter of learning a set of associ-

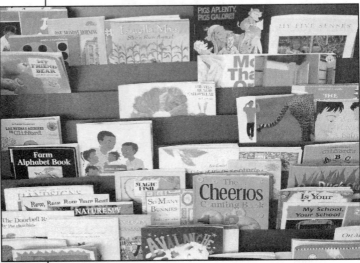

ations between sounds of the spoken language and printed squiggles on a page, learning to read would be relatively easy, because it would involve little that is new to the would-be reader with the exception that language will now be presented through the visual modality. The process involved in reading acquisition, however, is far more complex than a simple transfer of meanings from oral to written language. (p. 33)

Most researchers would agree that 80 percent of children in elementary schools learn to read adequately (Catts and Kamhi, 1999; Fey, 1999). The 20 percent who struggle do so for many reasons. They may have sensory impairments, have developmental or language disabilities, or be second-language learners to name a few common situations (Snow, Burns, and Griffin, 1998). These students require explicit systematic instruction in the areas outlined by Lyon (as cited in Snow, Burns, and Griffin,

1998) to be successful (see sidebar for areas of instruction for successful readers). "Reading proficiency is an important goal for virtually all students who receive special education" (California Department of Education, 1999b, p. 7) and students with moderate to severe disabilities can benefit from literacy instruction (Kliewer and Landis, 1999; Koppenhaver and Yoder, 1993). Students who have developmental disabilities that affect cognitive organization, memory, language processing, and physical manipulation of print are often not taught reading in their self-contained classrooms (Erickson and Koppenhaver, 1995). Developing their literacy skills is often a challenge for speech-language pathologists and an important focus of intervention programs (ASHA, 2000d; Goldsworthy, 1996; van Kleeck, 1998; Yoder and Koppenhaver, 1993).

Roles and Responsibilities in Reading

Roles and responsibilities for speech-language pathologists to be involved in literacy develop-ment were identified in three sources. They were (1) national literacy recommendations, (2) state guidelines in special education and reading, and (3) ASHA guidelines for roles and responsibilities for speech-language pathologists in facilitating literacy.

The National Council on Preventing Reading Difficulties in Young Children noted in its findings that identification of and service to children with language problems by speech-language pathologists was the second in a long list of critical recommendations for prevention (as cited in Snow et al., 1998). It reported that identification of preschool children who were at risk for learning to read was based on these research-derived indicators:

1. In infancy or during the preschool period, significant delays in expressive language, receptive vocabulary, or IQ

2. At school entry, delays in a combination of measures of readiness, including:

   • Letter identification

   • Understanding the functions of print

Areas of Instruction for Successful Readers

In testimony to the U.S. House of Representatives, Committee on Education and the Workforce, July 10, 1997, G. Reid Lyon, Chief, Child Development and Behavior Branch of the National Institute of Child Health and Human Development (NICHD) said: "To learn to read, a child must integrate phonemic skills into learning phonic principles, must practice reading so word recognition is rapid and accurate, and must learn how to actively use comprehension strategies to enhance meaning" (as quoted in Snow, Burns, and Griffin, 1998, p. 41).

- Verbal memory for stories and sentences

- PHONOLOGICAL AWARENESS

- Lexical skills, such as naming vocabulary

- Receptive language skills in the areas of SYNTAX and morphology

- Expressive language

- Overall language development

Many states have robust literacy programs that address the issues of prevention of reading difficulties, philosophies of reading acquisition, the selection of reading books and educational materials, and university teacher education programs. States have documented that 80 percent of the children referred for special education programs exhibited reading problems (Kavale and Reese, 1992). The vast majority of goals and OBJECTIVES on IEPs address needs in reading and writing. Poor reading skills were preventing these children from accessing meaningful instructional content in their classrooms. For 85 to 90 percent of poor readers, effective prevention and early intervention can increase their reading skills to within average levels (Lyon, 1998). Speech-language pathologists and other special educators have a role to play in service delivery to students with reading and language disabilities as described in *The California Reading Initiative and Special Education in California: Critical Ideas to Focus Meaningful Reform* (California Department of Education, 1999b). Service delivery in reading

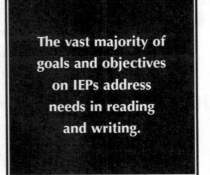

The vast majority of goals and objectives on IEPs address needs in reading and writing.

was heralded as "professionally exciting for all special education teachers and specialists, including school psychologists and speech and language specialists *[sic]*" (p. 3).

The ASHA (2000d) guidelines for speech-language pathologists' roles and responsibilities in promoting reading and literacy in school-age children (see sidebar) expand the initial technical report and the profession's position paper on reading and writing. Collaborative approaches with other school-based professionals are urged throughout the ASHA guidelines, along with close adherence to state and local policies, procedures, and regulations on the subject of reading and literacy. Service delivery for children with a combination of reading difficulties and language disabilities should include prevention, identification, assessment, intervention, coordination with other professionals, and contributions to future research and information. The ASHA document that outlines each of these areas in highly practical detail is almost 60 pages long, which attests to the importance of service delivery in this expanded model (ASHA, 2000d). This document will likely serve as a major resource for graduate courses in speech-language pathology. The guide is available on the ASHA Web site (*www.asha.org*).

Many speech-language pathologists working in schools now, or contemplating doing so in the future, may not have had university coursework in reading or literacy. They may wish to

ASHA Guidelines for Speech-Language Pathologists' Roles and Responsibilities in Promoting Reading and Literacy

1. Prevention

Joint book reading

Environmental print awareness

Concepts of print

Concepts of phonology

Alphabetic letter knowledge

Sense of story

Adult modeling of literacy activities

Experiences with writing materials

Other activities

2. Identification

Children at risk for reading and writing
   problems

Individual and cultural differences

Early identification

Older students

3. Assessment

Formal assessment

Emergent level

   Family literacy

   Phonological awareness

   Print awareness

   Oral language

Early elementary level

   Phonological awareness

   Rapid naming

   Letter identification

   Invented spelling

   Reading

   Writing

   Oral language

Later level (4th grade and up)

   Reading

Writing

Curriculum-based assessment

Metacognitive functioning

Oral language

Using published tools

4. Intervention

Targeting literacy

   Individual plans

   Individual implementations

   Expectations of the curriculum

Research-based interventions

   Strategic literacy goals

   Knowing the literature

   Characteristics of good and poor readers

Balanced intervention

Culturally appropriate intervention

Developmentally appropriate

   Early childhood programs

   Early elementary programs

   Later elementary and secondary
      programs

   Students with multiple or severe
      developmental impairments

Needs-based curriculum-relevant intervention

   Basic principles of curriculum planning

   Modifications for special needs

5. Other roles and responsibilities

Assistance to general education teachers

Curricular responsibilities on behalf
   of all students

Extending the knowledge base
   for students and colleagues

From *Roles and Responsibilities of Speech-Language Pathologists with Respect to Reading and Writing in Children and Adolescents,* by the American Speech-Language-Hearing Association (ASHA), 2000d, Rockville, MD: Author. © 2000 by ASHA. Adapted with permission.

take weekend courses, conference seminars, and other continuing education offerings to build their knowledge in this area of nationwide concern.

The guidelines provided in *Roles and Responsibilities of Speech-Language Pathologists with Respect to Reading and Writing in Children and Adolescents* (ASHA, 2000d) are intended to clarify that speech-language pathologists have the expertise and responsibility to play important roles related to literacy. They can ensure that all children gain access to instruction that helps them learn to read and write as well as to communicate orally, manually, or with augmentative and alternative techniques and devices. The fact that language problems are both a cause and a consequence of reading disabilities, and that written language capabilities are critical to academic success makes it not only appropriate, but essential, that speech-language pathologists accept responsibility for these roles.

Special educators, including speech-language pathologists, have investigated the myths and misconceptions that have revolved around teaching reading to students with mild, moderate, and severe disabilities. Many have concluded that a large number of these students were never taught to read using explicit, systematic instruction or effective books and materials. Special techniques, often lacking in empirical validation, were thought to be necessary because students were labeled "special" or experienced significant disabilities (Simmons and Kame'enui, 1998). Special educators involved in literacy instruction need to:

- Have a comprehensive knowledge of spoken and written English

- Understand the process of reading as both comprehension and decoding

- Know the early indicators of reading difficulty

- Intervene using research-based strategies

- Encourage all children to read often in authentic situations

- Know how to measure progress and make instructional adjustments when needed (Simmons and Kame'enui, 1998)

Comprehension and decoding may affect students' reading behaviors in different ways. One skill group without the other is not true reading; however, students with special needs will often acquire them unevenly. Balancing the teaching of comprehension (e.g., listening, narrative, and retelling skills) with decoding (e.g., sound-symbol matching, and pattern-recognition skills) must be a collaborative effort between speech-language pathologists and other educators. Speech-language pathologists provide intervention services in both components of reading (ASHA, 2000d).

Readers of this text are urged to expand their knowledge and skills in literacy instruction (see sidebar for a list of instructional and therapeutic strategies). Many excellent literacy Web sites are available. Periodic articles in the Special Interest Division #1 Newsletters from ASHA and ASHA's (2000d) *Roles and Responsibilities of Speech-Language Pathologists with Respect to Reading and Writing in Children and Adolescents* are also informative.

Instructional and Therapeutic Strategies

Speech-language pathologists report using similar instructional and therapeutic strategies in all settings. Frequently these are strategies created by speech-language pathologists working with students in schools. Although this list could be considerably longer, we chose only a few to highlight. Communication Lab (Pritchard Dodge, 1994) is a total class activity, addressing individual goals as well as general classroom discourse. It develops pragmatic skills and useful classroom social skills and interactions. Successful interventions for narratives and expository text development are the hallmark of *The Story Grammar Marker* (Rooney-Moreau and Fidrych-Puzzo, 1994) and *ThemeMaker* (Rooney-Moreau and Fidrych, 1998). *The Magic of Stories* (Strong and Hoggan North, 1996) uses classic children's literature for teaching text comprehension and narrative skills. *Conversations* (Hoskins, 1997) allows speech-language pathologists to target and monitor planned discourse for students in small groups. Successful strategies for these therapeutic environments are available to speech-language pathologists in many forms, including audiotapes (e.g., Nelson and Hoskins, 1997).

Phonological Awareness

PHONOLOGICAL AWARENESS is critical to the development of reading (Adams, 1999; Catts and Kamhi, 1999; Gillon, 2000; Goldsworthy, 1996; Snow, Burns, and Griffin, 1998). Yopp (1995) concluded that this overall awareness of how sounds are separate yet connected to each other in the speech stream is necessary to learn to read and the result of learning to read. Speech-language pathologists have highly relevant training and clinical experience in this area and can incorporate it into their service delivery (ASHA, 1999c; Gillon, 2000; Goldsworthy, 1996, 1998).

Phonological awareness can be defined as sensitivity to the patterns of spoken language that recur and can be manipulated without regard to their meaning (Snow et al., 1998). Goldsworthy (1998) offers a very useful hierarchy of skill development from less difficult sentence-level phonological activities, to word-level skills, and finally phoneme-level skills. Using this three level approach, speech-language pathologists reported immediate changes in students' reading skills confirmed by classroom teachers. Developing phonological awareness skills in students with significant language disabilities has become an effective service delivery approach for speech-language pathologists (Gillam, 1999b; van Kleeck, 1998).

Collaborative partners need to use each other's professional vocabulary with ease and be able to explain standards and BENCHMARKS to parents and policymakers. Some confusion exists for reading terms that seem to overlap with speech-language terminology. Speech-language pathologists need to know general education, special education, and speech-language terminology for phonological awareness. Figure 6.2 (page 188) provides some clarification for speech-language pathologists who follow their state guidelines to provide support in phonological

Figure 6.2

Phonological Terms Used in Reading

Phonological Processing is using information about the sound structure of speech to process oral and written language (Hodson and Edwards, 1997). These skills are used in aural and oral modalities.

↓

Phonological Awareness is the general ability to attend to the sounds of language distinct from its meaning, including rhyming, counting syllables, segmenting words, and recognizing onset and rime in words (Snow et al., 1998). Skills are used in aural and oral modalities.

↓

Phonemic Awareness is the explicit understanding that words are composed of segments of sound smaller than a syllable (phoneme) plus the knowledge that these individual phonemes have distinctive features (Torgesen, 1999). These skills are used in aural and oral modalities.

↓

Phonics are instructional practices that educators use to emphasize how spellings are related to speech sounds in systematic ways (Snow, Burns, and Griffin, 1998). These skills are used in aural, oral, and graphemic modalities.

↓

(Phonological) Decoding is a method to derive a pronunciation for a printed sequence of letters based on knowledge of spelling-sound correspondence (Adams, 1999). These skills are used in aural, oral, graphemic, and motoric modalities.

From *Inclusive Practices in the Middle School* [Handout], by J.K. Montgomery, 2000b, presentation at Hewes Middle School, Tustin Unified School District, Tustin, CA. © 2000 by J.K. Montgomery. Adapted with permission.

awareness as an extension of their speech-language interventions.

Serving Students in Preschool

Assessing and providing therapy for children under 5 years of age was a permissive program under the EDUCATION FOR ALL HANDICAPPED CHILDREN ACT (EAHCA) of 1975. A permissive special education program is one that federal law approves to be funded but does not mandate. Some states immediately began serving very young children, with Michigan offering programs in schools, preschools, and daycare settings for children aged 2 years. In other states, parents of children with long-standing conditions, such as hearing loss, cerebral palsy, developmental delays, or syndromes, waited for their children's fifth birthdays to have them assessed by the school district, so that they could receive services free and in the vicinity of their neighborhood school. Unfortunately, lack of intervention through the formative preschool years only made the task of appropriate programming that much more difficult in kindergarten.

School districts without preschool intervention found a need to know the number of children with disabilities, and which disabilities, would arrive in their kindergartens each year. Once they knew the children and families, they could prepare suitable programs and have staff hired or trained when necessary. The best reason for early intervention programs was, of course, that successful ones ameliorated children's disabilities and enabled them to be a part of a general education class sooner. Since these youngsters would spend the next 12 to 16 years in the school system, schools had a big stake in early and effective intervention.

With the amendments to the EAHCA (1975) in P.L. 99-457 (1986), preschool programs became a part of the full special education spectrum offered by schools. Preschool programs were included in Part B of the EAHCA, to include services for children with special needs beginning at age 3. Districts sought space to set up classes and offer center-based services (i.e., children come to a school facility to receive services), sometimes nudging out privately run preschools that were leasing empty classrooms in schools. In the late 1980s, large preschool programs were created in many states (e.g., Texas, California, and Maryland), including transportation systems for very young children and a full staff of specialists to assess children; counsel families; and provide occupational, physical, and speech-language therapy. Communication disorders quickly became the most commonly identified disability and its intervention the most frequently requested service in preschools. Most preschool children with identifiable impairments and disabilities demonstrate some type of communication disorder (Donahue-Kilburg, 1992; Hanson, 1984; Polmanteer and Turbiville, 2000).

Since children are still developing their language throughout preschool, delayed communication development can masquerade as simple immaturity. Children's communication skills are not yet stabilized and many children are still acquiring the last few motorically complex sounds of their first or second languages. Researchers have described the literal explosion of new vocabulary that a child acquires between the ages of 4 and 5, when school begins for most of them (van Kleeck, 1998; Vygotsky, 1978). In the preschool setting, it is particularly important for speech-language pathologists to have two well-developed bases of knowledge:

1. Normal acquisition of speech and language, so that children are not overidentified

2. Appropriate intervention models for this age group that are not merely scaled down versions of similar services for school-age children

Assessment and Eligibility for Preschoolers

Children aged 3 to 5 with suspected communication disabilities must be assessed by speech-language pathologists. Preschoolers are referred by parents, community agencies, physicians, private preschool administrators, or others outside the school. There is no cost for the assessment even if a child has not previously been known to the school. The assessment may take place at the neighborhood school, a central assessment center, or a child's home.

Young children should be assessed informally as well as formally using tools that are designed for their age group only. If a child's language or culture is different from that of a speech-language pathologist, the professional needs to be sensitive to the child-rearing practices of the family, listen carefully to what family concerns are, and use an interpreter if needed. For example, a speech-language pathologist must be cautious not to mistake a 3-year-old's

shyness while speaking to a stranger for a communication problem. Family members are often the best resource for the speech-language pathologist to learn about a child's typical performance.

There are separate preschool eligibility criteria in most states because of the importance of early intervention. The paucity of STANDARD-IZED TESTS at this level, the difficulty getting responses from a young child on demand, and the interplay of cognition and language at this age are accounted for in less stringent criteria at this level. Most criteria refer to developmental levels of children rather than test scores. States and school districts recognize the relatively short amount of time available to reach students during this critical stage of development and do not wish to delay or deny services by setting strict entrance criteria.

Individual Family Service Plans (IFSPs)

If a child is found to have a speech-language disability, services may be provided in a variety of places, such as a daily preschool for children with disabilities, the typical preschool the child already attends, a daycare center, a HEAD START PROGRAM, a typical public school, or in the child's home. An IEP or, as it is called at this age, INDIVIDUAL FAMILY SERVICE PLAN (IFSP) is developed by the team that has assessed the child, plus parents, and any other adults who know the child well. Usually, the child is too young to attend this meeting; although it does bring a real sense of authenticity when the child attends.

An IFSP states all the services needed, the person responsible for each, the location of the services, and the specific roles and responsibilities parents or caretakers will have. In this way, the IEP for preschoolers differs from the conventional IEP for school-age children. Preschoolers are part of their families and cannot be authentically discussed or planned for outside of that strong network. Often parents have specific questions about how to communicate with their child that should be addressed in the assessment and the service plan (Polmanteer and Turbiville, 2000). The IFSP is written for a year or less, whichever is appropriate for a particular child. Functional outcomes are incorporated into the planning, and accommodations for the language and culture of the family are integrated into the IFSP (see "Functional Outcomes and the School-Based Speech-Language Pathologist" in Chapter 5 for a discussion on functional outcomes). Some of these are family outcomes rather than direct child outcomes. The use of lay language rather than professional jargon is a marker of a family-responsive plan (Polmanteer and Turbiville, 2000).

> Speech-language pathologists need to devote larger blocks of time to serve preschoolers; maintain close contact with caregivers and teachers; and allow for children's regular recharging.

Caseloads and Scheduling

The models of service delivery and corresponding samples of speech-language pathologist's schedules discussed earlier in this chapter (see pages 164–165) have some application for preschoolers. However, preschool models and schedules often include a wider variety of settings and models.

Home-based programs are appropriate for some children, while center-based ones may be more effective for others. Natural environments for preschoolers vary depending on their families' child-rearing practices and preferences. Caseloads and scheduling of services for preschoolers in either setting should follow child-directed guidelines.

Speech-language pathologists need to devote larger blocks of time to serve preschoolers; maintain close contact with caregivers and teachers; and allow for children's regular recharging through naps, snacks, and a mixture of fine- and gross-motor activities. Speech-language pathologists work directly and indirectly in the preschool classroom, meeting with teachers and parents; using recess, snack time, and animal-petting time; and incorporating children's interests and friends to generalize new skills.

Preschoolers can be high energy one moment and too tired to keep their eyes open the next. Usually mornings are better times for teaching and learning new skills; however, afternoon preschools can be equally beneficial if time is used wisely. Center-based programs often run a morning and an afternoon class. Speech-language pathologists will serve students in preschool classrooms, others who are brought to centers for therapy only, and some in inclusive neighborhood child or preschool programs. Some preschool classes are taught by speech-language pathologists, enabling these professionals to thread language activities throughout the curriculum.

Preschool Schedules

Preschool schedules need to incorporate some elements that differ from school schedules due to the children's young age, the role of families, and the types of services offered. Frequently, the following elements are on preschool schedules:

- 10–15 minute individual treatment sessions

- Joint sessions with parent and child

- Group activities scheduled at the playground, art area, water table, clay sink, animal cages, and so on, that integrate gross- and fine-motor skills with language

- Snack or nutrition time

- Bathroom schedules

- Parent meetings

- Home visits

- Nap or rest time if more than 1½ hours of instruction

- Travel time to agency preschool sites, Head Start programs, or private facilities

Not all speech-language pathologists will need to schedule all these options. Some speech-language pathologists work exclusively with preschoolers; others work with preschoolers, infants, and toddlers; and others work with preschoolers along with a school-age population.

ASHA (2000b) recommends a caseload of 24 preschoolers for a speech-language pathologist working exclusively in this setting. This is a guideline that many schools have followed; however, caseloads are determined by state agencies, so there are fluctuations in this (e.g., Ohio, Florida, and Kentucky vary greatly). Providing comprehensive preschool services to 24 young children, their families, and other support personnel is a challenge. Keeping up-to-date on educational, therapeutic, and legal issues when dealing with families is equally important. Speech-language pathologists need to be culturally competent (see "Students Who Are Culturally/Linguistically Diverse (CLD)" in Chapter 7) and sensitive to families' interests and preferences (Brice, 2000; Cheng, 1999b). Even though it is children who are on the caseload, at this age, working with families is the key to success.

Developmentally Appropriate Programs for Children 5 and Under

Too many early intervention programs have been operated like school pullout programs. It is inappropriate for a 3-year-old child to sit across a table from a speech-language pathologist in a room separate from a preschool environment and learn new skills through drill. This situation offers virtually no opportunity for the preschooler to incorporate speech-language acquisition into play, experimentation, or ongoing physical and cognitive trial-and-error efforts. Therefore, artificial environments should be avoided.

Despite the predominance of the pullout model with preschoolers (ASHA, 1998d; Paul-Brown and Caperton, in press), speech-language pathologists have also used classroom-based and collaborative/consultative models. Advantages to these models include greater relevancy, generalization, frequency of intervention, and opportunity to assist other children who are at-risk but not receiving services (Cirrin and Penner, 1995). Initially, educators and families wanted children to be served in disability-focused programs. Administrators found it more cost-effective to serve all preschoolers in one building or complex. More and more speech-language pathologists were being trained as experts in working with children under 5 years of age, and they often chose to work with other similarly trained professionals exclusively. There were some advantages to having the expertise all in one place, but public policy and public pressure began to create a demand for programs that remained within the general education environment, including the natural environment for children not yet in formal schooling (Power-deFur and Orelove, 1997).

Effect of Inclusive Practices

INCLUSIVE PRACTICES for educating all children, including those under age 5, have not been defined in IDEA (1997) legislation. Instead, organizations have published statements about the effects of including students in general education environments. ASHA (1996b) produced a position statement on inclusive practices that, although it addressed all children, had a dramatic effect on the service provision for 3 to 5 year olds with speech-language disabilities (Paul-Brown and Caperton, in press) (see the sidebar on page 131 in Chapter 5 for the full text of ASHA's inclusive practice statement). Inclusive practices in preschools for children with communication disabilities set the tone for subsequent interventions in school. Speech-

language pathologists played a vital role in integrating communication skill building into children's days—a big departure from pullout sessions or therapy isolated from the normal activities of children's days.

The ASHA (1996b) document was philosophically situated between the liberal and conservative positions of other organizations. The Association for Severe Handicaps (TASH, 2000) concluded that all students should be included while others suggested very few children with LEARNING DISABILITIES could be educated full-time in the classroom (e.g., Learning Disabilities Association of America [LDA], 1993; CEC, 1997a; National Center for Learning Disabilities [NCLD], 1994). This vision had a great impact on preschool services at a time when preschools were being closely examined to determine functional outcomes and whether these programs were successful and enabled the children they served to enter general education programs (Valdez and Montgomery, 1997).

Paul-Brown and Caperton (in press) identified several service delivery factors that either supported or prevented inclusive practices in preschools. They compared the features of three service delivery models—pullout, collaborative/consultative, and classroom-based—described elsewhere in this chapter with five aspects of service delivery for children ages 3 to 5. The features were service setting, manner of service, content/curriculum for service, service-provider roles, and direction of service. Parents requested maximum direct service plus maximum peer contact (inclusion). See Table 6.6 for the comparison. The comparison shown in Table 6.7 is a tool that

Table 6.6

Compatibility of Service Delivery Models with Features of Inclusive Practices

Features of Inclusive Practices	Features of Service Delivery Models		
	Pullout	Collaborative/ Consultative	Classroom-Based
Service Setting	Provides services in typical educational setting	Separate intervention room	Classroom	Classroom
Manner of Service Delivery	Uses the natural environment to provide opportunities for peer interactions	Speech-language pathologist and child interact	Teacher and peer interactions in classroom	Teacher, speech-language pathologist, and peer interactions in classroom
Content/ Curriculum for Service	Integrates speech-language intervention within the classroom curriculum and activities	Uses classroom curriculum or separate content	Infuses speech-language goals with classroom curriculum and activities	Infuses speech-language goals with classroom curriculum and activities
Service-Provider Roles	Fosters collaboration among speech-language pathologist, teachers, parents, and others	Direct service by speech-language pathologist; could coordinate with teachers, parents, and others	Indirect service by speech-language pathologist; collaborative consultation (in contrast to unidirectional expert consultation)	Direct service by speech-language pathologist and teacher in classroom; ongoing collaboration
Direction of Service	Brings speech and language services to a child rather than taking the child to a separate treatment room	Brings child to services	Brings services to child	Brings services to child

From *Treatment Settings and Service Delivery Models for Children with Communication Disorders in the Context of Early Childhood Inclusion* (p. 441), by D. Paul-Brown and C.J. Caperton, in press, in M.J. Guralnick (Ed.), *Early Childhood Inclusion: Focus on Change*, Baltimore: Brookes. © 2001 by Paul H. Brookes. Adapted with permission.

Table 6.7

Factors Supporting or Inhibiting Inclusive Preschool Activities

Factors:	Supporting Inclusion	Inhibiting Inclusion
	Legislation	Resistance to change
	Society and public policy	Professionals' limited skills
	Social-interactive theory of language	Little administrative support
	Child outcomes in research	Family preferences
	View of language as social acts	Lack of planning time
		Little efficacy data available
Settings:	**Classroom Models**	**Therapy Models**
	Which ones?	Which ones?
	For how long?	For how long?
	For which children?	For which children?
	With which other professionals?	With which other professionals?

From *Treatment Settings and Service Delivery Models for Children with Communication Disorders in the Context of Early Childhood Inclusion*, by D. Paul-Brown and C.J. Caperton, in press, in M.J. Guralnick (Ed.), *Early Childhood Inclusion: Focus on Change*, Baltimore: Brookes. © 2001 by Paul H. Brookes. Adapted with permission.

could be shared with parents of preschoolers and, perhaps, the school IEP team. It is relatively jargon free and points out service differences without making value judgements. Objectivity can be hard to maintain when families request less intrusive services to allow their youngsters to enjoy childhood but still have maximum results. Speech-language pathologists recognize how little time there is to try one model after another.

Paul-Brown and Caperton (in press) concluded that segregated settings do not offer any advantages in terms of frequency of social interactions or other aspects of peer relations. They also suggested that limited research funds not be spent on comparing the effectiveness of various settings but rather used to improve services to young children who have communication disorders in inclusive settings.

Preliteracy and Literacy Acquisition

PRELITERACY and literacy skills develop in preschool. Many children who exhibit later reading problems had speech-language disabilities identified in preschool (Boudreau and Hedberg, 1999; Catts and Kamhi, 1999; Center for the Improvement of Early Reading Achievement [CIERA], 2000). Speech-language pathologists need to know how reading is acquired and how children begin to acquire PRINT MEANING and PRINT FORM between the ages of 3 and 5 (van Kleeck, 1998). Phonological awareness skills are informally taught and reinforced by parents in this time period (Torgeson, 1998). These are important precursors to reading and are frequently delayed in children who struggle with reading (Boudreau and Hedberg, 1999). Speech-language pathologists have an important role to play in literacy development since it includes reading, writing, speaking, listening, and thinking skills (Montgomery, 1998). The breadth of print-related activities that young children need is staggering (van Kleeck, 1998), and literally all these activities can be used by speech-language pathologists as language-based activities and objectives for preschoolers with communication disabilities. Models of reading that emphasize balanced reading and literacy instructional programs, such as those described by van Kleeck (1998) or Adams (1999), are advocated by many state departments of education.

Typical preschools are often rich in early auditory and visual patterning skills connected to reading, and children who have communication disabilities need to have the same opportunities to learn these patterns as their peers. They probably need even more exposure to and reinforcement of the patterns to be successful (Boudreau and Hedberg, 1999). Working with preschoolers requires speech-language pathologists to be constantly looking forward to the next stage of learning, no matter what the current performance level of a child might be. Low expectations at this early point can impede a child's ability to learn and grow in the mainstream of education. A disability or label does not indicate how much the child can achieve. Research has shown that diagnosis cannot be correlated with the child's ability, socialization, eventual employment, or motivation (Centers for Disease Control [CDC], 1999). Many professionals believe that preschool is the time to keep all the future academic options open (Marvin, 1994; van Kleeck, 1998). All preschool children should be considered potential readers and writers, so speech-language pathologists who provide services to preschoolers must acknowledge and plan for this eventuality.

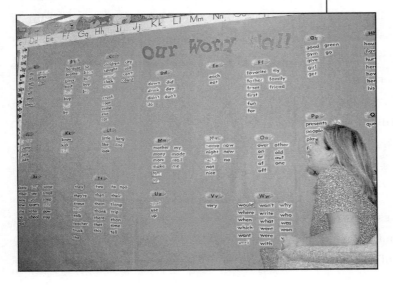

Feeding and Swallowing Problems in Preschool Populations

Children under 5 years of age who have feeding and swallowing problems may be eligible for services in preschool programs (O'Toole, 2000; Whitmire, 2000b) and usually present with fragile medical health, neurological disorders and syndromes, or related etiologies that place them at risk (Kurjan, 2000). An IFSP or IEP may have goals and objectives with a school team and family members that address a child's nutrition, eating habits, and skills at home and in a school program or center. Speech-language pathologists have been responsible for these specialized issues in preschools, using an MDT approach, including cross-training and co-treatment (Kurjan, 2000). Homer, Bickerton, Hill, Parham, and Taylor (2000) found that a large suburban school district in Louisiana needed to have specially trained speech-language pathologists, called a swallowing action team (SWAT), to ensure that preschoolers and school-age students had safe nutrition and hydration during school hours. Preschool programs often require speech-language pathologists to have skills, such as working with swallowing problems, that extend beyond the education traditionally received in undergraduate or graduate programs plus an understanding of scope-of-practice statements for state licensure and ASHA certification (Kurjan, 2000; O'Toole, 2000; Whitmire, 2000b).

The Clock Is Ticking!

One of the troubling realities of working with preschoolers is the brief time available. All the assessment and intervention with children and families must be accomplished within a mere 24 months because the ages of 3 to 5 have an established beginning and ending time. One cannot continue preschool services for just a few more weeks or months. The clock starts running immediately at age 3 and stops when children are old enough for kindergarten. From time to time, there may be a 5-year-old in preschool, but it is unusual and not encouraged. Assessment must be prompt and accurate, contacts with other service providers must be on-going, and intervention must be targeted and results driven. It is clear that speech-language pathologists who wish to work in preschool settings will need to know all the service delivery models and intervention techniques, be well versed in the development of 3- to 5-year-olds, be innovative and flexible to meet family and child needs, and devote their energies to assuring that a majority of the children who are served in preschool programs do not need continued communication services once they start school. Creating and maintaining preschool programs focused on maximum outcomes in 24 months or less is a major responsibility and an exciting area for speech-language pathologists.

Services for Secondary Students

IDEA (1997) mandates special education services for individuals from birth to age 22, but adolescents are "a population of students who have long been ignored," and few speech-language pathologists have attempted to support "the language they need to achieve academic and social success" (Apel, 1999, p. 229). Although speech-language services may not typically be organized by the age of clients, the interaction between a speech-language pathologist and a student is strongly influenced by the student's class and building assignments.

Characteristics of Adolescents

As students get older, they spend greater amounts of time with their peers and often appear to dislike or be uncomfortable in the company of adults. Intervention programs need to align with the interests, tastes, and motivation of a consumer to be effective in any setting (Larson, McKinley, and Boley, 1993; Nelson, 1992; Singer and Bashir, 1999). Students aged 13 and older frequently have well-defined interests and motivations (Apel and Swank, 1999). Their academic programs are typically departmentalized, including walking from class to class; working under several teachers; and increased personal responsibility for rules, regulations, homework, time schedules, and deadlines. They have more unscheduled time before and after school and are often exploring student groups, competitive athletics, clubs, service activities, and social time.

Apel and Swank (1999) reminded speech-language pathologists working with older students that "the self-concept and motivational level of these students must be recognized and addressed in their intervention program or success may be unattainable" (p. 239). Planning a

service delivery program at middle and high schools must take these factors into account.

Adolescents with communication disabilities also experience related academic difficulties. Their language deficits may adversely affect their comprehension skills, attention, organization, and writing ability. Speech-language pathologists should recognize some of the unique characteristics of older students who have LANGUAGE DISORDERS as described by Larson and McKinley (1995b) in Table 6.8.

Academic-Centered Goals for Adolescents

Many students with communication disorders need continued assistance from speech-language pathologists and other special educators to be successful in upper grades. The TRANSITION process (i.e., preparation for postsecondary employment or education) for students with special education needs must be carefully planned and implemented. On average, a student aged 13 or older who is receiving services has been in speech-language programs for several years. The goals and objectives have changed for the student, but he or she continues to need support to be successful and access the curriculum. There is a close connection between intervention and academic achievement in middle school, and by high school, therapy is often completely integrated into academic standards. In secondary schools, students are no longer learning underlying skills; instead, they must apply strategies to increase their comprehension, retain needed information, and produce acceptable written work. Spelling, constructing

Table 6.8	Characteristic Problems of Older School-Age Students with Language Disorders	
Category	**Expectations**	**Problems**
Cognition	To be at the formal operational level	They often remain concrete operational thinkers.
	To observe, organize, and categorize data from an experience	They make chaos out of order.
	To identify problems, suggest possible causes and solutions, and predict consequences	They may not recognize the problem when it exists; if they do, they do not know how to develop alternative solutions.
	To place concepts into hierarchical order	They often cannot place concepts in a hierarchy.
	To find, select, and utilize data on a given topic	They have limited strategies for finding, selecting, and utilizing data.
Metalinguistics	To demonstrate conscious awareness of linguistic knowledge	They have difficulty bringing to awareness categories and relations in all aspects of language.
	To talk about and reflect on various linguistic forms	They do not know the labels for talking about language during formal education.
	To assess communication breakdowns and revise them	They do not have awareness of breakdowns and, if they do, they lack repair strategies.
Comprehension and Production of Linguistic Features	To comprehend all linguistic features and structures	They misunderstand advanced syntactical forms.
	To follow oral directions of three steps or more after listening to them one time	They may not realize that they are being given directions and/or have difficulty following them.
	To use grammatically intact utterances	They often use sentences that are fragmented and that do not convey their messages.
	To have a vocabulary sufficient for expressing ideas and experiences	They have word-retrieval problems as well as a high frequency of low-information words.
	To give directions with clarity and accuracy	They often leave their listeners confused.
	To get information or assistance by asking questions and to respond appropriately to questions asked of them	They may know what questions or answers to give, but they do not know how to do so tactfully.

Continued on next page

Making a Difference
for America's Children

Table 6.8—*Continued*

Category	Expectations	Problems
	To comprehend and produce the slang and jargon of the hour	They do not comprehend or produce slang/jargon, thus they are ostracized from the group to which they most desire to belong.
Discourse	To produce language that is organized, coherent, and intelligible to their listeners	They use many false starts and verbal mazes.
	To follow adult conversational rules for speakers	They consistently violate the rules (e.g., maintaining a topic, initiating a topic).
	To be effective listeners during conversation without displaying incorrect listening habits	They often have poor listening skills.
	To make a report, tell or retell a story, and explain a process in detail	They often leave their listeners confused.
	To listen to lectures and to select main ideas and supporting details	They often do not grasp the essential message of a lecture.
	To analyze critically other speakers	Their judgments are arbitrary, illogical, and impulsive.
	To express their own attitudes, moods, and feelings and to disagree appropriately	They have abrasive conversational speech.
Nonverbal Communication	To follow nonverbal rules for kinesics	They violate the rules and misinterpret body movements and facial expressions.
	To follow nonverbal rules for proxemics	They violate the rules for social distance.
Survival Language	To comprehend and produce situational phrases and vocabulary required for survival in our society	They do not have the necessary concepts and vocabulary needed in places such as banks, grocery stores, and employment agencies.
	To comprehend and produce concepts and vocabulary required across daily living situations	They do not have the necessary concepts and vocabulary needed across daily living situations such as telling time, using money, and understanding warning signs.
Written Language	To comprehend written language required in various academic, social, and vocational situations	They do not consistently and/or efficiently process information obtained through reading.
	To produce cohesive written language required in various academic, social, and vocational situations	They do not consistently and/or efficiently generate written language that conveys their messages.

From *Language Disorders in Older Students* (pp. 78–79), by V. Lord Larson and N. McKinley, 1995b, Eau Claire, WI: Thinking Publications. © 1995 by Thinking Publications. Reprinted with permission.

sentences, expanding vocabulary, developing and describing ideas, plus locating pertinent information and writing about it dominate the intervention process at this level (Graham and Harris, 1999). In addition, many students need assistance with pragmatics and social language to engage in the reciprocal friendships and working relationships so critical at the secondary level (Donahue, Syzmanski, and Flores, 1999).

Transition Plans

IDEA (1997) requires that for all students with disabilities, beginning at age 14 (or younger, if appropriate), an IEP include a statement about the transition service needs of a student that focuses on his or her course of study (34 C.F.R. § 300.347 [b] [1]). Beginning at age 16 (or younger, if appropriate), an IEP must include a statement of needed transition services including, if appropriate, a statement of "interagency responsibilities or any needed linkages" (34 C.F.R. § 300.347 [b] [2]).

INDIVIDUALIZED TRANSITION PLAN (ITP) development is often a part of an IEP process but may be a separate assessment and meeting in a given school or district. The purpose of an ITP is to begin planning for a student's integration into the world of work and independent living. For many students, communication skills are critical to be successful in a job situation. Speech-language pathologists may find themselves designing role-plays of job interviews or working collaboratively with job coaches to help students achieve ITP goals (Montgomery, 1997a).

Functional outcomes are the best tool for evaluating adolescent services. The model chosen by speech-language pathologists and school teams is appropriate if students learn to function at a higher level on meaningful school-based or quality-of-life indicators. In middle and high school, these indicators should be a part of an IEP and be observable beyond the speech room. Transition goals may help all educators focus on functional outcomes instead of limiting their focus to helping students earn credits for graduation. Older students can help keep track of their own progress in many secondary school environments (Montgomery, 1997a). Apel and Swank (1999) were convinced that programs for older students could be successful when speech-language pathologists were strongly committed to "second chances" (p. 231). Eger (as cited in Bland, 1999)—an audiologist, speech-language pathologist, and administrator in a large urban cooperative school district—offered the following summative statement:

> If we focus on outcomes or end products, our intervention strategies will be much more integrated into the rest of the child's educational program. For example, teaming and having the educational team, not the speech-language pathologist alone, set communication priorities for each student will be the routine. Success will be judged by how well the student communicates in class, in the lunchroom, on the playground, and at home, not in the therapy room. (p. 10)

Making a Difference at the Secondary Level

Larson and McKinley (1995b) have presented educational, social, ethical, and fiscal arguments for providing services to adolescents in unique and meaningful ways. Reversing patterns of failure and refocusing previously undirected students toward finishing high school and pursuing career or job opportunities become important functional outcomes for adolescents (Nelson, 1996). Students, with the assistance of speech-language pathologists and other IEP team members, can develop highly practical, personally motivating IEPs for themselves. IDEA (1997) lists students as members of IEP teams, if appropriate. The law requires that students be invited to IEP meetings whenever transition services are considered, and if students do not participate in meetings, the district must take other steps to ensure that students' preferences and interests are considered. It is hard to imagine how an effective IEP for an adolescent, transition-related or not, could be written without that student's input.

Some students with significant disabilities will continue to receive speech-language services in middle and high school if an IEP team agrees that improvement or progress is expected for a student within a year. Maintaining the student's functional level does not require intervention; it requires practice with the skill in an authentic setting. This type of practice may be carried out by other educators. All intervention should be directly tied to an observable improvement in the students' daily activities. An IEP for students in grade six or above should include one or more of the following goals written in measurable terms:

- Increased literacy (i.e., reading, spelling, and writing) skills

- Increased social language skills

- More appropriate peer interactions

- Progress on a transition plan

- Progress toward a vocational goal

- Improved organization, attention, or study skills

- Progress toward emotional control and stability

- Greater independence or interdependence than the previous year

Models That Match Students and School Settings

Selecting one or more service delivery models to encourage these important outcomes will depend on the factors presented in Chapter 5 plus the ages and interests of adolescents. Older students are more likely to be grouped, seen for periods of time that mirror the academic schedule, and held accountable for their own progress. Many speech-language pathologists teach a class called Communication Skills, so that students can receive academic credit for working on IEP goals. Others arrange to award grades, so that student work can be figured into the grade-point average. A class must be approved by a school board for students to receive credit. Other speech-language pathologists report that co-teaching is the most effective way to support students in classes that have challenging subject matter and high student expectations (Creaghead, 1992; Hoskins, 1995; Montgomery, 1997a; Nelson, 1996). Larson and McKinley's (1995b) models are included in Figure 6.3 as they present six ways that speech-language pathologists can structure service delivery for adolescents. Of these, the prototype model (i.e., offering speech-language service as a course for credit) is usually the most palatable to adolescents (Larson and McKinley).

Students with various types of special education needs will receive attention from a high school IEP team. Service delivery models will need to be changed from time to time during the school year to accommodate students' changing needs or to intervene, to avert, or to recover from, a crisis situation (Sanger and Moore-Brown, 2000). Students who are fully included in high school may need speech-language

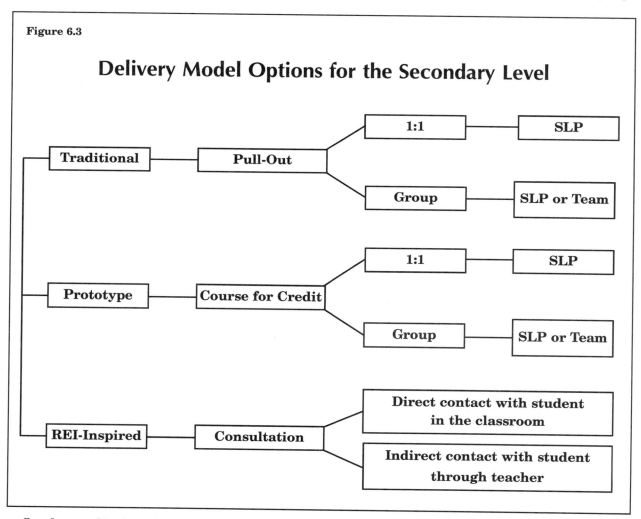

Figure 6.3

Delivery Model Options for the Secondary Level

From *Language Disorders in Older Students* (p. 154), by V. Lord Larson and N. McKinley, 1995b, Eau Claire, WI: Thinking Publications. © 1995 by Thinking Publications. Adapted with permission.

pathologists' support. These students often fall into one of two categories: students with mild to moderate learning disabilities who require ongoing assistance to succeed or students with severe disabilities who require extensive supports—such as one-to-one aid, ASSISTIVE TECHNOLOGY, modified physical environment, and other communication skills—to flourish in a general education PLACEMENT (Montgomery, 1997a; Wallach and Butler, 1994). Students who are fully included do not automatically require speech-language intervention; however, adequate communication skills often determine whether students are successful socially and academically (Wallach and Butler, 1994)

CHAPTER 7

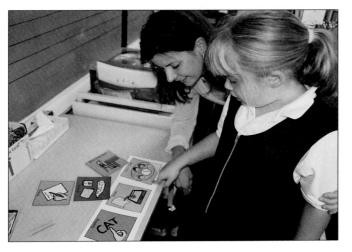

Expanded and Specialized Services

Many school-based speech-language pathologists are called on to provide expanded or specialized services extending beyond the general education curriculum. Students with communication disorders may present characteristics on the autism spectrum. Some individuals will be English language learners, some will use assistive technology or augmentative and alternative communication, and still others may be infants or toddlers who were identified at birth with a hearing loss. Some students must be temporarily educated at home or in hospitals, rehabilitation units, or detention facilities. Increasing numbers of these students with special needs are served in school-based programs, necessitating highly flexible service delivery models to accommodate their location and unique needs. Speech-language pathologists must be ready for expanded or specialized practice in the schools.

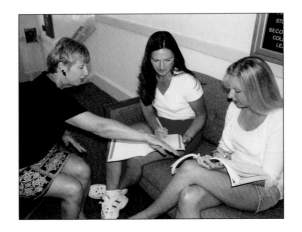

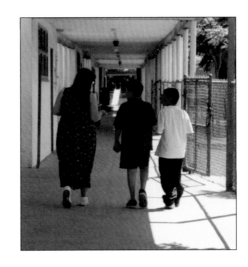

1. Describe the important elements of working with the families of students with communication disorders whose culture or language is different than the speech-language pathologist's.

2. Explain the difference between accent and dialect and how the speech-language pathologist can help other educators and administrators to differentiate both from communication disorders.

3. Why is it important to know the various definitions of autism spectrum disorder to provide the services parents and administrators request in the schools? What role does the speech-language pathologist's professional judgement play in the decision making?

4. Compare and contrast AT and AAC. What does it mean to "consider" technology according to IDEA?

5. Explain the universal newborn hearing screening mandated by law, and how it has an impact on the school service delivery programs for speech and language.

6. What are the educational rights of students who are serving time in prison during their school years? What impact does this have on the speech-language pathologist?

7. Locate a speech-language pathologist in the schools who has responsibilities as a lead speech-language pathologist. Interview this person about the advantages and disadvantages of this type of service delivery. Examine his or her weekly and monthly schedule to appreciate the increased and varied responsibilities.

Students Who Are Culturally/Linguistically Diverse (CLD)

School SERVICE DELIVERY in the expanded model for students who are CULTURALLY/LINGUISTICALLY DIVERSE (CLD) has four distinct aspects: (1) selecting the language of instruction—including special factors to consider from the INDIVIDUALS WITH DISABILITIES EDUCATION ACT (IDEA) AMENDMENTS OF 1997, (2) using interpreters in intervention, (3) being aware of accents and dialects, and (4) working with families who are culturally/linguistically different from the speech-language pathologist.

Individuals with limited English proficiency are the fastest growing population in our nation, and some of them will need SPECIAL EDU- CATION, including speech-language services. Special education REFERRALS of students who are English language learners (ELLs) have been reported to be inappropriately high in some parts of the country (Garcia and Ortiz, 1988). Students learning English frequently struggle with academics until their English language skills are more highly developed. (See the dis- cussion on the increase in diverse populations in schools under "Children and Families in the Twenty-First Century" in Chapter 1).

Years ago, speech-language pathologists were told, "Multicultural research and continued development of techniques and materials for assessment and intervention need to be pri- orities of professionals who provide services to these populations" (American Speech- Language-Hearing Association [ASHA], 1985, p. 32). These needs are ongoing. To serve the needs of children who are CLD and have communication disabilities, approaches to assessment and intervention must change (Quinn, Goldstein, and Pena, 1996). School- based speech-language pathologists have reported that their monthly CASELOAD consisted of a high percentage of students who were CLD (ASHA, 1997b). The ASHA school survey (1998d) presented this distribution of students served by race or ethnicity during 1995:

66.94% White

17.88% African American

10.96% Hispanic

2.22% Asian Pacific Islander

1.51% Native American

.49% Unknown ethnicity

Almost a third of the children served in speech- language programs are CLD in a nationwide sample, not in just a few border states as once thought.

Second-language issues were prominent on the list of challenges that speech-language pathologists in schools ranked in ASHA's (1998d) survey. "[L]anguage diversity is one of the most discussed and possibly contentious areas among educators concerned with students' academic achievement" (Cheng, 1999a, p. vii). Butler (1999) reminded us that there are far-reaching effects of language diversity on reading and other academic performance in students today:

No longer may those who deal with chil- dren or adults as teachers or clinicians [sic] assume that they will be working with speakers, readers, or writers of Standard English. The current focus on phonological awareness as the core deficit of a reading difficulty, while based upon research that has been undertaken in many countries and many languages, may require that we learn considerably more about first and second language acquisition than is currently the case (p. iv).

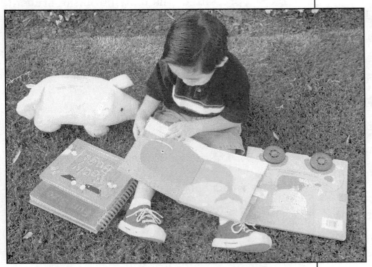

IDEA (1997) added a requirement to INDIVIDUALIZED EDUCATION PROGRAM (IEP) development: "In the case of a child with limited English proficiency, consider the language needs of the child as such needs relate to the IEP" [§ 614 [d] [B] [ii]). An IEP team must carefully consider and document its consideration of the effect of a student's being a second-language learner on his or her achievement and ability to be involved and progress in the general education curriculum. The IEP team must also consider what supports will be needed for the student to benefit from special education.

Choosing the Language of Instruction

When choosing the language of instruction and service delivery for a child, the IEP team must consider where on the continuum the student's language skills are within both his or her primary language and English. Speech-language pathologists play a role in this decision for the team and must consider the student's pragmatic, social, or interpersonal communication skills instead of the structural accuracy of the language. The key is to distinguish between errors made because of lack of exposure to the curriculum and insufficient opportunity to master the language. Although English may be the language of instruction in the school, the child may have more advanced skills in a primary language used for social interaction. This would suggest that the home language should be used for instruction initially or concurrently.

Consideration of special factors is necessary for the assessment, ELIGIBILITY, and IEP phases of the special education process. A communication limitation can make it very difficult to determine if a student is primarily struggling with second-language learning or has one or more disabilities. Once eligibility is determined, the speech-language pathologist may work with the student because of communication disabilities related to a disorder or condition. Selecting the language for service delivery cannot be based on what skills the speech-language pathologist possesses, but rather on what skills the student needs, and in what language. Suggestions from Ortiz and

Garcia (1988) to determine language proficiency were used to create these questions that may guide the IEP team in their decision-making:

- What is the student's dominant language in various settings?

- What is the student's level of proficiency in both the primary language and English for social and academic language?

- What are the styles of verbal interaction used in the primary language and English?

- How much exposure has this student had to styles of verbal interaction in English?

- What is the extent and nature of exposure in each language? (family, peers, TV, stories, etc.)

- Are the student's language behaviors characteristic of second-language learners?

- What types of language intervention has this student already had and for how long?

"The literature in bilingual education of the last two decades suggests that children who are learning two languages may benefit from a bilingual approach in intervention" (Gutierrez-Clellen, 1999, p. 299). Gutierrez-Clellen emphasized that no studies were able to show that English-only was a preferable intervention approach for students with communication disabilities. She stated that achievement and performance were maximized when the student's first language was used as an organizational framework. In addition, speech-language pathologists need to help students identified with special needs learn pragmatic and social-cultural aspects of language (such as eye contact, facial expression, nonverbal messages, and tone) that will enable them to participate in the activities of the classroom (Cheng, 1999b; Fung and Roseberry-McKibbon, 1999). Service delivery for children who are CLD must take the form of multidimensional, interspersing sessions in the therapy room, in the classroom, and in small interactive groups that encourage conversation (Battle, 1998). The speech-language pathologist will need to move easily from one setting to another to encourage the adaptation necessary to fit into the dominant culture (Brice, 1993).

Using Interpreters/Translators in Intervention

When the child's primary language is not English, speech-language pathologists must either speak the child's language or use an interpreter/translator. (Note that *interpretation* refers to oral language and *translation* refers to written language.) Less than 4% of the professionals belonging to ASHA report speaking a language in addition to English (ASHA, 1999d). Some states have many more bilingual speech-language pathologists than others. In some large states and some border states (e.g., Florida, Texas, California, and New York), bilingual speech-language pathologists are in great demand and can command salary bonuses, previously unheard of in school settings.

Using an interpreter/translator is the method of choice for those who are not fluent enough to provide therapy in both languages (ASHA, 1999d; Langdon, 1999). Langdon (1999) and others have pointed out both the cautions and the value of working with interpreters/translators when serving students. A resource titled *Working Successfully with Interpreters and Translators in Speech-Language Pathology and Audiology* (Langdon and Cheng, in press) describes effective service delivery and gives guidance specific to the speech-language pathology field.

Accents and Dialects

Accents and dialects, used both by speech-language pathologists and by students who speak languages in addition to English, have been controversial in the field of speech-language pathology. Although bilingual or multilingual speech-language pathologists have been in great demand in this country, many of them have reported facing bias in graduate education programs and in the job market (Montgomery, 1999a). Public school students with accents or dialects that are different from that of the mainstream culture of their school have been referred for special education services, speech services, or viewed as low achievers (Roseberry-McKibbon and Eicholtz, 1994). In the late 1990s, an effort to dispel these misguided concerns and avoid potential discriminatory behaviors resulted in a position statement and supporting technical report entitled *Students and Professionals Who Speak English with Accents and Nonstandard Dialects: Issues and Recommendations* (ASHA, 1998c). In this statement, accent was defined as a phonetic trait from one's first language that was carried over to one's second language (Wolfram, 1991). The listener can hear some of the patterns of sound production found in the person's first spoken language that are not in the second language. Persons who use English as their second (or third or fourth) language may have accented English, depending on their age and the circumstances under which they learned English.

Dialect was defined as a set of differences, wherever they may occur, that make one English speaker's speech different from another's (Wolfram and Fasold, 1974). Each dialect has distinguishing linguistic characteristics (phonological, morphological, semantic, syntactic, and pragmatic), although the majority of linguistic features of the (American) English language are common to each of the varieties of (American) English (Montgomery, 1999a).

The concluding statement of ASHA's (1998c) position statement issues a clear directive:

> All individuals speak with an accent and/or dialect; thus, the non-acceptance of individuals into higher education programs or into the professions solely on the basis of the presence of an accent or dialect is discriminatory. Members of ASHA must not discriminate against persons who speak with an accent and/or dialect in educational programs, employment, or service delivery, and should encourage an understanding of linguistic differences among consumers and the general population. (p. 28)

Speech-language pathologists working in the schools must recognize that "no dialectal variety of English is a disorder or pathological form of speech or language. Each social dialect is adequate as a functional and effective variety of English" (Cole, 1983, p. 25).

Dialects and accents are often called language varieties to emphasize that they are accepted differences in speech (Cole, 1983). The educational, emotional, political, and economic controversies related to these language varieties continue in many settings. Service delivery for students who are CLD must be grounded on what they need for academic success, not on accent or dialect differences falsely perceived as disabilities. School-based speech-language pathologists must provide appropriate service delivery options for these students along with information for colleagues and families. Reasoned judgments based on current research should guide decision-making and service delivery. Speech-language pathologists must model respect for the children who offer the richness and variety of their accented speech.

> Service delivery for students who are CLD must be grounded on what they need for academic success.

Working with Families

Families are often the basic social unit for students who are CLD, and they should be included in the context of the child's intervention program as much as possible for best results (Roseberry-McKibbon, 1999; Wyatt, 1999). For example, according to Seymour, Bland-Stewart, and Green (1998), determining difference versus deficit in children's use of African American English (AAE) is more accurate, and more appropriately treated, when there is family contact. Including the family in the intervention process shows respect, increases carryover, and knits the school and community together in the same cause.

Family LITERACY is a common school-related activity for children, parents, and extended families. The read-aloud aspect of family literacy has considerable appeal and effectiveness for families that are CLD. The speech-language pathologist may consider taking an active part in organizing such communication-related programs as Family Reading Night, Grandparents Read-Aloud Program, or Everybody Read Together. These activities are especially meaningful to families, encourage respect, and are extensions of the collaborative service delivery process described in Chapter 6.

Infants and Toddlers

IDEA (1997) and state special education programs provide intervention for identified infants and toddlers in collaboration with developmental disability services, mental health agencies, or similar health-care entities. Programs for infants and toddlers in schools are covered in Part C of IDEA, which attempts to link families, communities, and schools with a program for children birth to 3 that is qualitatively different than Part B. Section 631 describes an urgent and substantial need:

1. to enhance the development of infants and toddlers with disabilities and to minimize their potential for developmental delay;

2. to reduce the educational costs to our society...by minimizing the need for special education and related services after infants and toddlers with disabilities reach school age;

3. to minimize the likelihood of institutionalization...;

4. to enhance the capacity of families to meet the special needs of their infants and toddlers with disabilities; and

5. to enhance the capacity of State and local agencies and service providers to identify, evaluate, and meet the needs of historically underrepresented populations, particularly minority, low-income, inner-city, and rural populations.

Each state must have a statewide system for services to infants and toddlers which meets all the requirements of Section 635 of IDEA (1997). Each state has developed systems with different kinds and numbers of agencies involved, their own guidelines, and service delivery that matches that state's infrastructure. They all share the concept of the INDIVIDUALIZED FAMILY SERVICE PLAN (IFSP) in place of the IEP for children under age 3. An IFSP may be also used for children ages 3 through 5 if agreed to by the family and school. (See Chapter 6 "Individual Family Service Plans [IFSPs].")

Settings for Infant and Toddler Programs

One of the qualitatively different aspects of serving infants and toddlers is the setting; they are typically served in their homes or daycare settings. Speech-language pathologists and other specialists work directly with families in these settings, showing them methods to encourage speech and language development and coaching families as they work with their infants.

Speech-language pathologists need special training to work with infants, toddlers, and families to be effective. This training is available from some graduate education programs, many state personnel development grants, some employers, and every major annual state speech-language association conference or ASHA convention. Journals that focus on the communication needs of infants and toddlers are available (e.g., The National Association for the Education of Young Children publishes *Young Children* and the Council for Exceptional Children, Division for Early Childhood publishes *Journal of Early Intervention* and *Young Exceptional Children*) as are videotaped continuing education courses and teleconferences offered by experts in the field.

Speech-language pathologists must work closely with medical staff, counselors, other therapists, and families when infants have multiple health and medical needs in the first two years of life. This is facilitated in center-based rather than home-based programs. While some school districts hire speech-language pathologists for these positions, others contract with county agencies, state Early Start or Even Start programs, or university clinical programs. Due to fewer families and reduced resources overall, smaller districts often assign the speech-language pathologists at K–12 schools responsibility for the infants and toddlers in their own communities. Although not ideal, this arrangement is financially feasible and helps prepare the school staff for some children's needs four years before the children enter school.

If babies are served in a center, the family members must come with them for training, contact with each other, support, and new ideas from other professionals. Direct therapy with a baby for prespeech development is highly unusual and not considered a PREFERRED PRACTICE PATTERN. ASHA has many documents and publications to assist the speech-language pathologist with family-focused therapy (ASHA, 1990; ASHA, 1997a).

> **Direct therapy with a baby for prespeech development is highly unusual and not considered a preferred practice pattern.**

Unique Aspects of Infant Programs

A program conducted in an infant's home with the family is the most common service delivery model (Donahue-Kilburg, 1992). Speech-language pathologists travel to the home weekly or monthly, often followed up by an assistant or support person for a later visit. The family is taught communication support techniques and encouraged to integrate them into their daily routines. The speech-language pathologist has the responsibility to be culturally competent, recognize and appreciate the child-rearing approaches the family uses, include all the relevant family members, and not present knowledge or techniques that may offend care providers or make them feel uncomfortable (ASHA, 1991b, 1997a; Brekken, Carr, and Cranor, 1988).

For example, the concept of RECIPROCITY is important (Guarneri, Carr, and Brekken, 1988). The speech-language pathologist recognizes that the child is a product of how the parents have raised him or her, and the way the baby has influenced the parents. It is a constant give-and-take relationship. Parents do not merely do things to babies; babies in turn shape parent responses. The speech-language pathologist goes into the home to help the baby develop communication skills with the parents, but also to help the parents develop a communication system with their child. Each must change and react to the other. Lewis (1984) outlined the following typical Infant Development Principles used to reach this goal:

1. Infants are active—They participate in their own development and act on their own environment. As early as 10 weeks, infants show interest and increased activity when their movements cause audio-visual stimuli to occur.

2. Infants are competent—Babies come well equipped. They are able to see, hear, smell, and respond to touch. They are very capable of signaling their caregivers through crying to provide them what they want.

3. Infants are social—Babies come with systems in place for carrying out interaction. At birth, their visual acuity is greatest at 8½ inches, which allows them to focus on a parent's face when feeding. They prefer the configuration of a face over random figures, and they prefer the higher pitch of a female voice.

Assessment of Infants and Toddlers

Speech-language pathologists use vastly different measures to assess for communication delays in infants and toddlers compared to school-age or even preschool children. There are a few STANDARDIZED TESTS, but most are rating scales, family inventories, structured observations, caregiver reports, and medical histories (Sparks, Clark, Erickson, and Oas, 1990). In the hands of competent and experienced speech-language pathologists, these are fine tools. The speech-language pathologist who has not worked extensively with infants, toddlers, and families, who has not taken appropriate coursework, or who has not been mentored by an experienced professional team is advised to seek out the many excellent resources in the communication field (e.g., Crais, 2000; Retherford, 1996; Rosetti, 1993; Wetherby and Prizant, 1992; Wilcox, 1997) before performing assessments independently. They should also be guided by section 12.0 Prespeech, Prelanguage, and Language Assessment for Infants and Toddlers in the ASHA (1997c) Preferred Practice Patterns for assessment, included in Appendix A.

One of the primary assessment measures for this population is to find the category of risk for a condition evident at birth, as listed in the sidebar. Assessment might begin at any of these risk categories, and may or may not lead to a diagnosis of a disability that requires special education support from the speech-language pathologist. The condition of at-risk does not immediately translate into identification or services (Sparks et al., 1990).

As described in Chapter 1, the changing composition of the family structure is a growing trend. Whenever intervention is planned for babies and young children, the speech-language pathologist will be working closely with a variety of individuals who care for and are a part of the child's life besides the parents. Those involved in a child's care, and therefore the intervention plan, can include grandparents, aunts, uncles, siblings, partners of parents, babysitters, nannies, and neighbors. Any one of these individuals may serve as the caregiver in a center-based program or participate in the assessment or intervention activity. They must all be taught to facilitate the child's development. Rather than being frustrated or surprised at having many different family members involved, the speech-language pathologist should appreciate the richness that many care providers can bring to the child's program.

Impact of Newborn Hearing Screening on Infant and Toddler Programs

SCREENING of babies at birth is a long established method of identifying risk conditions as soon as possible, so medical or other intervention can begin before the baby starts to develop. Infants have been screened for PKU, Tay-Sach's

Categories of Risk for Communication Disorders in Newborns and Infants

Conditions of established risk:
1. Chromosomal disorders, Fragile X, Down syndrome
2. Single gene disorders—Hunter/Hurler syndrome, Tay-Sachs disease
3. Environmental disorders—fetal alcohol syndrome, AIDS

Conditions of unknown expectations of risk:
1. Congenital hearing loss
2. Cerebral palsy
3. Neural tube defects
4. Clefting

Conditions that may result in a disability:
1. Anoxia
2. Maternal infections—syphilis, rubella, herpes
3. Maternal diabetes
4. Blood group incompatibility
5. Maternal alcohol and drug ingestion
6. Lack of prenatal care
7. Prematurity
8. Low birth weight
9. Respiratory distress syndrome
10. Hyperbilirubinemia
11. Anesthetic intoxication
12. Neonatal medications
13. Acute or chronic disease of the central nervous system
14. Failure to thrive
15. Otitis media
16. Seizures
17. Head injury, accidents, abuse
18. Neglect
19. Iatrogenic disorder
20. Exposure to toxic agents

Conditions of care-giving that have implications for disorders:
1. Mentally, physically or drug-impaired parenting
2. Mother under 19 years old
3. Parents with very little education
4. Parents who have experienced recent loss of infant or loved one
5. Parents with low self-esteem
6. Parents with unrealistic expectations for an infant
7. Parents who abuse or neglect
8. Parents who did not want the pregnancy
9. Single parent without a support system
10. Parents experiencing grief for an existing risk condition
11. Poverty
12. High stress
13. Separation of parents from infant

Source: Sparks et al. (1990)

disease, and Rh incompatibility for many years. Hearing loss has typically not been discovered until age 2½ to 3 years, when auditory behavioral testing is more dependable. This has meant that hearing loss in babies could go undetected during the critical first years of their lives (Herer and Glattke, 2000; Smith Lang, 2000).

This wait-and-see situation changed dramatically in 1997 when the National Joint Committee on Infant Hearing in conjunction with the National Institutes of Health Consensus Panel agreed that all newborns in this country should have their hearing screened before they leave the hospital. Screening a baby's hearing can now occur as early as nine hours after birth (Herer and Glattke, 2000). New technology, called *oto-acoustic emissions*, has allowed sleeping babies to be tested in about three minutes using a small ear probe to record the "echo" of the cochlea's response on a computer. Preliminary data from three years of screening indicate that the technology is reliable, relatively inexpensive, and can identify babies with hearing loss at birth (Herer and Glattke, 2000; Smith Lang, 2000).

Infant hearing screening has a profound effect on families, early intervention programs, and school-based infant and toddler programs. Speech-language pathologists must develop the skills to work with 3-month-old babies wearing hearing aids, teach parents multiple communication systems, and help parents choose educational interventions for their child during the critical early years when speech and language skills are acquired. There is great potential for these children to be in fully inclusive settings, working at grade level with appropriate supports (Herer and Glattke, 2000). Early intervention plays a unique role to ready these families to put all the necessary support in their first three years, and not have to catch up or rehabilitate later. Prevention is the essence of the IDEA (1997) philosophy (U.S. Department of Education, 1999). COMMUNICATION DISORDERS may be one of the first disciplines to demonstrate the value of preventive intervention.

A UNIVERSAL NEWBORN HEARING SCREENING (UNHS) PROGRAM, designed and supervised by an audiologist, is implemented by trained technicians in a birthing hospital. Protocols for universal programs do not screen only at-risk babies or those with familial histories of deafness or hearing loss. Rather a UNHS program screens all newborns. Any baby who is not screened faces the potential of reduced auditory input during the speech, language, and cognitive development time (Herer and Glattke, 2000).

Herer and Glattke (2000) examined results based on over 10,000 babies tested in a UNHS program in 1998-1999. They concluded that the incidence rate confirms the figure reported in the literature; that babies with conductive losses can also be identified early for medical interventions; that more than half of the babies did not have risk factors and would not have been reported to the High Risk Registry; and that if they only screened the Neonatal Intensive Care Unit, as some have suggested, they would have missed 93% of the babies with hearing loss born in those hospitals during the three years of the study.

Identification of Hearing Loss (HL) in Newborns

- 2.3 babies per 1,000 identified with HL at birth

- 1 per 1,000 had mild to severe bilateral sensorineural HL

- 0.3 per 1,000 had bilateral conductive HL

- 0.6 per 1,000 had unilateral sensorineural HL

- 0.4 per 1,000 had unilateral conductive HL

- 45% of those identified had risk factors present

- 55% did not have risk factors

- 93% of the babies with HL were in the well-baby nursery

- 7% with HL were in the Neonatal Intensive Care Unit (NICU)

Source: Herer and Glattke (2000)

The impact on services that speech-language pathologists provide in school districts has just begun. Audiologists are currently working with several school districts to develop appropriate IFSPs for toddlers who were identified at birth with moderate to severe sensori-neural hearing losses, wear hearing aids, and are now developing speech and language skills within normal limits. The toddlers wear hearing aids, attend typical preschools, and receive family-centered therapy from their local school districts. There are great changes ahead in these programs as audiologists and speech-language pathologists work closely with families of infants and toddlers (Herer and Glattke, 1998).

Outcomes for Infants and Toddlers

The history of service delivery for infants and toddlers with communication disabilities is a fairly recent one. Speech-language pathologists and special education administrators anticipated a rapid change to family-focused models and improved service delivery for children under age 5 (Angelo and Lowe, 1993; Ferguson, 1992; Montgomery, 1993a). Functional outcome data have confirmed that evaluation requires a number of different strategies to examine impact, outcome, and the overall effectiveness of early intervention (Mullen, 2000). Sometimes changes in babies can be measured. Effectiveness is often judged most authentically by families, the consumers of services for infants and toddlers.

Perhaps the most cogent source of evaluation is family satisfaction with the program. If families feel that they have been supported in their efforts to provide the best possible environment for child development, the program has had a positive impact (Donahue-Kilburg, 1992, p. 273)

Children with Autism Spectrum Disorders (ASDs)

One of the most demanding areas of school-based speech-language service delivery is meeting the needs of students identified with AUTISM SPECTRUM DISORDERS (ASD), formerly called autism. The awareness of ASD as an educational problem has skyrocketed in recent years, with research indicating that it is being diagnosed in 1 in 500 children (Maugh, 2000). Communication is a primary issue for children with ASD and speech-language pathologists play a prominent role in programming in school and home. School districts in every state have added comprehensive professional development courses for their special education staff, and many districts report that they have selected speech-language pathologists to be trained as experts in the area.

Services have been created rapidly in the last decade. They vary from private or state-administered schools, to 40-hour-a-week intensive behavior modification DISCRETE TRIAL TRAINING sessions, to general education PLACEMENTS with PULLOUT sessions with the speech-language pathologist, to full inclusion programs with one-to-one aide support in the general education classroom (Moore-Brown and Montgomery, 1999). Perhaps educational and therapeutic programming for children with ASD is so diverse because ASD itself is so diverse, presenting in so many different forms and degrees of ability.

Speech-language pathologists need to be well informed on this topic through coursework, independent study, reading recent literature, and experience working with children who present with ASD. Wetherby (2000) has stressed the great need to examine the efficacy of interventions being used across the nation. Speech-language pathologists in school programs are expected to know what set of services is best for a child and then make continual adjustments for age and progress (Greenspan and Wieder, 1999). Speech-language pathologists in the schools must be well acquainted with ASD and the service delivery options that schools and parents request.

Multiple Definitions of Autism

Autism has been defined several ways in medical and educational literature. Definitions and the perceived nature of a disability may affect how services are delivered in schools. For the purposes of this book, three definitions will be briefly examined: the classic autism definition from the Autism Society of America (1996), the mental health/psychology definition from the *Diagnostic and Statistical Manual of Mental Disorders (DSM-IV)* (American Psychiatric Association [APA], 1995), and IDEA's (1997) definition.

The classic definition from the Autism Society of America (1996) is as follows:

> Autism is a severely incapacitating, lifelong, developmental disability that typically appears during the first three years of life. The result of a neurological disorder that affects functioning of the

brain, autism, and its behavioral symptoms occur in approximately fifteen out of every 10,000 births. Autism is four times more common in boys than girls. It has been found throughout the world in families of all racial, ethnic, and social backgrounds. No known factors in the psychological environment of a child have been shown to cause autism. (p. 1)

According to the Autism Society of America (1996), some behavioral symptoms of autism include:

• Disturbances in the rate of appearance of physical, social, and language skills.

• Abnormal responses to sensations. Any one or a combination of senses or responses is affected: sight, hearing, touch, balance, smell, taste, reaction to pain, and the way a child holds his or her body.

• Absence or delay of speech and language, although specific thinking capabilities may be present.

• Abnormal ways of relating to people, objects, and events.

The definition from the *DSM-IV* (APA, 1995) begins with a list of the five diagnostic categories:

1. Autistic disorder

2. Asperger's disorder

3. Pervasive developmental disorder—not otherwise specified

4. Childhood disintegrative disorder

5. Rett's disorder

The term *spectrum* used in the context of Autistic Spectrum Disorders suggests a range of related qualities or activities. The same term used in reference to the Pervasive Developmental Disorders (PDDs) means the PDDs share related characteristics (i.e., that each specific PDD disorder, although different, shares some similarities. ASD is a class of related developmental disorders that overlap but are clinically distinct and separately diagnosed. It is generally conceded that autistic disorders (AD), or classic autism, is the prototypical and most severe form of ASD. With careful assessment, the PDDs can be differentially diagnosed (APA, 1995).

The IDEA (1997) definition is as follows:

Autism means a developmental disability significantly affecting verbal and nonverbal communication and social interaction, generally evident before age 3, that adversely affects a child's educational performance. Other characteristics often associated with autism are engagement in repetitive activities and stereotyped movements, resistance to environmental change or change in daily routines, and unusual responses to sensory experiences. The term does not apply if a child's educational performance is adversely affected primarily because the child has an emotional disturbance, as defined in paragraph (b)(4) of this section. A child who manifests the characteristics of "autism" after age 3 could be diagnosed as having "autism" if the criteria of this section are satisfied. (34 CODE OF

FEDERAL REGULATIONS [C.F.R.] § 300 [c] [1] [i] [ii])

This statement allows school-based teams to make the diagnosis of autism without reverting to either of the other two definitions; however, it is based on the information contained in the earlier more extensive explanations that should also guide the team's decisions. States have also developed definitions of autism to assist their school districts in determining eligibility for special education and RELATED SERVICES, rather than for the purpose of a medical or psychiatric diagnosis of an ASD.

Planning for Long-Term Services

Because ASD and PDD all include specific speech-language characteristics, the speech-language pathologist is always involved in the assessment, planning, and intervention for students who are so identified. The condition is so pervasive, long lasting, and disruptive to learning that professionals will need to consider many service delivery approaches over time to be sure that the programming remains suited to the child (Scott, Clark, and Brady, 2000). It is important to weigh program options, work closely with families, and be exceptionally creative. Mindful of Blosser and Kratcoski's (1997) premises for service delivery in the 2000s (see Table 5.2 in Chapter 5), the sidebar provides guidelines for school service teams serving students with ASD.

Intervention Approaches

The approach that works best for the child with ASD is the one that is the most specific to a given child's needs. Children with ASD demonstrate highly individualized learning styles (Schreibman, Koegel, Charlop, and Egel, 1990). Functional approaches (which tend to be behaviorally oriented) and developmental approaches (which need not be mutually exclusive nor competitive with behavioral methods) constitute the primary choices made by teams and parents (Greenspan and Wieder, 1999). Some children may respond best to applied behavior analysis methods, which are highly structured teaching and speech-language intervention in a controlled environment (Lord, Bristol, and Scholper, 1993; Palacio, 2000). Others benefit from play therapy (Wolfberg and Schuler, 1993) using socio-drama, peer interaction, and child-led interactions.

The speech-language pathologist may have a professional philosophy regarding therapy for children with ASD that may or may not mesh with the team's or parents' ideas. Because intensive speech-language intervention with the child and training for the family may be viewed as the core of the program (Greenspan, 1992), the way communication services are provided is a critical decision. Several approaches that school-based speech-language pathologists have used successfully in different circumstances are summarized in Table 7.1 (page 222). It is helpful when the speech-language pathologist knows the entire range of choices the parent may be considering.

Guidelines for the Service Planning Process
for Students with Autism Spectrum Disorders

1. Have timelines been met? Was staff responsive to referral or request for service?

2. Has team planning been thorough and coordinated?

3. Was the multidisciplinary assessment team qualified and knowledgeable in all areas?

4. Did the report document determination, behavior implications, assessment in all areas of suspected disability, child's developmental levels?

5. Are required components of IEP, IFSP, and transition plans documented?

6. Have services addressed all areas of need?

7. Are service options provided by qualified, specifically trained personnel?

8. Does the program provide for coordination, collaboration, ongoing training, and supervision of providers and parents?

9. Does the documentation include all necessary information and data collection?

10. Are timelines and decision-making criteria established?

11. Have all responsibilities been assigned?

12. Are there dates set for further program planning and evaluation?

Source: California Department of Education (1999a)

The intervention approaches for children with ASD stress the functionality of language for these students. In addition to balancing the providers, activities, and contexts of service delivery decisions, the speech-language pathologist will need to consider the belief system of the educational team and parents, and the availability of comprehensive training for all service providers (Crais, 2000). Due to the nature of ASD, and its overwhelming impact on language and social contacts, these students will need strong communication intervention (Scott et al., 2000).

Information on effective intervention with ASD continues to develop (Wetherby, 2000).

Guidelines for ASD screening by pediatricians during well-baby checks have been proposed (Maugh, 2000). Filipek and others have drawn up specific probes and questions that physicians will need to ask parents to screen for ASD (Maugh, 2000). The American Academy of Neurology announced its plans to adopt the early-screening guidelines in the summer of 2000. Parents have typically waited for identification until services were sought from the local school system, but in the future, first-level screenings would be conducted on all children from infancy (Maugh, 2000). The guidelines are heavily influenced by the early speech-language characteristics of ASD as seen in these questions (Maugh, 2000):

Table 7.1

Intervention Methods for Students with ASDs

Method	Description
TEACCH Treatment and Education of Autistic and Related Communication Handicapped CHildren	Highly structured teaching and accommodations in the learning environment, includes parents as teaching assistants. Picture schedules are posted for children, and visual cuing is used in instruction. Applies to many settings. Source: Lord et al. (1993)
IBI Intensive Behavior Intervention	One to five years of structured learning opportunities for 37–40 hours per week address all significant behaviors in all of child's environments by all significant persons. Emphasizes speech and language in early years, and one-to-one training sessions are most effective. Requires specialized training. Source: Lovaas (1996)
Natural Language intervention	Using procedures similar to those for typically developing children, language targets are taught in a variety of social settings using natural reinforcers with a communication partner. Useful in pullout and classroom-based settings. Source: Camarata (1996)
PRT Pivotal Response Training	Based on IBI approach, teaches a cluster of stimulus cues that will trigger simple or complex behaviors (like speech). Increases motivation of students, broadens opportunities for child to respond, increases generalization. Useful in many settings. Source: Koegel, Schreibman, Good, Cerniglia, Murphy, and Koegel (1989)
PECS Picture Exchange Communication System	Teaches children to initiate communication in a social context by giving pictures to adults to request an object or action. Useful in many settings. Source: Bondy and Frost (1994)
AAC Augmentative and alternative communication	Using an AAC system suited to child's cognitive and academic level facilitates social interaction and communication. Useful in many settings. Source: Williams (2000)
DIR Developmental, Individual-Difference, Relationship-Based approach	Emphasizes the differences between students with ASD, and the relationships that can be built with the child and the family. Source: Greenspan and Wieder (1999)

- Is the baby babbling before 12 months?

- Is the baby pointing by 12 months?

- Does the baby have a first word by 16 months?

- Has the baby or child lost language skills he or she once had?

Needless to say, parent responses to these questions could also signal a language impairment or related developmental disability. Since the pediatrician's questions are being proposed as a screening tool, the intent is to collect information early and have evaluations conducted by the appropriate professional team. Parent responses to these speech-language questions would raise the awareness of doctors to this condition, trigger earlier evaluations if needed, and bring treatment to these children sooner (Maugh, 2000).

Appropriate Benefit

Parents and teachers of students with ASD are brought into contact with many medical and educational professionals. Some are brief encounters while others are ongoing. Key members of the team are the speech-language pathologist and audiologist. Their roles have been typically diagnostic in nature; however, they have become increasingly related to intervention in many states (Scott et al., 2000). Speech-language pathologists must be aware of the ongoing controversy when schools serve students with ASD. School programs can be effective interventions for students; however, their underlying treatment premise varies from the private sector. Families and school teams can disagree heartily on what the school can or should do for students with ASD. Speech-language pathologists need to understand why service delivery recommendations appear to clash.

Since appropriate (not best or maximum feasible) benefit remains the federal standard for students with disabilities, a fairly modest set of expectations is fostered in special education. This frequently comes into conflict with the culture of autism. Many parents of children with autism are well aware of and believe they should expect the best education and related services shown to be effective. Perhaps it is the pervasiveness of autism, coupled with the startling progress some students make under optimized programs, that drives families to seek BEST PRACTICES rather than settling for less. In response to the advocacy efforts of families and professionals, several states have gone beyond the federal minimum and have raised their standards and commitments to all students with disabilities in their state constitutions. (Scott et al., 2000, pp. 108–109)

Professionals in communication disorders continue to play a very active role with the treatment of ASD, including the development of interdisciplinary clinical practice guidelines for ASD (Interdisciplinary Council on Developmental and Learning Disorders [ICDL], 2000). This approach uses a cross-disciplinary, comprehensive, and functional developmental intervention system for students and families. Developmental

Individual-Difference Relationship-Based (DIR) approach is designed to meet the unique needs of children and families. The model is built on research that shows that while students with ASD have common characteristics, they are not all alike. Their interventions must be matched to personal characteristics, interests, and family strengths. The speech-language pathologist is required to build a relationship with the student and experience the world the way he or she does (Greenspan and Wieder, 1999). For example, the ICDL Guidelines state that 45% of the sample of 200 children with ASD use limited speech, while 55% have virtually no speech. Speech-language pathology proponents of the ICDL intervention guidelines question how any communication program can be proscribed for students with ASD if half of the population is known to have vastly different speech and language behaviors (ICDL, 2000).

DIR is based on building a relationship with each child and working on "all essential functional developmental capacities (regulation and attention, engagement, two-way purposeful interaction, problem solving, interactions, the creative uses of ideas, and logical thinking), individual processing differences (auditory, language, visual spatial, motor planning, and sensory modulation), and child-caregiver interactions and family functioning as well as additional cognitive and learning skills" (ICDL, 2000, p. 26). DIR has 10 major principles: (1) floortime, semistructured, and structured learning; (2) all day and evening programs; (3) intensive individual therapies; (4) integrated play opportunities; (5) appropriate IEPs; (6) tailored biomedical approaches; (7) technology-based learning matched to the child's potential; (8) mental health consultations; (9) no delays or waiting periods if a child is found to have

interruptions in relating, communicating, or thinking; (10) continuity of programming as the child grows. Speech-language intervention, conducted by qualified and specifically trained speech-language pathologists plays a major role in carrying out each of the 10 principles (ICDL, 2000).

Contrasting Perspectives

Some interventions for students with ASD that were considered highly controversial in the 1990s continue to be the focus of carefully constructed and appropriately controlled research (Biklin and Cardinal, 1997; Creaghead, 1999). Facilitated communication, auditory integration training, sensory integration therapy, and intensive, computer-assisted auditory temporal processing programs have all been interventions difficult to validate using conventional procedures (Calculator, 1999; Creaghead, 1999; Duchan; 1999; Gillam, 1999a; Griffer, 1999; Madell, 1999; Mauer, 1999; Tharpe, 1999; Veale, 1999). The speech-language pathologist has the educational background and the professional resources to make valid communication intervention decisions for students with ASD. Whitmire (1999) offered a systematic series of questions the speech-language pathologist should use to evaluate treatment procedures, products, or programs in school settings, including:

- "What are the stated uses of the procedure, product, or program" (p. 427)?
- "To which client/patient population does it apply" (p. 427)?
- "To what other populations does it claim to generalize" (p. 427)?
- "Are outcomes clearly stated" (p. 427)?

- "Are there publications concerning this procedure, product, or program" (p. 427)?

- "Is there peer-reviewed research that supports or contradicts the stated outcomes or benefits" (p. 427)?

- "What is the professional background of the developers" (p. 428)?

- "Are there similar procedures, products, or programs currently available? How do they compare in performance and cost" (p. 428)?

- "Is it within my profession's scope of practice" (p. 428)?

- "Have you checked to see if there are any ASHA statements or guidelines on this topic" (p. 428)?

- "Is the cost reasonable and justifiable" (p. 428)?

- "Is the use justifiable" (p. 428)?

- "What are potential risks/adverse consequences" (p. 428)?

- "What is recommended as sufficient training to be considered a qualified user" (p. 428)?

Students Who Use Assistive Technology (AT) and Augmentative and Alternative Communication (AAC)

In 1992, Congress recognized the importance of ASSISTIVE TECHNOLOGY (AT) devices and services as tools to assist students with disabilities to lead more independent and productive lives (Rehabilitation Act Amendments). AT had been used in schools before this time (ASHA, 1991a), but use was sporadic and often overlooked by busy school special education teams. At times, knowledge about AT was thin, and staff did not feel confident about what equipment was available, how it was used, and how it could augment the communication and/or education of a child. Concerns about cost and lack of funds also caused teams to avoid the AT discussion. Speech-language pathologists and others lobbied Congress heavily to include specific wording in IDEA to assure that these service delivery problems would be addressed and resolved. Many students with severe physical and neurological disabilities could not communicate with speech and they needed alternative, often technological, methods to communicate and learn. The addition to the law in 1992 was crucial to the field, and further refinements occurred in the reauthorization of IDEA in 1997: "Assistive technology device means any item, piece of equipment, or product system, whether acquired commercially off the shelf, modified, or customized, that is used to increase, maintain, or improve functional capabilities of a child with a disability" (34 C.F.R. § 300.5).

> Assistive technology service means any service that directly assists a child with a disability in the selection, acquisition, or use of an assistive technology.
>
> The term includes—
>
> (a) The evaluation of the needs of a child, including a functional evaluation of the child in the child's customary environment;
>
> (b) Purchasing, leasing, or otherwise providing for the acquisition of assistive technology devices by children with disabilities;

(c) Selecting, designing, fitting, customizing, adapting, applying, maintaining, repairing, or replacing assistive technology devices;

(d) Coordinating and using other therapies, interventions, or services with assistive technology devices, such as those associated with existing education and rehabilitation plans and programs;

(e) Training or technical assistance for a child with a disability, or, if appropriate, that child's family; and

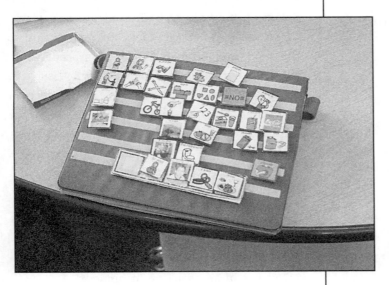

(f) Training or technical assistance for professionals (including individuals providing education or rehabilitation services), employers, or other individuals who provide services to, employ, or are otherwise substantially involved in the major life functions of that child. (34 C.F.R. § 300.6)

IDEA (1997) requires that technology be considered at every IEP meeting. Schools must consider, on a case-by-case basis, the use of school-purchased assistive technology devices in the child's home or other settings if the IEP team determines a device is needed to ensure FREE APPROPRIATE PUBLIC EDUCATION (FAPE). To comply with IDEA requirements, many school districts have hired or trained personnel to be AT specialists and have provided in-service education for special education staff. Some professionals embraced the concept easily, while others have remained somewhat intimidated by technology and reliant on other team members to handle this part of special education.

Many speech-language pathologists are well equipped by education and experience to become AT specialists in their districts. Some have been using AT systems for many years, and are able to "think outside the box" to support a student who struggles with the motoric aspects of reading, writing, speaking, and listening. Hearing aids and other ASSISTIVE LISTENING DEVICES (ALD) are well known to speech-language pathologists, and many have used communication boards or computer software as intervention strategies (Glennen, 2000).

AT and AUGMENTATIVE AND ALTERNATIVE COMMUNICATION (AAC), though closely related, are not the same. Assistive technology can be used to support students with many types of disabilities. AAC may be a type of AT for students who need to have their communication supported so they can access the curriculum and take part in their daily life activities. AT and AAC can be either low-tech or high-tech.

Low-tech examples include: equipment and other supports readily available in schools, including off-the-shelf items to accommodate the needs of students that can be provided by general or special education through the STU-DENT STUDY TEAM or IEP process. Low-tech items include items such as calculators, tape recorders, pencil grips, school constructed language boards, and TV captioning.

High-tech examples encompass equipment and other supports for students who may need more specialized equipment and support services beyond basic AT (often students with low incidence or severe disabilities), which requires more in-depth assessment and customizing. Examples of high-tech items include closed circuit television, FM systems, augmentative communication devices, sound field systems, computer access devices, and specialized software.

When considering AT, teams should begin by considering low-tech adaptations that may be appropriate for the student and easily obtained. The term *technology* suggests highly sophisticated equipment, but that was not the intent of the law. A team needs to be sure the student needs it and will use it. Table 7.2 (page 228) lists AT devices organized by the academic task that would be adapted or modified for the student. AAC is listed under the activity of speaking; however, there is considerable overlap with writing, reading, and other curriculum-based school tasks since communication intersects with so many daily activities.

The awareness and use of technology has greatly increased in the general population in the last few years, making it easier for necessary technology to reach students in schools. Computers are an expected part of every classroom and school. A student's curriculum and learning strategies incorporate computers as learning tools, providing better access for students with severe speech disabilities to AT necessary for literally all of their communication. In some cases, a student with LEARNING DISABILITIES may use AT for writing (spell checker) or mathematics (calculator) unrelated to his or her communication skills, and the speech-language pathologist will simply incorporate this technology into speech services if needed. In other cases, communication will be such a critical component of the child's needs that the AAC will dictate all the other parts of the education program. Training teachers, family members, peers, and communication partners to use the AAC with the child is also the responsibility of the speech-language pathologist and is listed on the IEP as a related service necessary for the child to benefit from special education.

Other texts (e.g., Buekelman and Miranda, 1998; Church and Glennen, 1992; Romski and Sevcik, 1996) are available to provide greater detail about the assessment and intervention services for students who need AAC. This section was designed to help speech-language pathologists recognize the scope of AT and AAC and the role that speech-language pathologists play in team decisions, parent training, equipment upgrading, and curriculum matching.

Table 7.2

Assistive Technology Organized by Academic Task

Academic Area or Task	Sample Assistive Technology Devices
Speaking	Communication boards
	Picture Exchange Communication Symbols, Bliss symbols
	Speech-to-speech telephone access
	Speech output augmentative devices
Listening	Assistive listening devices
	Variable speech control tape recorder/player
	Conventional tape recorder
	Loop amplification system
Writing	Word processor, spell checker
	Proofreading programs
	Outlining software
	Abbreviation expanders
	Speech synthesis screen reading programs
	Word prediction programs
Reading	Optical character recognition speech synthesis
	Speech synthesis for books on tape
	Variable speech control tape recorders
	Audio-taped books
	Picture Story software
Organization and Memory	Classroom schedule frame on wall
	Personal data organizer software
	Free form data base, calendar programs
	Tape recorder/player
Mathematics	Talking calculators, conventional calculator
	Onscreen computer-based calculator
	Drill and practice software programs with scoring
Daily Activities	Adaptive eating devices
	Adaptive drinking devices
	Adaptive dressing devices
Mobility	Walker, grab rails, manual wheelchair
	Power chair, powered mobility toys and appliances
	Easy access switches to operate equipment

From *Assistive Technology for Children with Learning Difficulties* (p. 25), by M. Raskind, (2000), San Mateo, CA: Schwab Foundation for Learning. © 2000 by M. Raskind. Adapted with permission.

Intervention using AAC is a big task that speech-language pathologists should not do alone. It is always more successful when the full team is involved (Blackstone, 2000), widening the circle of potential communication partners for the student, and vastly increasing the number of daily opportunities for practice and reinforcement.

Successful AT/AAC services in schools can generally be examined by using five critical elements. Speech-language pathologists are not responsible for all the elements, but they frequently play a large role in the coordination of this effort and the linkage with parents and other agencies. If the AT is an AAC system, the speech-language pathologist usually functions as the team leader or CASE MANAGER and will likely be involved in all five elements:

> **Intervention using AAC is a big task that speech-language pathologists should not do alone.**

1. Assistive technology evaluation

2. Training and technical assistance

3. Acquisition and use of devices

4. Maintenance of devices

5. Coordination of services

Each element is described below as it relates to an AAC device, mindful that the same would be true of any other AT device. Use of low-tech devices may take less time to implement, since they are easier to obtain and their effectiveness can be evaluated more quickly. Training and technical assistance are important, even for low-tech devices, as an appropriate tool can be rejected if the professionals do not know how to implement the technology, or if the student's use is inconsistent. High-tech devices require a slower pace for decision-making and have greater consequences for the student and the school's resources if found unsuccessful. Assessments do not have to entail long test batteries or trips to a distant rehabilitation center. Teams who are willing to work with AT and learn what to do will become accomplished at making all low-tech decisions. Some teams can also handle high-tech decisions or make them in conjunction with another agency or regional support center which has access to equipment for trials.

Assistive Technology Evaluation

States have regulations and procedures for assessment, and districts may have selected resources to use for this purpose. The assessment must be both developmental and functional and at least partially conducted in the student's customary environment. A series of questions may be asked at the IEP meeting to determine what types of technology would be helpful. A speech-language pathologist within the district, or a Tech Center outside the district, could be used. Technology centers may be set up by nonprofit agencies to enable families to try out various systems, which are often too expensive to rent or buy outright. Usually an occupational or physical therapist assists with seating and positioning if that is an issue.

Making a Difference
for America's Children

There should be a written report and recommendations based on the student's trial with a device or devices. A student has changing needs, so the evaluation may need to be updated from time to time, either by the educational team or by an outside team. Newer technology is constantly becoming available, so re-evaluation will allow the team to focus on better interventions as they become available.

Training and Technical Assistance

Training is a critical key to success with all AT. Training is an organized, scheduled event with specific GOALS and topics for the participants (e.g., educators, the AAC user, parents, and peers). Technical assistance, on the other hand, is more informal, involving an ongoing relationship between the persons on the team and the family, including troubleshooting, discussions, and moral support.

The speech-language pathologist typically provides student instruction during therapy or collaborative sessions in the classroom. The SPEECH-LANGUAGE PATHOLOGY ASSISTANT (SLPA) often continues this instruction until the next level of skills are needed. The classroom teacher may assist with AT instruction that is connected to the curriculum. All three of these people may need education themselves to be proficient enough on a device to teach the student. Sometimes, the classroom aide or a personal assistant assigned by the school will help to encode new vocabulary to expand a device, teach new access skills, or practice an oral or written report with a child. The more people who are involved in the instruction, the more communication partners the AAC user will have (Blackstone, 2000).

Technical assistance for the speech-language pathologist will likely be needed if the device malfunctions or if adjustments or modifications need to be made. Some of these can be done by the speech-language pathologist or assistants, but many are time-consuming or require special tools. The technical support person must be a part of the team and easy to reach. Technical assistance may be listed on the IEP as a support for either the trainer or the trainee.

Both training and technical assistance need to be set up ahead of time, so that the student can begin using the communication system without long delays or interruptions. There are some costs involved here, and the speech-language pathologist needs to be sensitive to how they are handled. IDEA (1997) requires that a member of the IEP team, called the LOCAL EDUCATION AGENCY (LEA) representative, be a person who is authorized to commit the district's resources as needed to carry out the IEP. If an AAC device is written into the IEP, the costs for training and technical assistance are absorbed by the school district. In some cases, the family or another agency will step in to assist with costs. Teams should discuss these training and technical assistance requirements at the IEP, so that all team members are aware of them. Technical support may be included in the purchase of a device, or it may involve an additional fee. The speech-language pathologist should encourage the team to arrange for such services to make the AT choice successful.

230

Acquisition and Use of Devices

An AAC device is used by students to communicate and thereby participate in and benefit from their educational program. This condition of educational benefit is necessary for assistive technology to be identified on the IEP as a related service. The AAC device often enables a student to engage in academics for the first time, have some control of his or her environment, and make personal choices. All of these lend themselves to a less restrictive environment, greater access to the general education curriculum, and improved academic progress and FUNCTIONAL OUTCOMES. AAC must be tied to these educational expectancies or the family becomes responsible for providing AAC through other funding sources.

Devices can be purchased, leased, loaned, or received as a gift or donation. They are listed either generically or specifically on the IEP with other related services. When school systems are responsible for acquiring the AAC system, devices purchased by the LEA remain the property of the school. At times, the family may choose to purchase the device so that the student has sole access to the device in all settings. Regulations state that the equipment must be procured in a timely manner, not delaying the implementation of the signed IEP. Insurance companies and Medicaid may also purchase equipment if it is found medically necessary for the student. The school makes AAC decisions based on what is educationally beneficial for the student. These two ideas can be in conflict at times, and the speech-language pathologist may be the only team member who can differentiate between health-care requirements and educational standards.

Students use their AAC device in school, but the IEP team may also determine that it can be taken home for educational purposes that allow the child to receive FAPE. A device may be used by more than one student at school, as long as it is available to each student whenever it is needed according to each student's IEP.

When students move from school to school, or from school to post-school environments, the ideal situation is for customized AAC equipment to follow them. As noted previously, the equipment is often the property of the school district. Ownership of a customized piece of equipment must be addressed in state and local policies, but the issue is often neglected at the local level until there is a relocation. The U. S. Department of Education issued a policy guidance statement on June 28, 1998, encouraging this transfer of devices to the person's new setting, but this guidance is not stated in IDEA (1997). The speech-language pathologist is in a pivotal position to be sensitive to the user's need for a personal communication system, yet recognize the financial commitments of the school district. The policy guidance statement may be helpful to avoid the public relations disaster likely if a school attempted to reclaim its device from a graduating student with disabilities. With the rapid turnover in high technology, most AAC systems have extremely limited resale value. Speech-language pathologists should seek advice from their supervisor early in the process to assure that an equipment transition will be smooth.

Maintenance of Devices

AAC devices are rarely ready for use right out of the box. They must be designed, fitted, programmed, customized, adapted, maintained, repaired, and replaced. The school might need to use technical assistance for fitting or customizing. The speech-language pathologist, teacher, and student may personalize the AAC system with identification, photos, taped messages using a friend's voice, and so on. The school district is responsible for maintenance and repairs of student-owned equipment, if it is used at school.

A list of approved repair vendors is invaluable. The speech-language pathologist may be the person who arranges for a substitute AAC device while the main one is being repaired. Substitute devices must allow students to maintain their communication skills and not jeopardize their educational activities or grades during a lengthy repair period. Though few states have specific qualifications for those who repair AAC equipment, the repair person should be knowledgeable and experienced with that equipment. The speech-language pathologist is rarely qualified to be the repair person.

Coordination of Services

AT needs to be coordinated with all other interventions or services the student receives. For example, typically one team member works directly with the student and AAC device; knows the technology well; and has contact with all the other members of the team, including the parents. This coordinator is usually not the AT specialist who is responsible for AT support for the entire district or region. The AT specialist serves the team better in technical assistance than in day-to-day coordination of services for each AT or AAC user.

Occupational therapists, physical therapists, or teachers may coordinate a student's IEP, but experience has shown that it is often speech-language pathologists who coordinate the AAC user's overall program, because of their education and skills and also because communication is so central to these students' school lives. The entire team will contribute to any brainstorming or problem solving necessary for the AAC user, but one team member has to see that the plan is completed, that each person follows through, and that parents and students have an informed role in the process. Misunderstandings between team members are common as the program is implemented.

The IEP should identify roles and persons to carry out these tasks. When AAC is coordinated, the IEP goals and OBJECTIVES will reflect how the technology serves as a support to the student's education program.

Has Technology Been Considered?

Figure 7.1 illustrates the steps a school district could take to select an AT service or AAC device when the team responds affirmatively to the IEP question "Has technology been considered?" and determines that AT or AAC is appropriate for the student. Notice how each step leads to one of the five elements of AT. Selection of functional outcomes and writing of goals and SHORT-TERM OBJECTIVES or BENCHMARKS leads to the expected progress. If the student shows lack of progress, the team returns to the

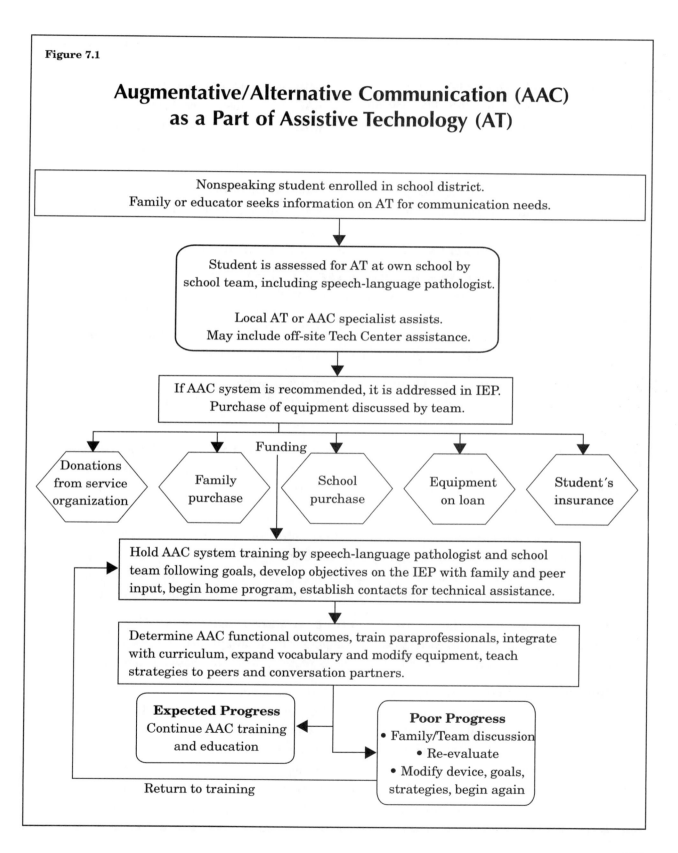

Figure 7.1

Augmentative/Alternative Communication (AAC) as a Part of Assistive Technology (AT)

Nonspeaking student enrolled in school district.
Family or educator seeks information on AT for communication needs.

Student is assessed for AT at own school by school team, including speech-language pathologist.

Local AT or AAC specialist assists.
May include off-site Tech Center assistance.

If AAC system is recommended, it is addressed in IEP.
Purchase of equipment discussed by team.

Funding

Donations from service organization

Family purchase

School purchase

Equipment on loan

Student's insurance

Hold AAC system training by speech-language pathologist and school team following goals, develop objectives on the IEP with family and peer input, begin home program, establish contacts for technical assistance.

Determine AAC functional outcomes, train paraprofessionals, integrate with curriculum, expand vocabulary and modify equipment, teach strategies to peers and conversation partners.

Expected Progress
Continue AAC training and education

Poor Progress
• Family/Team discussion
• Re-evaluate
• Modify device, goals, strategies, begin again

Return to training

decision-making process and tries again. All AAC decisions are complex and have many possible results, largely because communication is a very personal act and because any method of communication must take multiple factors into account.

Working with AT can be a challenging part of the speech-language pathologist's job that requires use of many diagnostic, negotiation,

prediction, therapeutic, educational intervention, and coordination skills. Since speech-language pathologists are often key IEP team members for AAC, they must learn techniques for working with students with significant communication needs, coordinating large numbers of people, obtaining and maintaining a relatively costly intervention device, and directing ever-changing sets of student skills and emerging technologies.

Frequently Asked Questions about AT and AAC

Q. Are schools required to pay for AT and AAC devices?

A. Yes, school districts have the responsibility under IDEA (1997) to provide equipment, services, training, and programs for students with an IEP who need AT in order to increase, maintain, or improve their functional capabilities. Other funding resources may include insurance companies, foundations, fraternal organizations, businesses, and individuals.

Q. Do students have access to AT or AAC if they are eligible for extended-year services?

A. Yes, if the IEP team decided that the student needed AT to access the curriculum in summer school or extended-year programs.

Q. Is a school district required to provide state-of-the-art equipment for a student?

A. No. The equipment needs to be appropriate for the student's needs to ensure FAPE. The IEP is guided by the assessment and is under no obligation to select a more or less expensive or sophisticated device.

Q. Under what conditions may AT or AAC be considered a related service?

A. AT equipment is a related service if it is a complementary service necessary for the student to benefit from his or her special education. Instruction or technical assistance for family members or staff to communicate with a student using AAC would also be an example of a related service.

Q. How can school districts use Medicaid funds to purchase AT or AAC?

A. Medicaid regulations vary in each state, but the parent must always give permission to access the funds. Funds can be used according to Medicaid regulations, which are based on medical necessity.

Q. How can school personnel locate AT and AAC resources?

A. Working with AAC resources requires more than the usual materials and supply catalogs. Many states have technology centers that may also function as assessment centers in some regions. The sidebar beginning on page 235 lists six national contacts that will put the speech-language pathologist in touch with state resources as well. AAC is available in every state and many countries around the world. Local manufacturing representatives have been known to visit schools, join planning teams if requested, or bring loaner equipment for students to try.

Home-Bound, Home-Schooled, Hospital-Bound, Suspended/Expelled, or Incarcerated Children and Youth

Students who are eligible for special education services, including speech-language services, may need to receive this support in locations other than the school for periods of time. This can occur for various reasons.

A student may be restricted to home due to a medical condition, such as severe allergies or autoimmune disorders, with education provided by a home-based teacher assigned by the school district. Students hospitalized for a period of time (the amount of time varies from state to state) may receive general and special education services from either their home district or the school district in which the hospital or rehabilitation facility is located. If they were eligible for speech-language services before the protracted hospitalization, students are entitled to continued services if they are physically able to benefit. This is usually coordinated with the provision of academic instruction. Speech-language pathologists who are employees of the hospital or rehabilitation facility may provide services, but there are often complicated fiscal issues to resolve between the school district, other funding sources, and service providers.

Resources for the Speech-Language Pathologist Using AT and AAC

The Alliance for Technology Access (ATA)

2175 E. Francisco Boulevard, Suite L

San Rafael, CA 94901

415-455-4575 • 415-445-0491 (TTY)

Email: *atainfo@ataccess.org* • Web site: *www.ataccess.org*

This is a national network of technology resource centers and technology vendors.

Assistive Technology Funding and Systems Change Project

1660 L Street NW, Suite 700

Washington, DC 20036

202-776-0406 • 202-776-0414 (fax)

Email: *atproject@uspa.org*

This project provides information and technical assistance on AT issues, through a consortium of six national organizations led by United Cerebral Palsy Associations.

Continued on next page

Continued

State Tech Act Programs

1700 North Moore Street, Suite 1540

Arlington, VA 22209-1903

703-524-6686 • 703-524-6630 (fax)

Email: *resnata@resna.org* • www.resna.org

This is a technical assistance project funded by IDEA and operated by the Rehabilitation Engineering Society of North American (RESNA) to help you reach the project located in your state.

State Protection and Advocacy Agencies

202-406-9514 • 202-408-9520 (fax)

Email: *napas@earthlink.net*

This agency will help parents and others with legal questions about technology and other education issues. There is a contact agency in each state, which can be located through this central number in Washington, DC.

United States Society for Augmentative and Alternative Communication (USSAAC)

P.O. Box 21418

Sarasota, FL 34276

941-312-0992 • 941-312-0992 (fax)

Email: *USSAAC@aol.com*

This is a national organization of professionals, consumers, and families who are experienced with AAC devices of all types. They provide technical assistance, advocacy, and training for users, their families, and their service providers and have national and regional conferences and newsletters.

Communication Aid Manufacturers Association (CAMA)

P.O. Box 1039

Evanston, IL 60204-1039

800-441-CAMA (2262) • 847-869-5689 (fax)

Email: *cama@northshore.net* • Web site: *www.aacproducts.org*

This is an organization of manufacturers who coordinate their efforts to match the student with the most appropriate communication aid. They sell, lease, or loan low-tech and high-tech devices and offer low-cost training to professionals and parents throughout the country.

In the cases described above, the school speech-language pathologist would provide speech-language services according to the specifications on the IEP. The IEP may be revised, however, to accommodate the student's medical situation. IEPs for students who are off site are written to provide adequate progress in the curriculum. Students typically spend much less time with a teacher than they would spend at school, since they are receiving intensive one-to-one support. Some districts require the speech-language pathologist from the student's school to travel to the home or hospital. Others have a home or hospital special education team that serves all students at temporary home or medical sites.

Students with an IEP for speech-language services who are suspended for more than 10 days or expelled from school may need to receive these services at home until another school can be found. Even after EXPULSION, students retain their right to FAPE, and the IEP goals must be pursued. Other students may receive special education services at a neutral site, usually due to safety or discipline concerns present at the school site. Special educators are expected to carry out such assignments, with adequate safety precautions provided.

Students who are incarcerated during their school years typically receive their special education at their youth detention site. The assessment and appropriate intervention for speech-language services can be done by the home district, but more densely populated areas or larger penal institutions usually have speech-language pathologists employed by the state's corrections agency. Incarcerated persons 21 years of age and younger are entitled to special education services if they were identified with a disability, and had an IEP before their incarceration, and they have not yet received a regular high school diploma.

All school-aged children who reside in a district must be included in CHILD FIND activities. This includes children who are home-schooled or who are enrolled in private education facilities. Schools must make parents and professionals aware of the availability of special education services and how children may be referred for evaluation. Speech-language services, as one of those programs, are frequently requested.

Under IDEA (1997), students who are enrolled by their parents in private school, are entitled to evaluation for suspected disabilities, but they may not be entitled to the full continuum of special education services provided to children in public schools. Speech-language pathologists should inquire how their school district deals with this regulation.

Schools may provide special education services to some of these children in a variety of locations. If the child is transported to a special location for services, including the public school, the school district is responsible for the transportation cost. From time to time, school-based speech-language pathologists may need to travel to a distant site to serve a student or have a student transported for services. Working in a school may require the practitioner to negotiate the best way to offer services or create a delivery model that includes an adjusted compensation for time or travel.

All children in America must develop communication skills as they are vital to children's success in life. Through the models described in this chapter, school-based speech-language pathologists have added several new dimensions to their work that have been well received by educators and communities. "Current perspectives propose an expansion of service delivery options based on a commitment to serving all children in the environment that best fits their individual needs" (Blosser and Kratcoski, 1997, p. 99).

CHAPTER 8

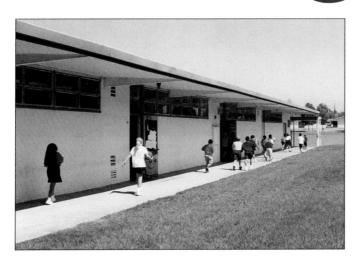

Procedural Safeguards and Other Protections for Children in Special Education

IN THIS CHAPTER

This chapter focuses on the procedural safeguards afforded to parents and children under IDEA (1997). In addition, the processes of mediation, due process hearings, and complaint procedures will be discussed. These processes are designed to ensure the due process rights of individuals with exceptional needs. Legal requirements are an important component of working within special education. The chapter will also address strategies for working with families to increase parent involvement and for dealing with difficult situations, including student discipline, which has specialized regulations for students with exceptional needs.

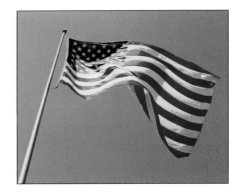

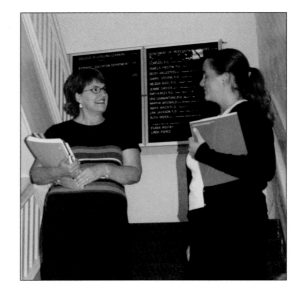

1. Review the rights and protections outlined in this chapter. Why do you think these specific rights were developed? What are the implications of implementing these rights? (Recall that Chapter 2 discussed the foundations of due process in the development of the EAHCA.)

2. Why is it important for speech-language pathologists to be familiar with student-discipline codes?

3. What role might speech-language pathologists take in dealing with the prevention of student violence? How might this role assist students on a speech-language caseload?

4. Locate and review a parental-rights document. Discuss the presentation of the rights. Is it understandable to the general reader? Would the reader know what to do if a disagreement develops? Where would the reader go for help in understanding these rights?

5. What procedures would a school-based speech-language pathologist want in place to ensure proper preparation in the event a case goes to mediation or due process hearing?

6. Reflect on how you, the reader, handle conflict. How might your reactions help or hinder a contentious interaction with a family? What skills might you need to learn?

7. What are the similarities and differences among the provisions of IDEA, Section 504, and the Americans with Disabilities Act (ADA)?

Parental Notification and Involvement

Special education laws, including the EDUCATION FOR ALL HANDICAPPED CHILDREN ACT (EAHCA) of 1975 and the INDIVIDUALS WITH DISABILITIES EDUCATION ACT (IDEA) AMENDMENTS OF 1997 are considered civil rights laws (See Chapter 2). Congress enacted legislation in 1975 that prevented situations in which parents were left out of the educational decision-making process for their child. Subsequently, the rights and protections afforded to parents and children through special education laws have been strengthened. Procedural safeguards that are written into these laws are the means by which parent involvement is ensured and defined. These safeguards are designed under constitutional principles known as DUE PROCESS of law. The requirements for due process of law are also applied in school discipline requirements for all students, with specialized requirements for students receiving SPECIAL EDUCATION. Turnbull (1993) explained due process passionately in his work *Free Appropriate Public Education: The Law and Children with Disabilities:*

> For those who pioneered the right-to-education doctrine, the procedures for implementing the right were as crucial as the right itself. Procedural due process is a means of challenging the multitude of discriminatory practices that the schools had habitually followed.... Without due process, the children would have found that their right to be included in an educational

program and to be treated non-discriminatorily (to receive a free appropriate education) would have a hollow ring. PROCEDURAL DUE PROCESS—the right to protest—is a necessary educational ingredient in enforcing every phase of the disabled child's right to an education.

> Procedural due process is also a constitutional requisite under the requirement of the Fifth and Fourteenth Amendments that no person shall be deprived of life, liberty, or property without due process of law. In terms of the education of disabled children, this means that no disabled child can be deprived of an education without the opportunity of exercising the right to protest what happens to him or her. (p. 207)

The legal requirements under IDEA (1997) can seem overwhelming to educators. Knowing the ramifications of these legal requirements is critical to the practice of special education and to the assurance of FREE APPROPRIATE PUBLIC EDUCATION (FAPE) for students. Violations can hold serious consequences for public agencies and the individuals IDEA (1997) was designed to protect.

PROCEDURAL COMPLIANCE questions have historically focused only on whether procedures had been followed correctly. Although IDEA (1997) shifted the focus of special education to quality programs and outcomes, procedural compliance and the assurance of due process of law remained the focus when compliance was questioned. A focus group of the National Association of State Directors of Special

Education (NASDSE) envisioned a system of balanced accountability built on three components: (1) rights, inputs, and processes to guarantee educational equity; (2) system results to guarantee program effectiveness; and (3) individual student learning to guarantee individual student achievement. When special educators base their decisions and actions on this three-part model, we should more fully realize "an educational system which is accountable for ensuring that all children, including those with disabilities, benefit from their educational experience" (Lieberman, 1995–1996, p. 47).

IDEA (1997) describes the processes and procedures that agencies and staff must follow to protect the rights of parents and children when delivering special education programs. Procedural safeguards are found in Part B, Subpart E of IDEA (1997); in Title 20 § 1415 of the UNITED STATES CODE (U.S.C.); and in Title 34 of the CODE OF FEDERAL REGULATIONS (C.F.R.). They include the following due process procedures: records examination and participation in meetings, INDEPENDENT EDUCATIONAL EVALUATION (IEE), notice requirements, and parental consent.

Records Examination and Participation in Meetings

Parents have a right to review all educational records and participate in all meetings that deal with their child's identification, evaluation, educational PLACEMENT, and FAPE provision.

However, Title 34 C.F.R. § 300.501 (b) (2) states that the requirement about parent involvement in meetings:

> [D]oes not include informal or unscheduled conversations involving public agency personnel and conversations on issues such as teaching methodology, lesson plans, or coordination of service provision if those issues are not addressed in the child's IEP. A meeting also does not include preparatory activities that public agency personnel engage in to develop a proposal or response to a parent proposal that will be discussed at a later meeting.

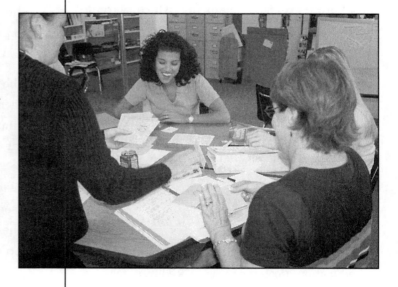

Parents must be involved in special education placement decisions about their child. It is critical that educators understand the provisions of this requirement. If parents are unable to participate, "the public agency shall use other methods to ensure their participation, including individual or conference telephone calls, or video conferencing" (34 C.F.R. § 300.501 [c] [3]). An individualized education program (IEP) team can make placement decisions about a student without the parent(s) only after several attempts have been made to involve the parents. These attempts must be documented according to standards set in 34 C.F.R. § 300.345 (d):

1. Detailed records of telephone calls made or attempted and the results of those calls;

2. Copies of correspondence sent to the parents and any responses received; and

3. Detailed records of visits made to the parent's home or place of employment and the results of those visits.

Independent Educational Evaluation (IEE)

The parents of a child with a disability have the right to obtain an IEE at public expense if they disagree with an evaluation obtained from a public agency (34 C.F.R. § 300.502 [b] [1]). If parents request that the school pay for the IEE, the district must inform them of the criteria for an acceptable evaluation and recommended service providers (34 C.F.R. § 300.502 [e]). If parents obtain a private evaluation that meets agency criteria and submit results to the school, an IEP team must consider the results of the evaluation as part of the IEP (34 C.F.R. § 300.502 [c] [1]). If parents submit a report from an evaluation they obtained, an IEP team meeting should be called to consider this information.

All special educators must know the rules regarding IEE. If parents request an IEE, educators must be cautious not to give any impression that such a request might not be honored. Such requests must be honored by the school team, and the resulting report must be discussed by an IEP team. Learning the appropriate protocol for the LOCAL EDUCATIONAL AGENCY (LEA) is necessary in the event that such a request is made. When parents request an IEE, notification of a supervisor, administrator, or program manager is highly advisable. Procedures will vary among school districts regarding the approval of and payment for an IEE. (See also Chapter 3, "Independent Educational Evaluation.")

Notice Requirements

The process whereby public agencies notify parents about proposed actions or refusals to act is highly regulated. Every time an action is being considered by IEP team members, written notice must be given to parents, including the items described in 34 C.F.R. § 300.503:

1. Parents must receive prior written notice whenever an agency proposes, refuses, or initiates a change regarding:
   - Identification
   - Evaluation
   - Educational placement
   - Provision of FAPE

2. The prior written notice must:
   - be in language understandable to the general public

- be in the native language of parents or translated orally for them

- describe the action proposed or refused

- explain why the agency is proposing or refusing the action

- describe other options considered and the reasons why those options were rejected

- describe the information used as a basis for the action

- include any other relevant factors used in making the decision

- include a statement that the parents have protection under the procedural safeguards of IDEA (1997) and, if the notice is not an initial REFERRAL for evaluation, include how a copy of the procedural safeguards can be obtained

- include sources of information to assist parents in understanding IDEA

Usually, LEAs have booklets for parents or have the notice of rights written on the back of an IEP document. The list of procedural safeguards is very long and complex under IDEA (1997) and may be daunting to parents attempting to understand it. Speech-language pathologists and other educators must be aware of their responsibilities under school policies for notifying parents of their rights and may be called on by parents to help explain the notice.

IDEA (1997) requires that parents be given notice (i.e., provided with written documentation and a verbal explanation) of their rights at each of the following times: when a student is initially referred for evaluation to determine ELIGIBILITY for special education, when a student is re-evaluated, when providing notice of an IEP meeting, and when filing a due process action. The responsibility for preparing the notice documents (i.e., parental-rights booklets or notice-of-meeting forms) belongs to educational agencies; however, under school policy, it may be the responsibility of special education service providers to ensure that parents receive and understand these rights and protections.

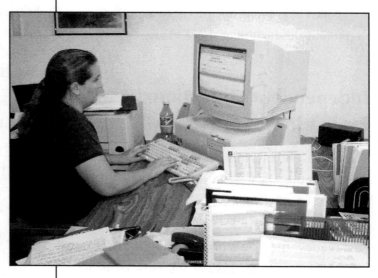

Speech-language pathologists who are new to public agencies should ask for assistance to learn how their employers want procedural safeguards to be explained to parents. Speech-language pathologists should review the procedural-safeguards-notice document, ask for clarification of questions they may have from administration in their agency, and be able to explain the document to families.

Parental Consent

Congress intended that decisions or actions never be taken with regard to a child's education without parent involvement. IDEA (1997) requires that parental consent be obtained before conducting an initial evaluation or a re-evaluation. To comply with this requirement, most agencies have a Consent to Assess form, also known as an ASSESSMENT PLAN or something similar. (See Chapter 3 for a discussion about when the assessment plan is needed.) The requirements for parental consent do not apply to reviews of files or data as part of an initial evaluation or a re-evaluation (34 C.F.R. § 300.505 [a] [3] [i]) or to the administration of testing done with all students in the school, such as group tests, unless consent is required from all parents (34 C.F.R. § 300.505 [a] [3] [ii]).

If parents refuse to sign an assessment plan (i.e., decline to have their child assessed to determine if the child has special needs), a public agency may choose to or may be required to pursue a due process action to proceed with an evaluation, depending on state law. (See "The Mediation Process" and "Impartial Due Process Hearings" for a discussion on mediation and due process.) Re-evaluations may proceed if parents do not respond to requests for consent. This section of the C.F.R. now gives the public agency the ability to conduct a re-evaluation without parental consent if reasonable steps to obtain these consents have been taken and the parents have not responded (American Speech-Language-Hearing Association [ASHA], 1999b).

IDEA (1997) requires documentation of attempts to obtain parental consent (consistent with the requirements noted earlier for attempts to involve parents in meetings, see page 243). Speech-language pathologists are strongly advised to consult with a supervisor or administrator before proceeding with a re-evaluation without parental consent.

IDEA (1997) prohibits denial of other services to a student based on parental refusal to consent (34 C.F.R. § 300.505 [e]). An example of this would be a student who is receiving resource-room services in addition to speech-language services. At the time of the triennial evaluation, the parents may agree to have the speech-language pathologist assess but not the resource-room teacher. In such a situation, all services to the child must continue, but the team should consult the supervisor or administrator for guidance on how to proceed.

Mediation, Due Process Hearings, and State IDEA Complaints

Due process of law is an element in both the FIFTH AND FOURTEENTH AMENDMENTS of the U.S. Constitution. Due process guarantees civil rights through procedural safeguards designed to protect individual rights (Pickett, 2000). Due process tends to be a phrase that is used in a variety of contexts in special education. Due process procedures include mediation, impartial DUE PROCESS HEARINGS, and state IDEA complaints. Procedural safeguards are part of due process. Due process also refers to the hearing process available when parents and LEAs disagree on issues related to a student's identification, evaluation, educational placement, or receipt of FAPE. Table 8.1 compares the procedures for resolving procedural complaints.

Mediation and due process hearings are utilized for disputes related to a student's IEP; that is, anything that deals with evaluation, GOALS and OBJECTIVES, program, placement, and services. The complaint process is designed for violations of procedural safeguards, such as timeline or implementation violations. These processes are available to parents and public agencies.

Most often, requests for hearings or investigations through the complaint process are actions taken by the parents. However, states are increasingly holding school districts accountable for ensuring a child's FAPE when there is a disagreement with parents. "FAPE belongs to the child, not the parent," advised attorney Melinda Maloney (1997). An LEA may later be held responsible for compensatory education for the student if a hearing officer finds that the school district failed to aggressively pursue the student's FAPE despite the disagreement on the part of the student's parents. It is for this reason that speech-language pathologists and other special educators must be very cautious when there are disagreements with parents regarding the recommendations and implementation of IEP procedures.

The Mediation Process

Under IDEA (1997), mediation is a voluntary process that at a minimum must be available whenever a hearing is requested (34 C.F.R. § 300.506 [a]). Mediation is a process of formal discussion with a neutral third party to resolve

Table 8.1

Due Process Procedures

Process	Who May Initiate	For What Reason	Example
Mediation or Due Process Hearing	Parents or LEA	Disputes in identification, evaluation, educational placement, FAPE	To assess or not, amount of service, if service is needed, goals and objectives
State Complaints	Any organization or individual	Perceived violations of the law	Service not provided, amount of service on IEP not provided, timeline violation, notice of rights not given

differences. At the point that due process procedures are being used, emotions may be running high on either side of the case, and the mediator can help parties refocus on the issues. Many states had mediation available prior to 1997, but the IDEA reauthorization made the availability of this process mandatory.

Mediation is a state-level process. Each state maintains a list of qualified mediators. LEAs may establish procedures to encourage mediation for parents who elect not to participate in mediation after requesting a due process hearing. Such procedures might include arranging a meeting for parents with a neutral party, so that the benefits of mediation are explained and parents are encouraged to use the process (34 C.F.R. § 300.506 [d] [1] [ii]). New Jersey and Wisconsin are examples of states that have put information about due process procedures on the Internet, increasing accessibility to this information for parents. (New Jersey Department of Education, 1999; Wisconsin Special Education Mediation System, 2001)

To attempt to resolve issues prior to entering into a mediation process, some regional and local agencies provide ALTERNATIVE DISPUTE RESOLUTION (ADR). This follows a win-win type of process, acknowledging desires and limitations on both sides. This is a local-level process that occurs before a state-level mediation agency is involved. Mediation and ADR procedures may never be used to delay or deny the right to a due process hearing (34 C.F.R. § 300.506 [d] [z]).

> Speech-language pathologists and educators should understand that mediation may result in agreements that are highly unusual.

The mediation process involves parties from the school district and parties from the family meeting with a mediator. Depending on agency procedures and the case, a speech-language pathologist may or may not be involved in the mediation process. Discussions occurring during the process must be confidential and cannot be used in a due process hearing (34 C.F.R. § 300.506 [b] [6]). Both sides have an opportunity to tell the mediator their perspective of the dispute and what it would take to solve the dispute. If a solution cannot be reached with both parties, in the same room, the parties caucus independently with the mediator. The mediator goes back and forth between the two parties, attempting to reach a mediation agreement. Such an agreement must be put in writing (34 C.F.R. § 300.506 [b] [5]). The agreement may resolve all of the issues being brought forward, or it may resolve only some of the issues. If issues are not resolved, either of the parties may choose to proceed to a due process hearing.

Speech-language pathologists and educators should understand that mediation may result in agreements that are highly unusual. These agreements should be considered individualized in all cases, not precedent setting. For example, a speech-language pathologist may be required to make up missed therapy sessions. Although not precedent setting, the agreement will often change the way services are offered or documented districtwide to prevent problems in the future. Implementation of a specialized program might lead to others deducing the outcomes of an agreement, but all mediation agreements are confidential.

Impartial Due Process Hearings

With or without voluntary mediation, parents, students who have reached the AGE OF MAJORITY (age 18 in most states), and school districts are able to request an impartial due process hearing (also referred to as a fair hearing). Issues that can be resolved in a due process hearing are limited to issues involving the IEP process: identification, evaluation, educational placement, FAPE, and placement of a student in an interim alternative educational setting as a result of a disciplinary matter (Gorn, 1997b). School districts and parents should try to work with each other to avoid going to a hearing. In a small percentage of cases, however, a hearing will be held to decide the dispute. Some states, such as New Jersey, may offer prehearing conferences to help parents clearly understand the options of mediation, develop a settlement agreement, or define the issues for the hearing (New Jersey Department of Education, 1999).

A due process hearing is a formal procedure with a hearing officer who presides and listens to evidence presented by both sides. Often both sides are represented by attorneys. Unlike the mediation process, where parties have a neutral third party attempting to assist in developing a compromise, a due process hearing is like a court proceeding where evidence is presented and, ultimately, one side prevails. The general feeling about due process hearings is that in the long run no one really wins as there are so many hard feelings after these events.

School districts are typically reluctant to use their power to file for (i.e., request) a due process hearing against parents. In California, the education code (56346) reinforces a school district's affirmative duty to file for a due process hearing if the district believes that the actions of parents are resulting in the denial of FAPE to students. As explained previously, the right to FAPE belongs to students, not parents, and cannot be denied by the school district based on parental wishes (Maloney, 1997). In California, a district's failure to take parents to a hearing in such a case may result in the district later being ordered to provide compensatory education to students. This can happen if students file for due process once they reach the age of majority and prevail in a claim that FAPE was withheld.

Attorneys often become involved in cases that could lead to a hearing. All STATE EDUCATIONAL AGENCIES (SEAs) and LEAs are required to provide parents with information about low-cost legal services and other relevant services when parents request a due process hearing (34 C.F.R. § 300.507 [a] [3]). This is the responsibility of an administration, not a speech-language pathologist. In any situation where parents mention an intent to seek counsel from an attorney or advocate, the speech-language pathologist should notify a supervisor. Such a comment is considered a "red flag," indicating that parents are unhappy about something. Hopefully, the speech-language pathologist is aware of the specific concerns of the parent and can inform the administrator about them. In that way, once the administration is notified, attempts to resolve the issues can begin prior to the situation escalating.

Under IDEA (1997), parents can no longer seek reimbursement from a school district for their attorney's fees for attendance at an IEP meeting unless the meeting is ordered by a hearing officer or administrative law judge. A court may award attorney fees to parents when the parents are the prevailing party in a due process proceeding, meaning that one or more of their points are upheld. In such a situation, the school district will be responsible for the cost of attorneys on both sides (if both sides have attorneys) in addition to any costs involved (e.g., the costs of equipment, staff, or training that is found to be necessary) in the educational request of the parents (34 C.F.R. § 300.513 [a]).

Depending on agency procedures and the case, a speech-language pathologist may be involved in a mediation process leading up to the hearing. If a case goes to a due process hearing, the speech-language pathologist may be asked to testify. The situation is much like testifying in court. When school personnel are called to testify, most attorneys for the school district will prepare them prior to the hearing. This means that the speech-language pathologist testifying will know what to expect to the best of the attorney's knowledge. Statements of training and evidentiary information about education, background, documentation on student progress, and the like will probably be a part of the testimony. This is one reason why speech-language pathologists and special educators should be sure that they keep detailed records about

> [S]peech-language pathologists and special educators should be sure that they keep detailed records about student progress.

student progress and build treatment plans that are grounded in research-based protocols. The speech-language pathologist should rely on ASHA's (1997c) PREFERRED PRACTICE PATTERNS as a rationale for assessment and intervention methods (see Appendixes A and B).

Speech-language pathologists should be aware that every time a due process hearing is requested by either side, the procedural safeguard known as STAY PUT goes into effect. Stay put means that a student will remain in the educational placement he or she was in when the due process hearing request was filed unless the parties agree otherwise (34 C.F.R. § 300.514 [a]). For example, if an IEP calls for speech-language services twice a week for 40 minutes per session and the parents request a due process hearing, the amount of service remains the same (i.e., at present educational placement) until the matter is settled unless both parties agree otherwise through a mediation agreement (Gorn, 1997b).

Timelines apply when due process is initiated. States are required by IDEA (1997) to ensure that due process decisions are reached within 45 days of receipt of a request (34 C.F.R. § 300.511 [a]; 34 C.F.R. § 300.511 [a] [1]). If mediation is used, the parties may agree to an extension. The decision of the hearing officer is final unless appealed. In some states, the first appeal is to the SEA; in others, the appeal is directly to a state court of competent jurisdiction or federal court.

State IDEA Complaint Procedures

Complaint procedures can be used by families, staff, organizations, or individuals when violations of special education law occur (34 C.F.R. § 300.660 [a] [1]). Examples of common reasons complaints are filed include failure to provide records when requested or failure to implement an IEP. When parents are advised of their procedural due process rights, they must also be advised of the state complaint procedures (34 C.F.R. § 300.504 [b] [14]). This information is typically preprinted on parental-rights forms (California Department of Education, 1999e) and may be available on the Internet (e.g., New Jersey Department of Education, 1999, *http://www.state.nj.us/njded/parights/prise _b_w.pdf*). To file a complaint, a written letter must be sent to an SEA outlining the alleged violation. The SEA is required to respond, investigate, and issue a written decision within 60 days of receipt of the complaint. The time limit may be extended only if an exceptional circumstance exists in respect to a particular complaint (34 C.F.R. § 300.660).

Behavior and Student Discipline

Discipline Procedures

Safe schools have been one of the top concerns of citizens in America following the tragedies on school campuses that have become all too familiar news stories. Guidelines regarding the discipline of all students in a school setting are founded on the principle of due process of law:

> All student discipline must be accompanied by due process (Goss v. Lopez, 419 U.S. 565, 95 S. Ct 729 [1975]). The level of due process necessary will be determined by the severity of the sanction. But, before any sanction is imposed, the student must know what offense is charged and be given an opportunity to tell his or her side of the story. In the case of a relatively light sanction, such as detention, this entire process may take only a few minutes. But it must be complied with, to assure the school's right to impose discipline. (Collins and Dowell, 1998, p. 35)

Students receiving special education can be disciplined yet must be afforded due process of law when involved in a disciplinary action (Yell, Katsiyannis, Bradley, and Rozalski, 2000). Goss v. Lopez (1975), referred to by Collins and Dowell (1998) above, was the U.S. Supreme Court ruling that put into law the necessary components of due process for all student discipline. Honig v. Doe (1988) was a later Supreme Court ruling that required a MANIFESTATION DETERMINATION for students receiving special education prior to EXPULSION or long-term SUSPENSION. This means that before a student in special education participates in a district's regular discipline procedures, an IEP team must determine if the behavior for which the student is being disciplined was a manifestation of the student's disability and whether the student's placement was appropriate (see "Manifestation Determination").

All schools, school districts, and states have a code of conduct for their students. Most are similar to California's discipline code (see sidebar on page 252). Consequences for inappropriate actions are administered at the classroom level, with consequences of increasing severity for more significant violations under the educational code or policy of a district. The goal is to shape student behavior, encouraging them to learn appropriate behavior that allows them and those around them to learn.

Two types of removals are typically common in schools: suspension and expulsion. Suspension is the removal of a student from a classroom or a school for a limited period of time, usually 1 to 5 days. Expulsion refers to removal from the educational programs of a school district for a lengthy period of time, usually two semesters or longer, and is imposed by a school board or other governing body. Suspensions can be imposed by teachers and school principals and require a minimum of due

Functional Behavioral Assessment (FBA) and Behavior Intervention Plan (BIP)

IDEA (1997) instituted specific requirements to guarantee that IEP teams and school-based personnel work to remediate problematic behavior in students with disabilities. (34 C.F.R. § 300.520) Speech-language pathologists must be aware of requirements for conducting a functional behavioral assessment (FBA) and implementation of a behavioral intervention plan (BIP), which are necessary components of the IEP when a student is experiencing behavioral and/or discipline problems. A FBA is a systematic method of analyzing a student's behavior, examining when a student acts inappropriately and what circumstances precipitate the behavior. Most often, a school psychologist conducts the FBA, but the MDT is involved, especially those members who work with the student on a regular basis. The purpose of the FBA is to reveal patterns that predict the student's misbehavior. The FBA will consist of observations in a variety of settings, as well as interviews with staff and the parent(s) of the child, and, if appropriate, the student. One of the goals of the FBA is to discover situations that are reinforcing for the student. These situations will eventually become part of the behavior intervention plan (BIP). When the BIP is developed, the team will identify skills and strategies that need to be learned by the student. Speech-language pathologists may feel that their training did not encompass strategies for dealing with difficult behavior. In fact, communication strategies are frequently needed by students with maladaptive behavior (Sanger and Moore-Brown, 2000).

The IEP team should conduct an FBA whenever a student's challenging behavior is persistent despite implementation of generally successful behavior management techniques. Additionally, an FBA should be conducted whenever a student's behavior is harming him- or herself or others, and if his/her behavior is placing him at risk of, or subject to, disciplinary action, such as repeated suspensions or expulsion. Once a BIP is developed, consistent implementation is critical, especially to insure student success (Deveres and Pitasky, 1999a; Deveres and Pitasky, 1999b).

Although FBAs and BIPs are intended for use with any students who is presenting behavioral issues, specific regulations apply for students involved in disciplinary matters. If the student has been suspended for more than 10 days, manifestation determination provisions of the IDEA go into effect. Under these circumstances, the C.F.R. directs teams to conduct a FBA and develop a BIP if one is not already in place for the student , or to review the BIP if one is in place, and determine if modifications are necessary (34 C.F.R. § 300.520).

Grounds for Suspension and Expulsion

a. Caused, attempted to cause, or threatened to cause physical injury to another person or willfully used force or violence upon the person of another, except in self-defense

b. Possessed, sold, or otherwise furnished any firearm, knife, explosive, or other dangerous object

c. Unlawfully possessed, used, sold or otherwise furnished, or been under the influence of, any controlled substance, an alcoholic beverage or an intoxicant of any kind

d. Unlawfully offered, arranged, or negotiated to sell any controlled substance, an alcoholic beverage, or an intoxicant of any kind, and then either sold, delivered, or otherwise furnished to any person another liquid, substance, or material and represented the liquid, substance or material as a controlled substance, alcoholic beverage, or intoxicant

e. Committed or attempted to commit robbery or extortion

f. Caused or attempted to cause damage to school property or private property

g. Stole or attempted to steal school property or private property

h. Possessed or used tobacco, or any products containing tobacco or nicotine products

i. Committed an obscene act or engaged in habitual profanity or vulgarity

j. Had unlawful possession of, or unlawfully offered, arranged, or negotiated to sell any drug paraphernalia

k. Disrupted school activities or willfully defied the valid authority of school personnel

l. Knowingly received stolen school property or private property

m. Possessed an imitation firearm

n. Committed or attempted to commit a sexual assault

o. Harassed, threatened, or intimidated a student who is a complaining witness or witness in a school disciplinary proceeding

Additional Grounds: Sexual Harassment § 48900.2

§ 48900.3   Hate Violence

§ 48900.4   Harassment, Threats, or Intimidation (Grades 4–12 only)

§ 48900.7   Terroristic Threats

Mandatory Expulsion & Referral: § 48915 (c)

i.   Possession, selling, or otherwise furnishing a firearm

ii.   Brandishing a knife at another person

iii.   Unlawfully selling a controlled substance

iv.   Committing or attempting to commit a sexual assault or committing a sexual battery

Mandatory Recommendation for Expulsion: § 48915 (a)

i.   Causing serious physical injury to another person, except in self-defense

ii.   Possession of any knife, explosive, or other dangerous object of no reasonable use to the student

iii.   Unlawful possession of any controlled substance, except for the first offense for the possession of not more than one avoirdupois ounce of marijuana, other than concentrated cannabis

iv.   Robbery or extortion

v.   Assault or battery

Source: California Education Code 48900 (2000)

252

process. However, the number of days a child with a disability may be suspended without any educational services is limited to 10 cumulative days in a school year (34 C.F.R. § 300.121 [d]). Therefore, cumulative suspensions over 10 days require an IEP team meeting to respond to the change in placement and consider changes to the behavioral intervention plan. Expulsion can be imposed by a school board only and requires more extensive due process procedures, including a hearing where evidence is heard. Children with disabilities who are expelled from school must continue to receive FAPE (34 C.F.R. § 300.121 [a]). See "Home-Bound, Home-Schooled, Hospital-Bound, Suspended/Expelled, or Incarcerated Children and Youth" in Chapter 7 for further discussion of how to serve students who have been suspended or expelled.

Manifestation Determination

For students receiving special education, IDEA (1997) provides protections designed to ensure that students are not penalized for behavior that is manifested as part of their disability. Discipline procedures were specifically addressed in IDEA to make clear that speech-language pathologists and all special educators do have responsibilities in these matters. This includes participation in IEP meetings to determine if a student's behavior was a manifestation of his or her disability.

In situations when expulsion is recommended or required (e.g., carrying a weapon into school or to a school function or possessing or selling illegal drugs or controlled substances), a manifestation determination review must be conducted immediately, if possible, or no later than 10 school days after the decision to take disciplinary action. The purpose of the review is to determine the "relationship between the child's disability and the behavior subject to the disciplinary action" (34 C.F.R. § 300.523 [a] [2]).

An IEP team and other qualified persons must consider relevant evaluative and observational data, an IEP, and a student's placement. They use this information to determine if the IEP and placement was appropriate in terms of the behavior subject to disciplinary action. They also determine if the special education program and behavior intervention strategies were carried out as described in the student's IEP and placement. The team then determines if the child's disability impaired his or her ability "to understand the impact or consequences of the behavior" or "to control the behavior" (34 C.F.R. § 300.523 [c] [2] [i–iii]).

If a behavioral intervention plan was in place at the time of a serious incident, an IEP team must review the plan and decide if adjustments are needed (34 C.F.R. § 300.520 [b] [1] [ii]). If a functional behavioral analysis had not been conducted before the incident and a behavioral intervention plan did not exist, the IEP team must develop an assessment plan with the goal of developing a behavioral intervention plan (34 C.F.R. § 300.520 [b] [1] [i]).

Educators who are called to be a part of a manifestation determination review must consider what they know about the student and what could have been predicted about his or her behavior. For example, for a student with documented attention deficit hyperactivity disorder (ADHD), which manifests in impulsive action, it may be found that his or her impulsivity was responsible for the inappropriate action. In this case, the team could determine that the behavior was a manifestation of the disability and may also decide to revise the IEP to more effectively assist the student in coping with his or her impulsivity. However, impulsivity is likely not responsible if the same student was involved in an action that was planned over a number of days. In that case, the team may determine that the behavior was not a manifestation of the disability. A student who stutters may not have previously done anything that would have led IEP team members to believe that he or she would bring a knife to school. But a student with a pragmatic disorder may predictably be involved in an incident of disrespecting authority that might lead him or her to a disciplinary proceeding.

If an IEP team and other qualified personnel determine that an IEP or placement was deficient, immediate steps must be taken to "remedy those deficiencies" (34 C.F.R. § 300.523 [f]). If the group determines that the behavior was not a manifestation of the child's disability, then the usual discipline procedures may commence.

A common complaint about special education is that students cannot be disciplined—this is not true. However, procedural violations on the part of staff will stand out glaringly when a determination is made that a student's IEP was not being implemented and, therefore, the student will not be disciplined accordingly. In all situations involving student discipline, the speech-language pathologists must work closely with administrators to ensure that laws are followed. The manifestation determination review process is summarized in the sidebar.

Conclusive data are not available regarding whether students with disabilities are suspended or expelled more than their nondisabled peers. IDEA (1997) established requirements for states to begin collecting data in these areas (U.S. Department of Education, 1999). Speech-language pathologists might be involved in discipline cases due to the relationship between communication and violence (Sanger, Moore-Brown, and Alt, 2000.) Students with disabilities not only run the risk of being the perpetrators of misbehavior and violence but may also be victims, especially those students with cognitive impairments, LEARNING DISABILITIES, and emotional disturbances (U.S. Department of Education, 1999).

Working with Families

IDEA (1997) put additional emphasis on the importance of and requirements for working with families. Speech-language pathologists will find that the experience of working with families can vary greatly. No one will argue that parents are a critical part of the special program design and implementation of an IEP. Certain realities provide perspective and may be helpful when dealing with challenging situations. One reality is that parents and children have rights; school districts and school district personnel have legal obligations to ensure those rights (Gilyard, 1999). Another reality is that children do not choose the circumstances into which they are born. This applies to any circumstance, including economic, physical, or familial.

Manifestation Determination Reviews

When are manifestation determination reviews conducted?

A manifestation determination review is conducted when a student receiving special education is subject to the following disciplinary actions:

* Has been suspended for 10 school days (consecutive)

* Has been suspended for 10 school days (cumulative)

* Is recommended for expulsion.

Who conducts a manifestation determination review?

The IEP team members and other qualified personnel (34 C.F.R. § 300.523).

What is the timeline for conducting a manifestation determination review?

"Immediately, if possible, but in no case later than 10 school days after the date on which the decision to take that action is made...." (34 C.F.R. § 300.523)

What does the review consist of?

(1) First consider, in terms of the behavior subject to disciplinary action, all relevant information, including:

(i) Evaluation and diagnostic results, including the results or other relevant information supplied by the parents of the child

(ii) Observations of the child

(iii) The child's IEP and placement

(2) Then determine that:

(i) In relationship to the behavior subject to disciplinary action, the child's IEP and placement were appropriate and the special education services, supplementary aids and services, and behavioral intervention strategies were provided consistent with the child's IEP and placement

(ii) The child's disability did not impair the ability of the child to understand the impact and consequences of the behavior subject to disciplinary action

(iii) The child's disability did not impair the ability of the child to control the behavior subject to disciplinary action (34 C.F.R. § 300.523)

What if the IEP team meets and determines that the behavior was related to the student's disability, or that the placement was inappropriate, or that the student was unable to determine right from wrong?

If the any of the review standards are not met, the behavior is determined to be a manifestation of the disability. The student cannot be subject to the relevant disciplinary procedure. If the public agency has identified deficiencies in the child's IEP or placement, it must remedy them immediately.

What if the IEP team determines that the behavior is not a manifestation of the student's disability and that placement was appropriate and the student was able to determine the consequences of his or her behavior?

Then the student can be disciplined in the same manner as nondisabled students, with the exception that FAPE must continue to be provided.

What other requirements exist?

If a behavioral intervention plan was in place at the time of the incident, then the IEP team must convene a meeting to review the plan. If a functional behavioral analysis had not been conducted prior to the incident, and a behavioral intervention plan did not exist, the IEP team must develop an assessment plan toward the goal of developing such a plan.

Speech-language pathologists will discover that there are a multitude of family situations. Communication impairments affect the entire family constellation. When working with children, considering the impact of their disability on their home lives, in addition to their school lives, helps speech-language pathologists understand the big picture of the impact of the disability. The role of school-based intervention is to improve educationally related difficulties. However, since communication is at the heart of relationships and learning, both at school and at home, expanded understandings can promote effective interventions.

Working with families can put speech-language pathologists in some trying situations, such as being the person who confirms the presence of a disability or having to share data with parents that presents a child as being more impaired than the family may be prepared to accept. When specialists are dealing with parents, the circumstances can be sensitive. Children are the most precious connection to a parent's being.

Dealing with difficult issues regarding children can be rewarding and challenging at the same time. A reality of the entire IEP process, including assessment, identification, eligibility determination, and intervention, is that educators participate in IEPs as a part of the professional team. For parents, this is a part of their personal life. Participation in this process is new, frequently confusing, and even intrusive. As a school professional, it is a speech-language pathologist's job to work with parents in designing and carrying out an educational program for a child. Attorney Lawrence Siegel, a special education attorney and advocate, advised parents as follows:

Advocating for your child is easy. You want the best for her. Still, there will be bumps along the way. The IEP process is maze-like, involving a good deal of technical information, intimidating professionals and confusing choices. For some families, it goes smoothly, with no disagreements; for others, it is a terrible encounter in which you and your school district cannot even agree on the time of day. For most people, the experience is somewhere in between. (1999, p. 1/3)

Speech-language pathologists may find that the circumstances in a home are not conducive to supporting education. There may be no one available to assist a child with homework; books or other printed material may not be available, or the parents may be illiterate or experience a disability themselves. A child's linguistic development may be adversely affected in a home where the primary language is other than English or where cultural differences exist. Low socioeconomic homes likely have limited or poor access to health care. This may mean that medical situations that might lead to learning disabilities or communication impairments are not treated, exacerbating the situation. These examples do not mean that all children from low socioeconomic or culturally diverse situations are at risk of developing COMMUNICATION DISORDERS, but when evaluating such children, it is important to distinguish difference versus disorder versus delay. (See Chapter 3 for a discussion of dynamic assessment and Chapter 7 for further information on students who are CULTURALLY/LINGUISTICALLY DIVERSE [CLD].)

Parent Involvement

Children have a wide range of family constellations; family can mean any number and relationship of people who are involved with taking care of a child. Regardless of the circumstances, speech-language pathologists must remember that only parents or legal guardians assigned educational rights can sign for permission to assess or consent to placement in an IEP. Even when children have been removed from parental custody, parents may still retain educational rights. This is regulated differently in each state, so be sure to check state laws for clarification on this.

If children do not have a custodial parent, LEAs will assign a surrogate parent. Surrogate parents are individuals who have received specialized training and are assigned by the school district to represent children in all matters relating to children's identification, evaluation, placement, and provision of FAPE (34 C.F.R. § 300.515 [e]). When children are placed through court action in a licensed child-care institution (e.g., a group home) or a foster home, birth parents may still have educational rights, even if children do not live with these parents. These situations can become very complex for care providers, school people, children, and birth parents. Additionally, the dynamics of these situations can be trying. Speech-language pathologists should enlist the assistance of a supervisor when questions arise regarding parental status.

Parents may react in any variety of ways when asked to be involved in educational planning for children. Speech-language pathologists may work with parents in any of the following situations:

- Parents who do not respond to phone calls or do not come to appointments or IEP meetings. These parents may seem not to care, but may also have other demands that prevent active participation. IDEA (1997) requires holding meetings at a mutually agreed on time when parents can attend but does not require undue hardship of staff. Teleconferencing is allowed if that is the only way that parents can participate in their child's IEP.

- Parents who are grateful for the help and appreciative of the assistance of the specialists involved with their child. These parents may even be too passive in their acceptance of the information shared. The goal in all situations is to make parents partners in evaluation, planning, and treatment. Parents of this type may at first seem to be the most cooperative with which to work but are likely not carrying through at home or recognizing their role in their child's education.

- Parents who are active team members and bring ideas and suggestions to planning sessions. These parents are usually actively involved in home programs established for their child.

- Parents who are active team members and bring ideas and suggestions to planning sessions but may bring ideas that are contrary to those brought forward by professionals. This type of situation may be more challenging for professionals. This can lead to a situation that may be on the path to mediation or a due process hearing. Under no circumstances should ideas brought forth by parents be dismissed or not discussed. Seek assistance as soon as a situation appears to be adversarial or one that will create dissent. In all cases, listen closely, seek more information, and document what parents are requesting.

• Parents who are adversarial or mistrustful of the IEP process and may be confrontational or uncooperative. These types of people are challenging in any walk of life; however, in special education, a federal law requires that parents and school people work together. The next section gives some suggestions on strategies to use in difficult situations.

These generalities are likely exaggerations of any situation but do represent differing types of situations that speech-language pathologists should be prepared to encounter. In any of these situations, strategies that focus a group on the needs of children can help to improve the situation. The U.S. Department of Education (1999) reports that school personnel behavior can influence parental participation in either a positive or inhibiting way:

Research indicates that the overwhelming majority of parents of children with disabilities are involved in their children's education through meetings with teachers, volunteering at school, helping

with homework, or other school- and home-based activities. Educators may enhance levels of parent involvement by establishing on-going relationships with parents, teaching parents about their rights under IDEA, and using specific strategies to promote involvement. (pp. I-11–I-12)

Strategies for Avoiding or Managing Conflict

Training programs and literature in the field often do not prepare speech-language pathologists for work situations that involve conflict. Working in special education can at times be sensitive and perhaps even contentious due to the trying nature of the work: parents are struggling to adjust to the nature of their children's disabilities; general educators are attempting to work with these children as students in their classrooms while attending to the needs of the other students and demands for improved student performance; and special educators are grappling with increased student needs, demands for accountability and outcomes, and paperwork that can seem overwhelming. Administrators are trying to balance all of these needs and be fiscally accountable. Stressors exist at every level.

In training programs, speech-language pathologists learn how to use a scientific method to approach the disabilities presented by students. In many ways, approaching difficult situations should be viewed in much the same manner while adding heart, understanding, and patience. IDEA (1997) provides for a team approach to planning for and working with children. In the best of all possible worlds, all people come to their roles in the team equally prepared to work together and use solid, up-to-date information and research-based methods to help students. In such a scenario, the team acknowledges the importance of each person's role, including the valuable role parents play.

IEP teams, like any other team, are made up of individuals who each bring differing backgrounds and experiences to their responsibilities. In such circumstances, difficulties can arise. Some of these are unique to the situation of special education, others are unique to education in general, and some are characteristic of working with difficult people. For the latter circumstance, speech-language pathologists may find taking a workshop on working with difficult people useful. For the other circumstances,

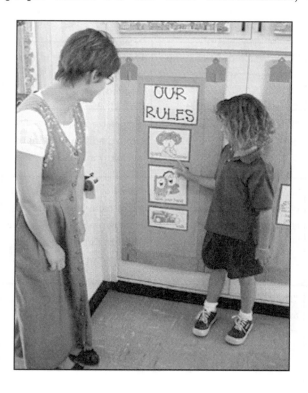

speech-language pathologists would be wise to watch and learn from those who have successfully worked under such situations for several years (e.g., fellow speech-language pathologists, mentor teachers, principals, or other administrators). These people have developed skills and abilities that can be learned and applied when necessary.

Chapter 4 describes an IEP as a process. Involving all parties as part of the process can help to achieve a "win-win" situation. All parties have a stake in the agreement reached with the IEP document. In an ideal scenario, all parties come to the process with something to contribute and respecting the input of others, and the process goes well. However, in some situations, this scenario does not occur. In these less than ideal cases, team members should examine issues that might confound successful teamwork to decide how to approach the process. Table 8.2 (see pages 260–261) offers some possible issues that speech-language pathologists may need to respond to when administrators, special educators, and other staff bring them to the IEP process. Some of these issues are hidden, while others are quite apparent. This table is certainly not exhaustive, but it encapsulates the types of situations that might arise.

Having a global perspective of how to approach difficult situations can provide team members with a method to deal with the types of issues and statements presented in Table 8.2. Alternative dispute resolution approaches were mentioned in the section on mediation (see page 246). Such strategies may be necessary in IEP meetings when the meetings necessitate negotiations. A successful business

Table 8.2

Strategies for IEP Team Member Issues

Disgruntled IEP Team Member	Possible Issue	Characteristic Statement	Suggested Strategy
General Education Teacher	Does not want to work with the student	"You know, I have 30 other students in my classroom."	Offer consultative support with specific times to meet
	Does not believe that it is his or her job to work with special education students	"It wouldn't be fair to the other students in the class if we made exceptions for Bobby."	Discuss "fairness," discuss and problem-solve issues of concern, have in-class support services to demonstrate methodologies
	Overwhelmed by other job demands	"I'm just not sure when I would have time to do this."	Discuss and problem-solve issues of concern, outline specific requirements, offer assistance with documentation
	Scared he or she does not know what to do with the student	"I'm not really the person who would know how to work with this type of problem."	Offer training, offer consultation, demystify the disorder and expectations
	Fearful of criticism/Lack of ownership	"We never receive any support when we do this."	Query what type of support is thought to be needed
	Cannot believe the referred student does not qualify for special education	"What am I supposed to do?"	Suggest accommodations/modifications/instructional methods to use
Special Education Teacher	High caseload	"It's hard for me to individualize with so many students to serve."	Assist with schedule; add extra time, if appropriate; review placement of other students in class
	Burnout/Not feeling supported	"They always give me the tough kids."	Acknowledge hard work

Table 8.2—*Continued*

Disgruntled IEP Team Member	Possible Issue	Characteristic Statement	Suggested Strategy
	Not having the skills to work with student's needs	"I've never had a student like this." "No one knows how hard my job is."	Offer training/staff development/program manager's support
Administrator	Concerned that special education takes too much time	"I have a whole campus to run."	Acknowledge how busy the administrator is
	Concerned about teachers	"I don't know how you can expect these teachers to do this."	Attempt to make concerns specific
Parents	In one of the grieving stages: shock/denial, anger (inward), anger (outward), depression, acceptance	"I don't believe you." "He can do that at home."	Remind parents that we are all on the same side, defuse the situation, remind parents that IEPs are temporary documents—they can always be rewritten
	Do not believe that anything can be done for their child	"My child doesn't belong in one of those classes." "My child is not like those children." "I'm the parent; I know my child the best."	Ask: "What part don't you believe?", discuss instructional methods and that there are different kinds of abilities/disabilities, agree that the parents are the experts on the child

book about negotiations, *Getting to Yes: Negotiating Agreement without Giving In* (Fisher, Ury, and Patton, 1991), provides an excellent methodology for working through such situations:

Any method of negotiation may be fairly judged by three criteria: It should produce a wise agreement if agreement is possible. It should be efficient. And it should improve or at least not damage the relationship between the parties. (A wise agreement can be defined as one that meets the legitimate interests of each side to the extent possible, resolves conflicting interests fairly, is durable, and takes community interests into account.) (p. 4)

These authors were not describing IEP meetings, but they might have been. Team members need to clearly understand everyone's roles (see "Who Comprises the IEP Team?" in Chapter 4) as involvement of parents, students, and general education teachers increases. When more people become involved in the team process, more perspectives are considered, which should be an advantage. Involvement of more people should mean more people focusing on what is needed for a student. When members do not have a common focus, the method outlined by Fisher et al. (1991) will be helpful. Their method, developed at the Harvard Negotiation Project, is known as Principled Negotiations, and is comprised of four primary parts:

> **Failure to find ways to implement appropriate IEPs can have serious consequences for school districts.**

People: Separate the people from the problem.

Interests: Focus on interests, not positions.

Options: Generate a variety of possibilities before deciding what to do.

Criteria: Insist that the result be based on some objective standard. (p. 10)

An IEP is not meant to be a contentious process. IDEA (1997) is silent on the conduct of the meeting, outlining only what should be addressed at the meeting (34 C.F.R. § 300.343). Siegel (1999) gives parents information on how to advocate for their children through an IEP process. Educators need to be equally informed on how to work through difficult issues and utilizing the Fisher et al. (1991) method may help. Failure to find ways to implement appropriate IEPs can have serious consequences for school districts, such as requiring reimbursement for the costs of private school placements, compensatory education, or damages (Bateman and Linden, 1998). When team members do not agree on IEP issues, what is sacrificed is the appropriate education of students.

In order to remove barriers and develop successful parent-school partnerships, the U.S. Department of Education (1999) recommended the following:

- Improve communication among parents, teachers, and administrators.

- Tap [into] parents' expertise.

- Involve families in community-based intervention/instruction. (pp. I-13–I-14)

Successful parent-school partnerships will contribute to IEPs that better identify student needs and methods to effectively meet those needs. When working through difficult IEP processes and implementing the methods of Fisher et al. (1991), speech-language pathologists and IEP teams may find the following strategies useful:

- Always check with participants about what is being documented. For example, if parents and school staff see a behavior differently, then document both points of view (e.g., "School staff report that Sally does not speak at school. She uses gestures to express her wants and needs. Parents report that Sally uses one- and two-word phrases at home to express her wants and needs.")

- Be sure that recommended goals and objectives or BENCHMARKS are founded on research-based practices, so that the rationale for their recommendation can be explained to other IEP team members.

- When team members disagree on recommended services or goals, attempt to agree on a short-term solution (e.g., agree to small group services three times per week for three months rather than a full year).

- Set a meeting time for two to three months in the future to address or re-address sensitive issues.

- Keep meeting notes for all IEPs. Always document parental comments and requests.

- Always begin meetings by identifying what issues are to be discussed and what process will be used. Always ask parents what issues they would like discussed at the meeting.

- Be sure everyone is comfortable with the language used (English or other) or have interpreter services available.

- Use a flip chart or white board to write issues and illustrate discussion items. This is particularly helpful when drafting goals, illustrating students' schedules, and writing topics that need to be covered.

- Make every attempt to resolve disagreements between professionals prior to a meeting. In other words, do not engage in professional debates in front of parents.

- Begin with one or two items everyone can agree on to set a positive tone.

- Offer to have weekly or bi-monthly (i.e., every other week) meetings of one or more members of the school team to check progress.

- If there is a time constraint for the meeting, identify it at the beginning. Keep track of the time throughout the meeting, as well as what still needs to be addressed.

- Write all decisions into the IEP document.

- If feelings run very high, suggest a five-minute break for fresh air, a drink of water, or a quick change of scene.

- Always thank everyone for being in attendance at the meeting.

- Remember that everyone has students' best interests at heart. There just may be different versions of how to achieve them.

- Smile, use a sense of humor (as appropriate), and shake hands.

Federal Laws That Prohibit Disability Discrimination

Section 504 and the Americans with Disabilities Act (ADA)

Two federal laws that are not specific to education have had an effect on school programs and facilities. SECTION 504 of the REHABILITATION ACT of 1973 was passed to prohibit discrimination against individuals with disabilities by any program receiving federal financial assistance. The AMERICANS WITH DISABILITIES ACT (ADA) was passed in 1990 to strengthen the access requirements of Section 504 and extend them to all public domains.

ADA (1990) and Section 504 (1973) issues frequently are related. ADA deals with access to buildings, facilities, and transportation and includes the provision of auxiliary aids and services to individuals with vision or HEARING IMPAIRMENTS. Provisions under Section 504 include anything required to enable access to an instructional program, including modifications to the learning environment and materials to meet the needs of students who have identified disabilities. ADA, Section 504, and IDEA (1997) overlap in places.

Until the 1990s, Section 504 (1973) was not commonly applied to students in schools. Since school districts receive federal assistance, however, this act applied to these agencies. Section 504 of the Rehabilitation Act of 1973 requires that:

No qualified handicapped person shall, on the basis of handicap, be excluded from participation in, be denied the benefits of, or otherwise be subjected to discrimination under any program or activity which receives Federal financial assistance. (Office for Civil Rights [OCR], 1999, § 104.4 [a])

Some children may receive speech-language services under Section 504 (1973) instead of special education. Speech-language pathologists who work in schools need to know the legal and procedural basis for this provision of services as it is quite different from special education. Both IDEA (1997) and Section 504 protect students' civil rights. IDEA, however, provides federal funding and describes the procedural requirements required to receive this funding at state and local levels. Section 504 does not provide funding, so schools must use local resources to provide any services or facilities that help students with disabilities access school programs.

A significant difference between the laws, in relation to school age students with disabilities, is the eligibility criteria. The IDEA protects only students who, by virtue of their disabilities, require special educational services. Section 504, however, prohibits discrimination against all school age children, regardless of whether or not they require special education services. (Gorn, 1997a, p. 11:2).

All individuals who are disabled under the Individuals with Disabilities Education Act (IDEA) are also considered to be disabled, and therefore protected, under Section 504/ADA. However, all individuals who have been determined to be disabled under Section 504 may not be disabled under IDEA. These children require a response from the regular education staff and curriculum. With respect to most students with disabilities, many aspects of the Section 504 regulation concerning FAPE parallel the requirements of the Individuals with Disabilities Education Act (formerly the Education of All Handicapped Children Act) and state law (Council of Administrators of Special Education [CASE], 1999b, pp. 1–2).

ADA (1990) deals with accessibility to public domains (including communication access) and "prohibits discrimination on the basis of disability in employment, programs and services provided by state and local governments, goods and services provided by private companies, and in commercial facilities" (U.S. Department of Justice, 1999, ¶ 1).

In communities and employment situations, ADA (1990) issues may become part of the work of speech-language pathologists in schools, particularly when dealing with TRANSITION to postsecondary settings. For example, a student who is DEAF may need a telephone decoding device (TDD) to communicate at a work site. Recent and future advances in telecommunications provide additional accessibility for individuals with communication impairments to be successful in the workplace and these must be made available by employers as they become reasonable to acquire. Schools

and public facilities must provide physical access for persons using wheelchairs or who have other mobility impairments (e.g., ramps and elevators); signs must be accessible to persons with visual impairments (e.g., Braille); safety features must be accessible to all (e.g., flashing lights on fire alarms); and facilities, such as water fountains, sinks, toilets, and light switches, must be accessible from various heights and clearances.

Responsibilities to Students under Section 504

Coverage under Section 504 (1973) is much broader than the eligibility criteria under IDEA (1997). An individual who is considered disabled under Section 504:

- Has a physical or mental impairment that substantially limits one or more major life activities, including "walking, seeing, hearing, speaking, breathing, learning, working, caring for oneself and performing manual tasks"

- Has a record of such impairment

- Is regarded as having such impairment (CASE, 1999b, p. 7)

To determine if a student is covered under Section 504 (1973), a data-gathering process that considers information from many available sources is used. The individuals involved with this evaluation process are those who are familiar with the student and the information considered and comprise the 504 team. The team then meets and determines if the student is considered disabled under the provisions of Section 504.

Section 504 (1973) requires public agencies (i.e., school districts) to provide FAPE in the LEAST RESTRICTIVE ENVIRONMENT (LRE) to any student with a disability that limits a major life function. "'Appropriate education' means an education comparable to the education provided to nondisabled students, requiring that accommodations be made" (CASE, 1999b, p. 8). A written plan is not required under Section 504 but is considered "good professional practice" (CASE, 1999b, p. 8). This accommodation plan should address five areas:

1. Nature of the student's disability and the major life activity it limits.

2. The basis for determining the disability.

3. The educational impact of the disability.

4. Necessary accommodations.

5. Placement in the least restrictive environment. (Gorn, 1997a, pp. 11:4–11:5)

As previously stated, students identified under IDEA (1997) automatically have the protections offered under Section 504 (1973) (CASE, 1999b, pp. 1–2). However, students who are identified as disabled using Section 504 procedures usually do not need the special education services offered under IDEA (Zirkel, 2000). Examples of such situations would be students with attention deficit disorder (ADD) who do not demonstrate a learning disability under IDEA, or who are not found to qualify under other health impairment or other eligibility criteria considered in IDEA. The accommodation plan would identify the necessary modifications and accommodations needed to allow the students to access their education. (See Table 8.3 for examples.)

If a student is found by an IEP team to be ineligible for special education, parents and teachers might advocate for the student to be identified as disabled under Section 504 (1973) with the goal of having the student receive special education and RELATED SERVICES through Section 504.

Technically, students identified under Section 504 (1973) cannot be denied special education services. However, if a student's needs are so significant that special education services are required, then an IEP team should identify that student under IDEA (1997). Accommodations and modifications, such as those identified in Table 8.3, do not need to meet IDEA eligibility for implementation, because they can be accomplished using general education staff and resources. Gorn (1997b) explained that "a speech impairment will not always trigger eligibility under either the IDEA or the more inclusive Section 504" (p. 1:9) due to the requirements for adversely affecting educational performance (under IDEA [1997]) or substantially impairing a major life activity (under Section 504 [1973]). A child with a tongue thrust, for example, would probably not qualify under either law, but only the school 504 team could make that determination.

Table 8.3

Section 504 Examples

Identified Disability	Major Life Activity Affected	Accommodations Provided
Attention deficit disorder	Learning	Shortened assignments Reminder prompts Learning center/Study carrel Timer Reinforcers Planning chart on desk Reminder binder Phone message from teacher to parent regarding homework assignments After-school tutoring Peer counseling
Asthma	Breathing	Adjusted physical education requirements, per doctor's orders Modified assignments for physical education Health plan developed for medication needs
Spinal tumor	Working, performing manual tasks	Extra time between classes Peer assistant to take notes Adjusted assignments (due to fatigue) Teacher calls at night to discuss assignments with parents, child, or both Homework club

CHAPTER 9

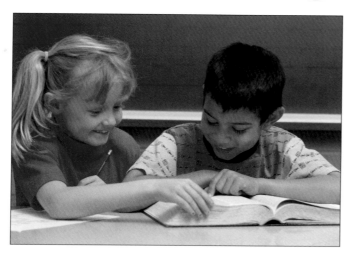

The Work World of Speech-Language Pathologists in Public Schools

IN THIS CHAPTER

The purpose of this chapter is to consider some of the practical and professional issues that impact school-based speech-language pathologists, to develop an understanding of the school environment and how it works, and to describe how to work effectively in a school environment. Topics include how to obtain a position, roles and responsibilities of speech-language pathologists and assistants, where to go for assistance, and a variety of professional and organizational issues that are characteristic of a public education system. This chapter is also intended to provide a school-based perspective to the speech-language pathologist exploring a career as an educational professional working in the child's natural environment.

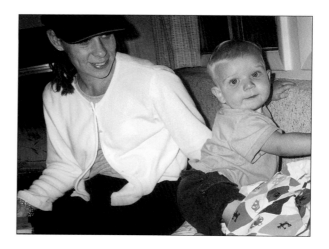

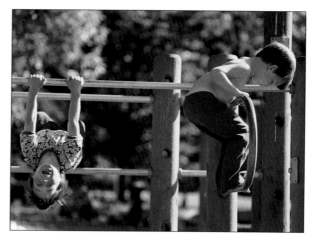

1. Discuss why providing private paid therapy for students from your school caseload on Saturdays would be unethical. What policies would be violated and which speech-language pathologist certifications could be endangered?

2. What does it mean to receive Medicaid payment for speech-language and hearing services in schools? If this is a practice in your area, invite a school-based speech-language pathologist to share the way the program works and how it can be structured as a benefit for children with disabilities, and for the speech-language staff in a district.

3. Review the licensing requirements for speech-language pathologists for your state. What do you need to know about your state license to practice in the schools?

4. Do your state's licensure rules address assistants or support personnel? Why or why not? What value might they provide to a school setting? How would you utilize their skills?

5. Why should school-based practitioners belong to more than one professional organization?

6. Does your state have labor unions in the schools? Why or why not? How are the school-based speech-language pathologists that you know represented in negotiations for salary and working conditions?

7. Practice answering the interview questions presented in this chapter.

8. Interview a speech-language pathologist from a local school system. Discuss the organizational structures in that school system. Who evaluates the speech-language pathologist? Where does the speech-language pathologist find help, assistance, support? Report your findings.

9. Review the list of roles and responsibilities (beginning on page 286) and discuss your impression of this list. What roles do you consider particularly interesting? Are there any that seem less familiar to you?

10. Discuss why the prudent professional carries liability insurance.

Certification and Licensing

The world of schools requires a specialized understanding of how "the system" works and what it means to be an employee in a public school. The system consists of national, state, and local regulations. Before being hired by a school, a speech-language pathologist applying for a job (see "Securing a Position" on page 274) must make certain he or she has completed all the necessary requirements and paperwork for CERTIFICATION, LICENSING, or both. Understanding the requirements of the school environment will help speech-language pathologists be more effective and make meaningful contributions to the students and staff there.

National Certification

The Certificate of Clinical Competence (CCC) was established in 1952 by the AMERICAN SPEECH-LANGUAGE-HEARING ASSOCIATION (ASHA). This national certification requires a graduate degree, 36 weeks of supervised clinical practice, and a passing score on the National Examination in Speech Pathology and Audiology through the Education Testing Service. Although ASHA certification is voluntary, it is recommended because holding the CCC indicates to potential employers that speech-language pathologists are committed to providing quality services since its holders have met the standards of excellence established by this national organization. ASHA certification is typically required in health care, private practice, or other settings that receive third-party reimbursement, since MEDICARE and Medicaid require ASHA certification for reimbursement. At a national level, the CCC permits its holders to provide independent clinical services and to supervise the clinical practice of students studying speech-language pathology and uncertified clinicians. States have the option to require the speech-language pathologist to have the CCC and hold membership in ASHA in order to supervise SPEECH-LANGUAGE PATHOLOGY ASSISTANTS (SLPAs), monitor a student teacher, participate in ASHA data collection projects, or oversee a colleague completing a Clinical Fellowship (CF). In addition, those who have earned the CCC in speech-language pathology have the verified knowledge and skills to work as speech-language pathologists in many settings worldwide including American schools and military schools abroad. Some countries (e.g., the United Kingdom) have reciprocity agreements that recognize the CCC.

While certification is important to establish credibility, licensing is required in many states to legally practice speech-language pathology. In most states, ASHA certification satisfies many of the state requirements for licensure. In fact, in several states, ASHA's certification standards are the only requirement for licensure (ASHA, 2000e).

State Licensing

A school district may not use ASHA's CCC as verification that the individual is appropriately qualified if the state department of education only recognizes its state's certification(s). Some school districts do require the CCC in addition to any state requirements.

Over 40 states require a license to practice speech-language pathology in nonschool settings. LICENSING is designed to serve as a protection for the public, assuring consumers that professionals in states requiring a license meet a minimum standard of education and preparation. Only Hawaii, Arizona, and Ohio have universal licensure, requiring that all speech-language pathologists in schools and health care be licensed. In these states, the license can also serve as a state teaching permit.

Teacher Certification

Each STATE EDUCATIONAL AGENCY (SEA) requires a credential that shows that a speech-language pathologist has completed a course of study in a university communication disorders program with certain elements, courses, and field experiences approved by that state. These state authorizations may be called teacher permits, teaching certificates, teacher licenses, or clinical service credentials. In this way, the SEA has final approval of all speech-language pathologists who work with students in that state.

Speech-language pathologists must have some type of state teacher certification to work in a public school setting. Some states have reciprocity with other states (e.g., New England states have reciprocity with each other), but most states only accredit their own state universities and their own teaching staff. Speech-language pathologists must have a state teaching or clinical license to bill a third party, such as an insurance company or Medicaid, for a student's services in schools.

Ideally, school-based speech-language pathologists should possess all three creden-

tials—ASHA's CCC, a state license, and teacher certification—in states that have licensure; however, the legal requirement is to hold whatever state certification is needed for providing speech-language services in a particular state's public schools. The requirements for the three credentials do overlap, especially academic requirements, clinical clock hour requirements, and the required professional year(s) of supervised practice. Simultaneously completing these national and state requirements early on is easier than trying to return to a university to complete one or more credentials later in one's career, since test scores often become outdated and logs of courses and hours can be misplaced or lost.

The current requirements for ASHA's CCC are available at the ASHA Web site (www.asha.org), as is an overview of teacher licensing requirements for each state and contact information for each SEA. Applications for a state teacher certificate must be requested from each SEA, and licensing applications must be requested from the state licensing panel or board, usually housed in a social services or health-care department. Although the requirements for certification and licensing might initially appear confusing, Table 9.1 should help school-based speech-language pathologists understand the details of certification and licensing and encourage them to acquire all three certificates.

An Ideal Timeline

Typically, candidates who intend to work in the public schools complete their bachelor's degree in COMMUNICATION DISORDERS, become full-time graduate students, attain their master's degree,

Table 9.1

Certification and Licensing Comparisons

Certification	Agency	Purpose	Academic Preparation	Test	Practica	Renewal	Required for School Services
Certificate of Clinical Competence (CCC)	American Speech-Language-Hearing Association (ASHA)	Recognize clinical competence	Graduate degree in the discipline	NESPA	250 hours clinical practicum, and 36 weeks of supervision on the job	Pay fee every year	No
Speech-language pathology license	Designated state agency	Protect the public from untrained practitioners	Determined by the state, many mirror the ASHA guidelines for the CCC	NESPA	1–2 years of supervision on the job	Pay fee every year or every other year plus obtain CEUs in 38 states	Only in states with universal licensure
Teacher certification	State Educational Agencies	Assure that students are taught by persons with uniform education	Varies from state to state, usually includes a fifth year or a graduate degree to acquire education courses	State teacher test of basic skills in some states	Student teaching—usually 12–18 weeks	Pay fee between 3 and 5 years plus obtain CEUs, develop a portfolio and a personal plan, or meet other needs depending on state	Yes

pass the national examination (e.g., the National Examination in Speech Pathology and Audiology [NESPA]), complete their CF during their first year on the job, meet ASHA's certification requirements, and apply for their other certifications by the end of their first year of work. This process may take longer for some candidates to accomplish than others. Some states do not require a master's degree in communication disorders for candidates to begin working in public schools; however, this is not endorsed by ASHA nor is it recommended by professionals in the field.

Some candidates choose to enroll in a master's degree program; apply for a teaching credential in their states; then work toward their CCC, license, and full state certification (a multiple-step process in some states) during their first three to five years of working in the schools. School-based speech-language pathologists may need to meet extra requirements for the state credentials and often must meet requirements of their school districts as well.

Speech-language pathologists must realize how important it is to schedule these personal benchmarks carefully and completely, with guidance from mentors in the school district and a graduate-school advisor. This scheduling may help speech-language pathologists avoid suddenly realizing that they cannot finish all the requirements in the first year and then lose the momentum needed to complete the academic preparation. Many candidates report that keeping the goal in sight can be hard, especially when others in the school community do not have to earn two more certifications after earning their teaching credentials. However, the CCC and the state license (in states with licensure) are critical steps in the preparation of a fully qualified speech-language pathologist. In order to work through a three- to five-year plan for completing these three certifications, speech-language pathologists will find it imperative to keep complete and accurate records of all courses, classes, clock hours, registered supervision plans, and test scores in a personal file for solid documentation. It is always the candidate's responsibility to provide proof of meeting all requirements.

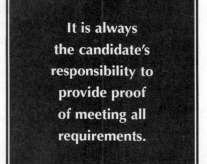

It is always the candidate's responsibility to provide proof of meeting all requirements.

Securing a Position

Shortages of special education teachers were documented in the *Twentieth* and *Twenty-First Annual Reports to Congress on the Implementation of the Individuals with Disabilities Education Act* (U.S. Department of Education, 1998, 1999). School districts throughout the country have testified to the need for speech-language pathologists. One of the challenges to school districts is that while substitute teachers can be put in SPECIAL EDUCATION and other classrooms, no one can substitute for a speech-language pathologist. The shortage issue was even the topic of the lead article, "How to Address the Shortage of Speech and Language [sic] Pathologists," in *The Special Educator* ("How to address the shortage," 1999), a newsletter commonly subscribed to by special education administrators. The article reports, "the nationwide shortage of speech and language [sic] pathologists has forced school districts to generate some unorthodox and creative ways to fulfill IEP requirements" (p. 1). The 1999 Workforce Study, commissioned by ASHA, projected that shortages would decrease by the year 2005 (1999d). This study did not, however, take into account employment areas, such as schools versus hospitals, nor did it account for rural, urban, or regional differences. Public school speech-language pathologists are still needed in many areas of the country, and many of these regions anticipate continuing shortages in the future.

The Application

Obtaining a job in a school setting is often a very formal process. Schools typically have an application process for all prospective employees that can be obtained from a personnel or human resources department. Before submitting an application to a LOCAL EDUCATIONAL AGENCY (LEA), the applicant may wish to determine if that agency has a speech-language opening. Such information can be discovered by calling the agency's personnel or human resources department, calling the special education department of the LEA, searching for job postings on a Web site (e.g., ASHA, your state speech-language-hearing association, the Council for Exceptional Children, your state department of education, local school districts, regional service agencies, or Web sites that specialize in posting employment opportunities), looking at job postings at a local university, or reviewing national or regional publications with classified advertisements.

Include a cover letter with all applications. In this letter, state what type of position is being sought, qualifications for the position (i.e., certification and licensing), and why there is an interest in that particular agency. This letter should be short, no more than one page, but should allow readers to see qualifications that might interest them as an employer. Emphasize interest and eagerness to work with children. Identify any specialized training received while in graduate school or any other unique experiences that show involvement with education or children.

In addition to the cover letter, most applications include an essay question. Such questions will typically be broad in scope, for example, "Describe your belief system about education," or "Describe some noteworthy experience you have had in the last three years," or "Who was the person who most influenced your decision to become a teacher?" Time and consideration should be taken in answering any essay question. The response is a prime opportunity to communicate interests, energy, and beliefs about education, special education, and speech-language pathology in the schools to the potential employer. The essay plays an important role in forming the first impression for those who are screening applications, so details, such as organization, clarity of ideas, spelling, and legibility should not be overlooked.

The Interview

Applications will be screened by one or more persons at the school district or agency prior to an invitation to interview. The interview process will vary from agency to agency, but candidates should expect to be interviewed by individuals who do not have expertise in speech and language. Candidates should expect a panel of two to five people to interview them. Additionally, there may be several different panels or meetings with various individuals. For example, the first-level interview might be with a building principal and staff members from a school site. Other special educators may or may not be included. Usually someone from the district special education department, such as the director or program manager, will participate as a member of the first interview panel. Second- and third-level interviews may be part of the process and may include other professionals, administrators, parents, PTA members, or teacher organization representatives.

Questions will vary depending on who is conducting the interview. Be prepared to answer questions of a technical nature about speech and language, including questions regarding SERVICE

DELIVERY and student ELIGIBILITY. Questions about student discipline and classroom management are likely to be included. It is also advisable to know something about the current educational issues in the local school or in the nation. Reading articles in recent issues of state speech-language-hearing association newsletters or ASHA publications or checking their Web sites are effective ways to prepare.

Personal presentation is very important in an interview. Practice responding to interview questions posed by familiar people a few days before the actual interview. Practice answering questions that are likely to be asked, such as, "Tell us about yourself, your background, and your educational training." The culture of schools can be very "student friendly" and interviewers will also want to know if you can provide this level of concern. Educators seek a caring and kind speech-language pathologist who is interested in students first, wants to be a member of their school team, and has a solid knowledge base in the profession so as to be a good resource for them. These traits should be communicated in an interview. With current requirements for access to curriculum, it is also critical that a candidate can explain the role of the speech-language pathologist working with a curriculum.

When interviewing for a school position, especially for the first time, do not be surprised if there are questions which are unfamiliar. Do not try to make up answers. Feel free to say "I do not know" or "I am not familiar with that area." When in an interview, remember that someone in the room wrote the question and does know the answer, so fabricating an answer is usually not successful. Another good answer is usually, "I don't know, but I am willing to learn." The most important advice for an interview is to relax and let personality and experience be guides. An example of common interview questions can be found in the sidebar. Use these as a starting point for practice.

There is usually a time in an interview when the candidate may ask questions. It is not advisable to ask questions about money or benefits at that time. It is considered appropriate to ask questions about working conditions, CASE-LOAD size, continuing education opportunities, and budget.

Accepting the Position

When an offer of employment is made, make sure all questions about employment conditions are asked and answered fully. Such questions should address the following topics:

- Salary
- Payment schedule (10 months or 12 months)
- Work calendar
- Benefits (including health, dental, vision, and other insurance)
- Union membership (required or optional)
- Site assignment(s)

If a candidate is in the enviable position of having two or more viable offers, he or she may be able to negotiate. However, be cautious so as not to lose both offers. It is acceptable to be straightforward and tell the prospective employer that another offer is being considered, describe the pros on that side, and see what the district will offer. Due to shortages, some districts are offering signing or incentive bonuses to entice candidates to sign on with their system.

Possible Interview Questions for Speech-Language Pathologists

1. Please begin by telling us about your professional training and experience, including your job-related experiences and education.

2. Describe how a student qualifies to receive special education services. What are the specific criteria to determine if a student is eligible to receive speech and language services?

3. A fourth-grade student has been referred for a language evaluation. How will you conduct the assessment? What tools and procedures will you use?

4. Describe your experience working with bilingual students. Discuss the issues related to students who come from a monolingual Spanish-speaking home but have received English-only instruction.

5. Review for us your experience with the following disorders. Discuss both assessment and intervention:
       Fluency
       Voice
       Articulation/Phonology

6. Describe your experiences with the following:
       Alternative and Augmentative Communication
       Assistive Technology
       Students with significant disabilities, including autism
       Oral motor disorders
       Literacy

7. Discuss the various types of service delivery models that you might use and how you would determine what is appropriate.

Organizational Structures

Schools in the United States are created under many different types of organizational structures. Schools themselves usually are part of a district, with names that may sound familiar: Jefferson County Public Schools (Louisville, KY); Rose Tree Media School District (Media, PA); Los Angeles Unified School District (Los Angeles, CA); and Sunnybrook School District (Lansing/Lynwood, IL). School districts vary by size, organizational structure, geography, historical events, and state fiscal procedures. The Los Angeles Unified School District encompasses a massive area not only in terms of land, but also in the more critical responsibility of educating nearly 800,000 children (nearly as many students as in the entire state of Wisconsin). And in Hawaii, the entire state encompasses only one school district, serving approximately 245,000 children.

The organizational structures that provide services to children with disabilities vary greatly from district to district and from state to state. Throughout this book reference has been made to local, regional, and state services. *Local* usually refers to a school district, but not always. For example, in a rural or smaller suburban district, special education services may be provided on a regionalized basis. Regional systems are typically cooperatives of smaller school districts that join resources together to provide services to children with specialized needs. State systems typically support schools for students who are blind or DEAF, and who require highly specialized forms of instruction. States may also run diagnostic centers. The federal law frequently refers to the LEA to denote the organizational entity that has responsibility for the provision of services to students with exceptional needs. Table 9.2 provides an overview of the organizational structures in 16 states and overseas.

Special education services may be provided through a variety of organizational structures. In some circumstances, the services are provided by speech-language pathologists and other service providers employed by the school district. In other circumstances, a regional area system may be the employing agency for speech-language pathologists or support personnel. In these situations, the service providers are then assigned to

schools or districts in the surrounding geographical area. When services are provided through a regional system, it may be that the school district is too small to support a full-time specialist staff or that there is a belief that a higher level of expertise can be maintained by supporting specialist staff through a regionalized service area. Both district and regional systems will have administrative and program support personnel. Depending on the size of the agency and the administrative structure within the local school system, the speech-language pathologist may or may not have much contact with the administrative regional and support staff.

Funding

Before trying to understand how funding occurs for special education, the prudent employee should have a basic understanding of how public education is funded in America. Education is compulsory for children through age 15, 16, 17 or 18, depending on the state. Each state constitution requires a comprehensive educational program to be created and funded, usually kindergarten (though not in all states) through grade 12. Some states have state-operated preschool, and some states have two-year post-secondary educational programs that are open to all high school graduates at little or no charge. Sometimes such systems articulate with a statewide university or technical college system, so costs are usually much less for residents than for persons from out of state.

Table 9.2

Public Education Organizational Structures

Responses of Council of State Association Presidents to November 1999 Survey

State	Organizational Systems for Public Schools
California	School Districts, County Agencies, Special Education Local Plan Areas (SELPAs)
Delaware	School Districts, Intermediate Units, County and Charter Schools
Georgia	School Districts, Regional Offices (Georgia Learning Resource Systems)
Hawaii	School District
Indiana	Special Education Planning Districts, Partners for Assistive Technology in Indiana (PATINS), Institute for Developmental Disabilities (ISDD at Indiana University)
Iowa	School Districts, Area Education Agencies (AEAs)
Louisiana	State Department of Education, Parish School Systems
Montana	School Districts, Private Cooperatives (provide contract services and serve rural areas)
Nebraska	School Districts, Educational Service Units
New York	School Districts, Board of Cooperative Educational Services Programs
North Carolina	Local Education Agencies, Raleigh Department of Public Instruction, Local County Units
North Dakota	School Districts, Local Education Co-operative
Ohio	School Districts, County Programs, Supervisory Network, Ohio Speech-Language Educational Audiology Coalition, Special Education Resource Centers
Oregon	School Districts, Educational Service Districts
Overseas/Department of Defense	Local DSOs, District Superintendent's Office, Early Developmental Intervention Services (EDIS)
Pennsylvania	School Districts, Intermediate Units
South Dakota	School Districts, Educational Cooperatives

Source: Moore-Brown and Montgomery (1999)

School Finance

The massive 1–12 or K–12 educational system is free to the citizens of all states, a concept found in few nations in the world. Revenue for school districts comes from a combination of local, state, and federal sources. Federal funds for education are quite limited and targeted to specific programs with strict usage guidelines. State taxes for education are derived from revenue sources that are relatively constant—income, property, and sales. These revenue sources are identified in the state constitution. Local funding is typically generated through levies on property values and sales tax charged in addition to state mandated taxes.

The actual dollars realized from each different revenue source can vary dramatically across states. In some states, city or county taxes are utilized for education, contributing to great variations between affluent and low income areas, urban and rural districts, and districts where property values are high versus low. Since the late 1970s, equity in state educational funding between school districts has been a controversial issue and the topic of many legal challenges (Picus and Wattenbarger, 1996).

Per pupil expenditures vary drastically from state to state. Table 9.3 provides a sampling of the great variations in where school funds come from and how much some states put into each child's education. The per pupil expenditure covers all costs of educational services, including teachers' salaries, materials, buildings and maintenance, and other related costs. Personnel costs always represent 80 to 85% of a school district's operating budget.

Funding for Special Education

Since the inception of the EDUCATION FOR ALL HANDICAPPED CHILDREN ACT (EAHCA) of 1975, the funding of special education has been one of the more controversial aspects of the whole school funding picture. When EAHCA was passed, federal funding for this program was originally promised by Congress at 40% of the total costs of special education in each state. This level of funding was never realized, and currently parents, professionals, and politicians are championing a renewed push for the full funding of the INDIVIDUALS WITH DISABILITIES EDUCATION ACT (IDEA) AMENDMENTS OF 1997. Special education is an unfunded mandate of the federal government, meaning that state and local entities are required to implement programs legislated by Congress for which they do not receive adequate federal funding. As his administration took office in January of 2001, President George W. Bush claimed to support the full funding of IDEA (Williams, 2000).

Categorical Funding

Special education funding is considered *categorical,* or restricted, meaning that the dollars in the special education fund are restricted to being spent on that category of services and related costs only. General education funding is considered *unrestricted* since those dollars can be spent on any program in the schools. The costs of special education programs represent approximately 12% of overall public budgets (Parrish and Chambers, 1996). The categorical dollars allocated to fund special education typically fall short of the true cost of the programs. There is an expectation

Table 9.3

State Revenue Resource Comparisons

State	Total Students Enrolled (1994–1995)	Federal Share of Total Revenues	State Share of Total Revenues	Local Share of Total Revenues	Per Pupil Expenditures
Alaska	132,123	11.8%	63.4%	22.2%	$9,097
California	5,803,734	8.2%	60.0%	30.8%	$5,414
Florida	2,294,007	7.4%	48.8%	40.0%	$5,986
Hawaii	189,887	8.1%	89.5%	0.4%	$6,144
Iowa	501,054	5.1%	52.0%	37.7%	$6,047
Massachusetts	949,006	4.8%	39.9%	54.0%	$7,818
Minnesota	853,621	4.3%	55.0%	36.9%	$6,371
Montana	162,335	9.4%	47.4%	39.0%	$6,112
Nebraska	292,681	6.0%	32.1%	56.4%	$6,472
Nevada	296,621	4.2%	31.9%	60.4%	$5,541
New Hampshire	201,629	3.5%	7.4%	86.6%	$6,236
New York	2,861,823	5.4%	39.4%	54.2%	$9,658
Tennessee	893,020	8.5%	48.5%	36.6%	$5,011
Wisconsin	881,780	4.3%	53.1%	40.5%	$7,398

Source: National Association of State Boards of Education (NASBE), (1999)

applied to most state special education funding formulas that the general education fund will contribute to the cost of special education programs. Rising costs and inequitable formulas for special education programs have created the need to increasingly draw on the general fund of most local education agencies. This underfunding of special education can be a serious disadvantage for the program. General educators, school board members, and parents may blame special education costs for the inability of their system to provide items for the students in general education. This polarization may make for challenging situations for special educators working in the school system.

Per pupil cost provides a more dramatic example of the cost of special education, especially in comparison to general education. In 1985–86, the cost of educating students in special education was found to be 2.3 times higher than the cost of educating general education students (Parrish and Chambers, 1996). Since that time, technology and other expensive resources have become more common, which increase the cost of special education and RELATED SERVICES even more.

Funding Systems

The Center for Special Education Finance (CSEF, 1999b) identified the types of funding systems that states use for special education:

- Pupil Weights—Funding is allocated on a per student basis, with the amount(s) based on a multiple(s) of regular education aid. Weights are generally differentiated on the basis of student placement (e.g. pull out, special day class), disability category, or a combination of these two factors.

- Resource-based—Funding is based on allocation of specific education resources (e.g., teachers or classroom units). Classroom units are derived from prescribed staff/student ratios by disabling condition or type of placement.

- Percent Reimbursement—Funding is based on a percentage of allowable or actual expenditures. That is, the amount of state special education aid a district receives is directly based on its expenditure for the program. Districts may be reimbursed for 100% of their program expenditures, or some lesser percentage.

- Flat Grant—Funding is based on a fixed funding amount per student or per unit. A variation of this approach, called a census-based approach, is based on the total number of students in a district, rather than the number of special education students.

During the 1994-95 school year, 38 percent of the states had a pupil weight funding system for special education. Twenty-two percent of the states have a percent reimbursement funding system, while flat grant and resource-based funding systems were being used by 20 percent of the states. (¶ 1–2)

Special education funding is complex and changing. When EAHCA (1975) was first passed, many children with disabilities were not receiving education (see Chapter 2). As a result, great efforts were required to locate children in the community to bring them into the educational system and provide them with needed services. The emphasis on CHILD FIND resulted in a funding model structured to pay districts and states for the numbers of children who were identified. As the numbers of children served in special education increased, the late 1980s saw funding systems being revised to move from child-count systems to census-based systems, with the latter being considered "incentive-free" (CSEF, 1999a, ¶ 4).

A census-based approach allocates funding using a fixed formula that is calculated according to the number of students in a school district, rather than providing funding based on the number of special education students served. In a census-based system, a school district will receive the same allocation regardless of the number of students identified. A census-based system should eliminate incentives to identify students for special education when the district can use prevention and intervention methods to reduce the severity of students' needs and thereby reduce the need for special education services.

Speech-language pathologists and other special educators need to understand how funding systems work for their state and local entity. Providers of special education services are frequently frustrated by the seeming lack of support or funding for the programs in which they work. Questions about why staff is not added or why supplies and materials or conference budgets are tight or nonexistent frequently plague service providers. In addition, pressures can be put on speech-language pathologists by parents and other educators to provide services when the resources to do so are not available. In these instances, speech-language pathologists may find themselves caught in the middle of the unfunded mandate quandary. Solving this quandary is clearly not the responsibility of

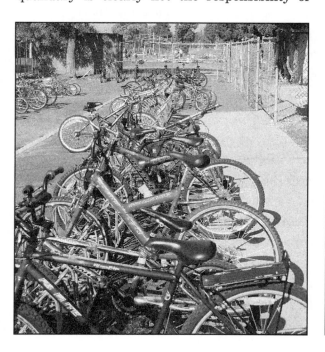

speech-language pathologists, but understanding the issues may help deal with the questions.

The number of students identified as requiring special education and related services continues to grow. Since the enactment of EAHCA (1975):

The number of students ages 6 through 21 served under Part B of the Individuals with Disabilities Education Act (IDEA) reached 5,541,166 in 1998–99, a 2.7% increase over the previous year. In the past decade, the number of students served grew 30.3%, from 4,253,018 in 1989–90 to 5,541,166 in 1998–99.

...The growth in the number of children with disabilities exceeded the growth in both the resident population and school enrollment. For this same period, growth in the United States resident population of children ages 6 through 21 was 9.7% (from 56,688,000 to 62,204,713). School enrollment grew 14.1%, from 40,608,342 to 46,349,803.

...In 1998–99, specific learning disabilities continued to be the most prevalent disability among students 6 through 21....Over half of the students with disabilities served under IDEA were categorized as having specific learning disabilities (2,817,148, or 50,8%. Speech and language impairments (1,074,548, or 19.4%), mental retardation (611,076, or 11.0%, and emotional disturbance (463,262, or 8.4%) were the next most common disabilities. (U.S. Department of Education, 2000b, pp. II-19–II-21)

The U.S. Department of Education (2000b) also reported significant growth in the prevalence of certain disability categories, notably other health impairment (OHI) (318.8 percent increase) and autism (243.9 percent increase) between 1989–90 and 1998–99. The increase in the OHI category is attributed to increased identification of children with attention deficit disorder (ADD) and attention deficit hyperactivity disorder (ADHD). Orthopedic impairment also showed a significant increase (44.6 percent) during this same reporting period.

While growth in the numbers of students receiving special education is reported to be staggering, examination of birth rates in this country demonstrate rising concern about the sheer numbers of students who will be entering the education system itself. "The next decade will usher in the beginnings of a steady and significant increase in the number of school-age children in the United States during the 21st century" (U.S. Department of Education, 2000a, ¶ 1). The increase in the student population is reported to be the result of the enrollment of children representing the Baby-Boom Echo, that is, the children born in or after 1977, who were children or grandchildren of the Baby-Boom generation or those born between 1948 and 1975. Based upon school enrollment of 52.8 million students in 1999, schools were expected to welcome 53 million students in the fall of 2000, representing "the highest enrollment in U.S. history and a net increase of 8 million schoolchildren in the last 15 years....Over the next five years enrollments at all levels of education will grow—to an estimated 53.5 million in grades K-12" (U.S. Department of Education, 2000a, ¶ 2).

This overall growth has provided stressors to the total funding system for education, with programs competing for the limited resources within the system as well for resources from external funding sources. At the same time, the special education population will continue to grow not only in numbers but in intensity of needs (Parrish and Chambers, 1996). Such factors will certainly impact the level of competence and skill required of school-based speech-language pathologists in order to be prepared to serve students in new and creative ways. (See "Speech-Language Pathologist Roles and Responsibilities," on the next page.)

Changes in Funding Systems

New federal funding formulas were enacted with IDEA (1997) amendments. Federal funding for special education comes to states in a number of different types of grants. These are allocation grants, not competitive grants, meaning that the states automatically receive the funds. These grants are distributed to states which then distribute the funds to local education agencies. The grant funds are to cover various costs such as personnel development, direct and support services to children in various age categories, administrative costs, and other related activities. In 1997, just over $3 billion was spent on Part B Grants, which are the grants for direct and support services to students. IDEA (1997) developed a new fund allocation formula to go into effect when the costs for the Part B Grants to states program exceeds $4.9 billion sometime between 1999 and 2005. The formula promotes flexibility in the ways that dollars can be spent. States have already reported utilizing the flexibility to provide technical assistance, support activities which will improve educational results for students with disabilities, and improve the mediation system (U.S. Department of Education, 1998).

IDEA (1997) strengthened the provisions for PLACEMENT of students with disabilities in the LEAST RESTRICTIVE ENVIRONMENT (LRE). For the first time, funding under IDEA (1997) was intended to be used jointly with funding from the TITLE I program of the Elementary and Secondary Education Act (ESEA) of 1965. The Title I program provides compensatory education for underachieving students at or below the poverty level. The joint use of Title I and IDEA 1997 funds is intended to provide coordinated prevention and intervention services that are not isolated or separate as was the case prior to this legislation. The new funding provisions require policies that eliminate incentives for restrictive placements, allow for benefits to nondisabled students, allow for schoolwide programs, and develop bridging services (e.g., summer preschool programs) for improved results. In addition, IDEA 1997 will not allow a decrease in a Local Education Agency's (LEA) financial contribution to special education programs as a result of the new formulas (U.S. Department of Education, 1998).

These funding changes mean that schoolwide plans may be developed that assign speech-language pathologists as a part of prevention or intervention programs. Speech-language pathologists may include nondisabled student peers in groups when working in class, and joint services may be provided to students who qualify for several programs. Speech-language pathologists in schools must know and understand local restrictions and allowances since each state and LEA will interpret these new regulations in slightly different ways. When doing joint work with team members, speech-language pathologists should ensure that supervisors are aware of any creative programming being done. Providing special education services to students on a consistent basis without appropriate parent notification, assessment, and determination of eligibility is not legal. Providing services through a service delivery model that benefit all students, such as COLLABORATION or co-teaching, is legal. Speech-language pathologists are funded out of special education dollars, which means that their services are considered special education. They may not, therefore, provide individual speech and language services to students without an IEP.

Speech-Language Pathologist Roles and Responsibilities

Primary Roles

The speech-language pathologist is responsible for a wide range of duties that vary from school district to school district but appear essentially similar in 50 states, the District of Columbia, and the Department of Defense Schools (DODS) for the U.S. military stationed in other countries. For this reason, ASHA was able to develop a fairly generic list in their *Guidelines for the Roles and Responsibilities of the School-Based Speech-Language Pathologist* (1999c), that has guided states as well as assisted individual ASHA members. The list, represented in the sidebar, was comprehensive and met the requirements for the changes in IDEA (1997).

To appreciate how the wording, the intent, and in some cases the spirit of school-based speech-language pathologists' roles change due

---

Core Roles and Responsibilities of School-Based Speech-Language Pathologists (SLPs)

Prevention SLPs, as educational team members, address the prevention of communication disorders, including consultation and active involvement for both primary prevention and secondary prevention for birth through age 22.

Identification SLPs participate as team members in identifying students who may be in need of assessments to determine possible eligibility for special education or related services; this includes prereferral, screening, and referral.

Assessment SLPs conduct thorough and balanced speech, language, or communication assessments; this includes collecting data and gathering evidence using appropriate, nonbiased tools, interviews, and structured observations.

Evaluation SLPs interpret the assessment, giving value to the data, including the nature and severity of the disorders and the potential effect on the student's educational and social performance. Clinical judgement is required to determine the communication disorder or difference.

Eligibility Determination SLPs, in cooperation with the educational team, determine the student's need and eligibility for special education or related services according to the eligibility criteria of each state.

IEP/IFSP Development SLPs assist a team in developing an individualized education program (IEP) or an individualized family service plan (IFSP) when students are found eligible for services. SLPs must take all special factors into account and help to design the IEP with all the required components (IDEA, 1997, § 614d (3) (a) (i–ii), 614d (1) (a) (i–viii).

Caseload Management SLPs assist the team in selecting, planning, and coordinating the appropriate service delivery using an array of services and inclusive practices. SLPs may serve as case managers for some students.

Intervention for Communication Disorders SLPs provide services for identified students using the most recent literature of the discipline, research-based intervention strategies, principles of effective instruction, and appropriate academic or developmental curriculum for each individual.

Continued

Intervention for Communication Variations SLPs must be knowledgeable about monolingual and bilingual language acquisition, the linguistic rules for social dialects and language differences, the use of interpreters and translators, and nonbiased assessment to assist the classroom teacher and others.

Counseling SLPs participate in honest and open communication regarding the recovery from, or adjustment to, a communication impairment using effective counseling techniques and coordination with other professionals.

Re-evaluation SLPs conduct reassessments of students receiving services at least every three years, when dismissal is considered, if special circumstances arise, or if parents request such. Re-evaluation is ongoing, thorough, and documented.

Transition SLPs participate with a team to assist students in transitioning from one setting to another, within school, or beyond school at all ages. SLPs may work directly with students on transitional goals.

Dismissal SLPs begin the consideration of dismissal when services begin, with a focus on achieving functional outcomes. SLPs weigh the factors for dismissal, including academic performance, state or local dismissal criteria, ASHA's guidelines for dismissal, or a combination of these.

Supervision SLPs may supervise other SLPs, support personnel, university practicum students, or volunteers. This supervision is conducted competently, ethically, and legally according to state licensing regulations and other procedures.

Documentation and Accountability SLPs keep clear comprehensive records to justify the need for and effectiveness of assessment/intervention. Performance appraisals, third-party billing, and risk-management records are maintained accurately, confidentially, and in accordance with federal, state, and local reporting requirements.

Additional roles and responsibilities that may be undertaken or assigned:
- Community and professional partnerships—research, grants, parent training
- Professional leadership—mentoring, specializations, school boards
- Advocacy—students, programs, legislative issues

Source: ASHA (1999c)

to state regulations, examples of similar lists from North Carolina and Connecticut are provided in the sidebar. Of course, state guidelines are state department officials' interpretations of federal laws within the funding and political structure of their state and consequently are more flexible and subject to more frequent changes than federal regulations. ASHA's guidelines are only suggestions from a national professional organization and are not binding

---

Roles and Responsibilities Defined by Two States

The North Carolina public school guidelines for speech-language programs (North Carolina Department of Public Instruction, 1985) describe the speech-language pathologist's major responsibilities:

- Planning and oversight of the local program of speech-language services
- Screening, testing, diagnosing, and advising of students and families served by the program
- Developing individual education programs for students with identified needs
- Managing and conducting intervention programs using effective interpersonal relations and appropriate tools and techniques
- Acting as a liaison with others for consultation, assistance, or referrals for the implementation of services (pp. 59–66)

This description is followed by 87 statements of sample evidence for each of the major roles for the speech-language pathologist in North Carolina public schools.

Some states defined the roles and responsibilities of speech-language pathologists according to each type of student they were serving. For example, Connecticut (1993) listed eight responsibilities for the speech-language pathologist who served the needs of middle and secondary school students, paraphrased as follows:

- Collaborating with students, families, and teachers to identify students at risk for or exhibiting communication disabilities;
- Using developing appropriate assessment and remediation strategies;
- Collaborating with students, families, and teachers to select the best service format for each student;
- Involving the student in his or her own service plan;
- Collaborating with others at the school on prevention issues related to noise exposure, drugs and alcohol abuse, traumatic brain injury;
- Collaborating with others to promote the general communicative effectiveness of adolescents to prepare them for post secondary experiences;
- Participation in developing and implementing transition plans;
- Providing information, training, and counseling as needed on later language development.

in any state. Local school districts, consortiums, and regional areas can also assemble such lists to guide their speech-language pathologists in a particular area. Many times school-based speech-language pathologists and their state professional organizations will help to write these lists so that they accurately reflect the professional aspects of the position that may not be known to education officers who are assigned these tasks (see "State Consultants," page 314).

Lists of roles and responsibilities may cast a longer shadow in school districts than they do in health-care or private practice environments because of employee unions. The conditions of work, the demands made on management on behalf of an employee, and most importantly the relative fairness of one employee's job responsibilities compared to another are critical issues. Therefore, lists of assigned, primary duties are important to know and follow in public education. Additional roles and duties, and who assigns them to the speech-language pathologist, are equally important.

Additional Responsibilities

Every work environment will place additional responsibilities on speech-language pathologists. These will vary according to an interesting set of criteria inherent in the individual school or school district and determined by school characteristics, such as the size, grade levels, ages of students, location (rural, suburban, or urban), degree of security needed, discipline codes, student transportation, teacher/staff relationships, community expectations, personal interests, and an administrator's style.

The following list of additional responsibilities and tasks represent those that speech-language pathologists have taken on voluntarily based on personal interests, because the previous speech-language pathologist did them, because the school was short-handed, or because everyone took on extra duties to cover the territory (see sidebar). It is easy to see how involved speech-language pathologists can get in their schools.

Additional Roles and Responsibilities of School-Based Speech-Language Pathologists

Recess duty	Bus duty	Morning duty
Play director	Bulletin board decoration	Club advisor
Athletics coach	Dance chaperone	Magazine sales coordinator
Social committee chair	Student government	Field trip assistant
Preschool monitor	Head Start read aloud	Parent education programs
Parent Teacher Association	Parent Teacher Organization	School accountability team
School discipline team	Curriculum committees	Triathlon coach
School newspaper	School yearbook	School Web site
Assessment team	Assistive technology	Candy sales
School store	School post office	Bilingual assessor
After-school care	Homework club	Internet pen pals
Literacy lab	Assistant principal	Department chair
Assessment Committee coordinator	Grant writer	School improvement committee
Administrator's designee	Principal's designee	Science fair mentor

Although taking on extra activities may not appeal to every speech-language pathologist, the authors engaged in one or more events each year and found that doing so enhanced their speech and language service delivery in unexpected ways. Additional school roles can increase the visibility of speech-language pathologists school-wide, offer opportunities to observe students communicating with their peers in a generalizing environment, build staff relationships, attract administrator support, and integrate speech-language pathologists into more aspects of the school and community.

Speech-Language Pathology Assistants (SLPAs) and Aides in Schools

Extending Service with Paraprofessionals

Professionals in many fields work with paraprofessionals who support professionals and enable them to accomplish more. Physicians work with physician assistants, attorneys work with paralegals, physical therapists work with physical therapy assistants, and occupational therapists assign duties to certified occupational therapy assistants. Speech-language pathologists can extend their services through the use of speech-language pathology assistants (SLPAs) and aides.

Support personnel in school speech-language programs may be called SLPAs, aides, assistants, technicians, paraprofessionals, and other related job titles. Some positions require entry-level skills; others seek applicants with advanced training, such as a postsecondary degree or a certificate to show educational accomplishments. More skilled support personnel take a greater responsibility for the instructional program and enable speech-language pathologists to be more effective and assume some or many of the tasks necessary to implement a single-school or multisite program. In some cases, SLPAs actually provide therapy and monitor student progress.

Although historically the use of untrained support personnel provided a valuable addition to speech and language programs, their contribution was constrained by their training, experience, and the limitations placed on them by regulations of the state or district (California Speech-Language-Hearing Association [CSHA], 1996). Today, however, SLPAs and aides are regulated by the state in which they work.

ASHA's Guidelines for SLPAs and Aides

In November, 1996, ASHA established the credentialing of support personnel in speech-language pathology (ASHA, 1996a). This included guidelines for training, credentialing, using, and supervising SLPAs and the less rigorous category of speech-language pathology aides. This was a comprehensive policy change for ASHA that took many years of discussion, review of state licensing laws, and development of procedures to assure that persons with communication disorders would still receive the services of fully qualified professionals. New service delivery models in health care and education demanded that support personnel be an integral part of the many new levels of service proposed to both reduce costs and compensate for the shortage of professionals (See "Securing a Position," page 274, for a discussion of personnel shortages). The U.S. Department of Education (1999) later identified a specific need for standards to be set for paraprofessionals working in the educational system, which is consistent with the actions of ASHA.

Under ASHA's (1996a) guidelines, there are two levels of support personnel in speech-language pathology: the aide, and the assistant (or SLPA). The complete text of the position paper establishing support personnel in all practice settings is available at the ASHA Web site *(www.asha.org/library/images/v3p112a.pdf)*. The discussion here will review the application of support personnel services in public school programs.

Aides are people with a high school diploma who have been trained by school-based speech-language pathologists to assist with programs. Aides are able to assist with contacting parents, locating and collecting identified students, developing materials, repairing equipment, and preparing a wide range of clerical work necessary for a school-based program. Aides do not

work with students but can be very helpful to busy speech-language pathologists. Aides may work in more than one general education or special education program and extend the activities of the speech-language pathologist to more corners of the school.

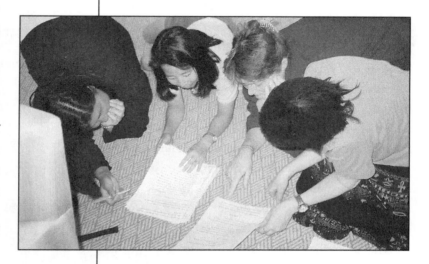

SLPAs, on the other hand, are persons with a minimum of an associate's degree or equivalent course of study in speech-language pathology. They work with students under the direct supervision of speech-language pathologists. They take coursework at community colleges or universities in child development and speech-language pathology and have the recommended number of hours of field experience with a variety of communication disorders. Although a bachelor of arts or sciences degree in communication disorders could be used as the coursework, the person would still need to take the practicum or field experience to be registered, or licensed in some states, as an assistant.

The strategic plan for full implementation of a speech-language pathology assistant program was approved by the ASHA Legislative Council in 1996; however, standards were still being written in 2000 by the Standards Council. According to existing ASHA guidelines, not standards, a speech-language pathologist should take a class in supervision to oversee assistants, and may supervise no more than three such support personnel. The school-based speech-language pathologist must be available 100% of the time but not necessarily on-site. This supervision, to meet ASHA guidelines, must be 30% for the first 90 days and then 20% thereafter, with at least 10% being direct supervision. The scope of responsibility for assistants allows them to do the following: screen students but not interpret results; help speech-language pathologists with evaluations; monitor routine therapy sessions; collect data; observe students in naturalistic settings for evidence of generalization of skills; check homework assignments; and follow through on computer-assisted interventions, communication labs, and similar guided group sessions. These comprehensive guidelines were developed by the Task Force on Support Personnel, then followed a careful process to be adopted by ASHA and are used as the basis for developing standards (ASHA, 1998b).

Aides and assistants can be utilized in school speech, language, and hearing programs if they are properly trained and appropriately supervised by a certified speech-language pathologist. Both the speech-language pathologist and assistant must follow their state licensing laws if they work in a state with licensure.

Speech-language pathology assistants and aides can make a significant difference in how

> Speech-language pathology assistants and aides can make a significant difference in how services are offered in many schools.

services are offered in many schools. Savvy speech-language pathologists need to know how to design quality programs that include these assistants and aides.

The Role of States in Regulating SLPAs

State licensing laws take precedence over ASHA guidelines (1996a) for the use of SLPAs. The ASHA guidelines (1996a) outline good clinical practice, responsible supervision, concern for students, and ethical conduct. Any direct conflicts between ASHA guidelines (1996a) and state laws need to be discussed at the state level with all involved agencies for the sake of students who need services. State speech-language-hearing associations often take the lead in these issues. In late 1998, of the 50 states and the District of Columbia, 31 had licensure laws that recognized support personnel, 16 had regulations that did not recognize support personnel, and 4 were without regulations (ASHA, 1999f).

There is wide variation in how states regulate aides and assistants in speech-language pathology (ASHA, 1999e; 1999f). According to ASHA (1999f), some require a high school diploma (Georgia, Nebraska, and Indiana) while others require a bachelor's degree (Arkansas, Kentucky, Rhode Island, and West Virginia). Kentucky's requirements for SLPAs apply to school-based settings only, while California's SLPA program addresses all work settings.

Maryland and Nevada are in the process of developing legislation to regulate this area of practice. Sixteen states have registration for assistants and 10 have licensing. Kansas has registration for audiology assistants only; in New Mexico, New Hampshire, and Wisconsin, assistants are monitored but not regulated. The most common title is *assistant,* with 18 states using that term alone or in conjunction with other terms. Louisiana, Maine, Arkansas, and Iowa have a two-tiered system that recognizes advanced preparation by some assistants. North Carolina and California require a two-year degree from a community college, plus clinical practicum hours in a variety of settings, one of which is the public school. Seven states require assistants to take from 8 to 12 continuing education hours each year to maintain their position. Oklahoma is in the process of developing its requirements. Any listing of support personnel guidelines or state requirements are subject to updating on a continual basis.

Speech-language pathologists in schools have the responsibility of knowing their state licensing regulations as well as ASHA's guidelines for support personnel to assure that students receive the most effective services from qualified personnel. IDEA (1997) amendments required paraprofessionals in special education programs to be trained and supervised. This includes aides or assistants who are assigned to school districts speech and language programs.

SLPA Responsibilities and Limitations

According to ASHA's *Guidelines for Training, Credentialing, Use, and Supervision of Speech-Language Pathology Assistants* (1996a), SLPAs may conduct the following tasks under the supervision of speech-language pathologists in schools:

- Conduct speech language SCREENINGS
- Provide direct intervention to students
- Follow documented intervention plans and IEPs
- Document student progress
- Assist during assessments
- Assist with informal documentation, prepare materials, and perform clerical duties
- Schedule activities and prepare charts, records, graphs, or otherwise display data
- Perform checks and maintenance of equipment
- Participate in research projects, in-service training, and public relations programs

In contrast, SLPAs are not authorized to:

- Perform standardized or nonstandardized tests, formal or informal evaluations, or interpret test results
- Participate in parent conferences, case conferences, or any INTERDISCIPLINARY TEAM meeting without the presence of a supervising speech-language pathologist
- Provide student or family counseling
- Write, develop, or modify an intervention plan
- Assist students without following the intervention plan prepared by a speech-language pathologist

- Sign any formal documents, reimbursement forms, or reports

- Select students for services

- Dismiss a student from services

- Disclose confidential information about a student

- Make REFERRALS for additional service

- Communicate with families or students without the specific consent of a supervising speech-language pathologist

- Represent themselves as speech-language pathologists

State laws may differ slightly from these guidelines in regard to the roles of SLPAs. How SLPAs are utilized will differ on a local or building level as well. SLPAs will be in contact with aides in the special education program who have vastly different duties. Some administrators may require greater uniformity at their schools and require that all support staff carry additional duties. SLPAs may be assigned by the principal to contribute to some of the overall activities of the school such as:

- Bus or recess duty
- Field trip assignments
- Office assignments
- Health monitoring
- Fire drill assignments
- School fundraising campaigns
- Homework correction

The primary function of SLPAs should be serving students. If schools assign SLPAs to duties that disrupt services to students on the caseload, speech-language pathologists may need to advocate for a change with the super-

visor. Each SLPA's role must be managed by the supervising speech-language pathologist with appropriate attention to other educators and administrators. The value of trained SLPAs, of course, is their knowledge of communication disorders, sensitivity to child development, and availability to continue therapy when speech-language pathologists must complete evaluations or visit another site or home. The SLPA can also maximize the use of the augmentative communication system during instruction. If SLPAs speak another language besides English or have a culture different from speech-language pathologists, SLPAs can be tremendous assets to programs. Many SLPAs represent the cultural and linguistic diversity of their communities and can be powerful extensions of the speech and language program into the community (Montgomery, 2000a; Moore-Brown, Cooper, and Ferguson, 1998; Moore-Brown, Robinson, Williams, Claussen, and Martinez, 1998).

Both high school and elementary speech and language programs with SLPAs can provide highly effective services. As seen in the photograph below, they may assist students with moderate to severe disabilities who require close monitoring in the classroom.

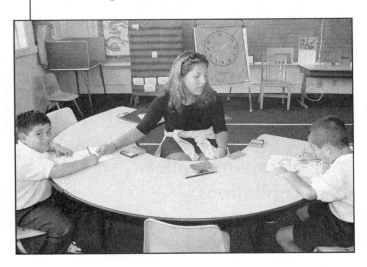

Frequently Asked Questions about SLPAs

Q. Will speech-language pathology assistants be used to replace speech-language pathologists?

A. No. Assistants cannot replace qualified speech-language pathologists. Rather, they can support clinical services provided by speech-language pathologists. ASHA criteria and guidelines were developed to ensure that speech-language pathology services provided to the public are of the highest quality and that speech-language pathologists continue to be responsible for maintaining this quality of service. According to ASHA criteria, guidelines and state licensure laws, no one can employ a speech-language pathology assistant without a speech-language pathologist as supervisor. ASHA guidelines and most state laws limit the number of speech-language pathology assistants a speech-language pathologist may supervise and define boundaries for how assistants are used.

Q. What are the advantages to the speech-language pathologist in using speech-language pathology assistants in his/her practice?

A. The speech-language pathologist may extend services (i.e., increase the frequency and intensity of services to patients or clients on his/her caseload); focus more on professional level tasks; increase client access to the program; and have more efficient/effective use of time and resources.

Q. Who is responsible for services provided by a speech-language pathology assistant?

A. The fully qualified, ASHA-certified speech-language pathologist is responsible for the services provided by assistants. In states that regulate speech-language pathology assistants, speech-language pathologists who hold full, unrestricted licenses assume these responsibilities for persons working under their direction.

Q. Does ASHA credential speech-language pathology assistants?

A. Yes, through a national voluntary registration process, that is effective January 1, 2003. Speech-language pathology assistants who wish to become registered with ASHA must submit an application for registration and meet the criteria set by ASHA's Council on Professional Standards in Speech-Language Pathology and Audiology.

Q. How does one become a speech-language pathology assistant?

A. ASHA's 2000 *Background Information and Criteria for the Registration of Speech-Language Pathology Assistants* calls for assistants to complete an associate's degree from an ASHA-approved technical training program.... Because the requirements for speech-language pathology support personnel vary across the country, persons interested in serving as speech-language pathology assistants should check with the state of intended employment for that state's specific requirements.

From *Frequently Asked Questions about Speech-Language Pathology Assistants,* by the American Speech-Language-Hearing Association (ASHA), 2000a, Rockville, MD: Author. © 2000 by ASHA. Adapted with permission.

Speech-language pathologists who use SLPAs report that it is "energizing," "more interactive during the day," "easier to reach more students," "refreshing," and that the speech-language pathologist's role "extends into many more classrooms and increases my visibility throughout the school" (Montgomery, 2000a).

ASHA's policy on support personnel, the Guidelines for SLPAs, and the list of states with AA degree programs can be found at ASHA's Web site *(www.asha.org)*. School-based speech-language pathologists may need to present this information to their school districts, directors of special education, and other administrators. These public education officials may be unaware of the way personnel are trained, hired, and compensated for their work in the comprehensive speech-language program. Speech-language pathologists may need to provide information on how SLPAs enhance the therapy program to parents who may be unaware of the training and skills of supervised SLPAs and may not recognize how beneficial such services can be. Speech-language pathologists need to constantly examine what all the students in a school need, how staff are attempting to meet those needs, and the possible advantages of one or more SLPAs to improve overall productivity and educational outcomes.

Ethics

Ethical behavior is expected of all professionals. Speech-language pathologists in public schools will find themselves in situations that call on an individual's ethical code of conduct. Speech-language pathologists who are ASHA members with a CCC or who are in a Clinical Fellowship (CF) are bound to abide by ASHA's (1994) Code of Ethics (see Appendix F). State speech-language and hearing associations also typically have a code of ethics that members are expected to uphold. While membership in professional associations is recommended, the code of ethics should serve as a guideline for any individual who practices as a speech-language pathologist, regardless of membership in these organizations. Under the code of ethics, speech-language pathologists have a reporting responsibility if they are aware of unethical behavior on the part of a fellow professional. ASHA's Ethical Practices Board responds to violations that are reported against ASHA-certificate holders.

In a *Communication Connection* article entitled "Professionalism and Ethics: How do you spell success? E-T-H-I-C-S," Frank C. Bucaro (2000) noted that each individual brings life experiences and moral beliefs to their daily decisions. According to Bucaro, training in ethical decision making should be addressed by employers and institutions of higher education so that instincts, emotions, and moral spirit are utilized appropriately in given situations. This is especially important because, "Every decision you make affects someone else, and we must always take that into consideration before making the decision" (p. 4).

Americans generally hold honesty and integrity as important values and do not anticipate situations that would compromise such values. In the everyday work world, unfortunately, situations may arise that create uncertainty regarding appropriate behavior. In more extreme situations, a speech-language pathologist may encounter people who do not behave ethically and who put the speech-language pathologist in a compromising position. In all cases, speech-language pathologists must follow federal and state regulations and laws. Consider Cooper's example given in the ASHA Ethics Roundtable (Moore-Brown et al., 1998) entitled "When Supervisor and Supervisee Disagree." In this case study, the speech-language pathologist makes recommendations for an intervention plan in her report and the supervisor changes the recommendations. In dealing with this type of a situation, speech-language pathologists may find themselves in an ethical conflict between doing the right thing for the student and possibly compromising their employment position, if questioning the supervisor presents a threat to employment.

Other situations that may arise in public schools include:

- A student needs a type of intervention that the speech-language pathologist does not feel competent to provide.

- A teacher or parent demands services when a student is not in need of such service.

- The speech-language pathologist believes that a student should be referred to a private speech-language pathologist for specialized treatment or evaluation services, but the school district will not pay for the referral.

- The speech-language pathologist believes that a student requires more intervention time than is available in the schedule.

If speech-language pathologists are challenged in this way, it is wise for them to seek advice from a mentor. Such a mentor could be another colleague or an administrator (including a principal, program specialist, or director). Be certain that whomever is selected will keep the issue confidential. Maintaining professionalism and confidentiality in communications regarding an ethical situation are equally important. Speech-language pathologists can also contact the state department of education or regional education agency for assistance.

State and national speech-language-hearing associations are good places to turn when situations arise that provide ethical challenges to the speech-language pathologist. Questions to these organizations are quite common. These organizations may provide guidance to those in the field regarding a variety of professional or ethical challenges, such as:

- Caseload size and management

- What to do when a supervisor directs an evaluation be conducted when the speech-

> State and national speech-language-hearing associations are good places to turn when situations arise that provide ethical challenges to the speech-language pathologist.

language pathologist has screened and indicated no evaluation is necessary

- What to do when a parent demands to be present during an evaluation

- Use of new therapy techniques that are controversial

One legal and ethical challenge that often faces speech-language pathologists in schools is the issue of providing services to children outside of the school setting in a private practice situation. If a speech-language pathologist is serving a student in the school setting, it would be considered a conflict of interest to provide that same student outside services that address his or her IEP GOALS. The reason for this is that IDEA (1997) calls for program, placement, and services to be provided to children through the IEP in order to provide FAPE. The parent would have recourse, through due process, to argue that the services provided outside the school should be provided or paid for by the school district. These are sticky situations, so it is recommended that speech-language pathologists avoid private practice with students who are being served in their employing school system under an IEP.

Another scenario that might present itself is a request for the speech-language pathologist to serve the student during the summer, or when the student is off-track in a year-round setting. Regulations pertaining to the provision of extended-year programming do not allow school districts to categorically exclude certain students from services during break periods. Therefore, while speech-language pathologists previously may have felt comfortable serving students on a fee-for-service basis during the

summer or over school breaks, the new regulations make it clear that some children may be eligible for school-funded summer programs if the service is required for the child to receive FAPE (34 C.F.R. § 300.309). It is recommended that the speech-language pathologists be very cautious about serving students in a private practice setting if they are also providing services to these students during the school year.

Professional Organizations

Professional organizations provide a needed link to current developments in the field, legislative information, and networking with others. Speech-language pathologists who work in schools have many professional organizations they can join. Speech-language pathologists typically want to affiliate with organizations that will keep them in contact with at least three aspects of their employment: (1) the discipline of speech-language pathology nationally, (2) their discipline within the state, and (3) the broader field of schools and education. In many cases, speech-language pathologists will also wish to become members of an organization for a specialty area within speech-language pathology, such as fluency, autism, or family counseling. Joining several organizations will provide speech-language pathologists with a more well-rounded view of controversial topics, more scholarly journals, access to conferences for up-to-date information, as well as a greater (or multiple) effect on regulatory agencies. Although there are some costs involved in maintaining one's membership dues and in attending conferences, professionals should view membership in more than one organization as a necessity, not a luxury. The following suggestions are designed to help speech-language pathologists decide which are the most appropriate organizations to join.

The National Organization: The American Speech-Language-Hearing Association (ASHA)

ASHA is considered the primary association for the professions of speech-language pathology and audiology. Since certification and membership are separate entities, speech-language pathologists who have their CCC need to request membership if they wish to join. Membership in ASHA should be viewed as a responsibility and a privilege of school-based speech-language pathologists. Working in a school district with many other ASHA members is a distinct advantage and increases each speech-language pathologist's professionalism. A school district with speech-language staff who hold ASHA membership will attract new professionals to complete their CF there in order to take full advantage of the valuable mentoring opportunities. Many other professionals who work in school settings do not have the opportunity to hone their new skills in a nurturing CF environment their first year on the job. Interestingly, related fields are seeking ways to do this, through externships for special educa-

> ASHA is considered the primary association for the professions of speech-language pathology and audiology.

tion teachers and through state sponsored mentor-teacher positions for more skilled educators to help new employees learn the ropes.

Membership in ASHA provides journals, newsletters, conventions, access to important lobbying and political action committees, position papers and technical resources for service delivery, the latest information on a clinical population or new assessment tools, and a code of ethics to guide one's practice and decision making. The network of over 100,000 professionals in speech-language pathology and audiology is a tremendous resource. The interests of each state are represented in the governing body of ASHA and in the work of national committees and task forces that influence school-based practice. Attracting school-based speech-language pathologists to ASHA committees is very important to the viability of the national organization, but it is even more important to the practice of speech-language pathology in public schools. National regulatory agencies, particularly the Office of Special Education and Research (OSERS), can interact directly with ASHA on key issues, access to policymakers that is nearly impossible for school district employees to get on their own. ASHA also provides its members benefits such as low-cost professional liability insurance, continuing education options to maintain a license or increase one's skills, and critical resources on FUNCTIONAL OUTCOMES and accountability for services.

Special Interest Divisions are an important part of the organizational structure of ASHA. Divisions allow for an in-depth professional connection around a particular aspect of the profession. ASHA has the following special interest divisions:

1. Language Learning and Education

2. Neurophysiology and Neurogenic Speech and Language Disorders

3. Voice and Voice Disorders

4. Fluency and Fluency Disorders

5. Speech Science and Orofacial Disorders

6. Hearing and Hearing Disorders: Research and Diagnostics

7. Aural Rehabilitation and Its Instrumentation

8. Hearing Conservation and Occupational Audiology

9. Hearing and Hearing Disorders in Childhood

10. Issues in Higher Education

11. Administration and Supervision

12. Augmentative and Alternative Communication

13. Swallowing and Swallowing Disorders (Dysphagia)

14. Communication Disorders and Sciences in Culturally and Linguistically Diverse Populations

15. Gerontology

16. School-Based Issues

Division 16 was established in December 1999 as the newest division, dedicated to school issues and service delivery. Division 1 also addresses the language and learning aspects of students in educational settings. School-based speech-language pathologists are likely to find that belonging to one or more divisions will provide them with a strong base of information about topics specific to their needs. Each special interest division has a newsletter that provides both scholarly and practical information for practitioners in that area. Divisions also sponsor or co-sponsor conferences and workshops for continuing education credits that are responsive to member needs. (Visit *www.asha.org/sidivisions/sid_list.htm* for more information.)

The National Student Speech-Language-Hearing Association (NSSLHA)

Prior to ASHA membership, students in communication disorders programs are eligible to become members of the National Student Speech-Language-Hearing Association (NSSLHA). Membership in NSSLHA allows students to receive journals and discounted conference rates. NSSLHA members can also belong to ASHA Special Interest Divisions and will receive a discount when they convert to full ASHA membership, upon completion of their education requirements. Joining NSSLHA affords students an opportunity to meet colleagues from the discipline, become knowledgeable about national issues, gain valuable insight into clinical and professional topics, and get a head start in their first job.

State Speech-Language-Hearing Associations

Another discipline-specific organization of interest to the speech-language pathologist in schools is the state speech-language-hearing association. Every state and the District of Columbia has such an organization, plus there is an organization for those who work overseas, mainly in American Schools and Department of Defense Schools (DODS) for dependents in the U.S. Armed Forces. The state associations and their Web sites are listed in Table 9.4 (pages 302–303).

State associations are independent entities, not chapters of the national association. They address their members' state concerns, represent them before legislative bodies, create continuing education opportunities, and determine their own membership criteria. Nearly all state organizations have student membership at a reduced membership rate. A state organization is also discipline-specific, but carries much more weight than does ASHA with state governance, funding sources, higher education agencies, and state licensing bureaus. In fact, many times a state organization is the only entity that can address inequities for speech-language pathologists in a school system, since public schools are state-funded enterprises. State associations vary in size from approximately 100 to 5,000 members and have a loose relationship with ASHA as "recognized associations." The state organizations can band together at times to push for federal changes, led by the Council of State Association Presidents (CSAP). Information about CSAP is available on their Web site, *www.csap.org.*

Membership in a state association greatly assists school-based speech-language pathologists with licensing requirements, continuing education offerings, state news, and connections with a network of professionals who work under the same state regulations. Some state organizations work very closely with their state departments of education, interpreting and influencing state policy. Being part of this process is important to speech-language pathologists and their school districts. Participating in special interest groups and committee work in state associations can enhance speech-language pathologists' effectiveness. Having held state association presidencies, both authors are convinced that membership in one's state association is critical for speech-language pathologists and for the profession.

Associations of Related Interests

Another association type is one reflecting general education, special education, or both. Some speech-language pathologists find that they can appreciate and be appreciated by their general education colleagues if they feel a connection with the greater education environment. Organizations listed in the sidebar on page 304 are popular choices for speech-language pathologists because they either combine educational approaches, or give another perspective on public schools. One speech-language pathologist compared joining the Association for Supervision and Curriculum Development (ASCD) to "finally finding the main highway that most of the cars were taking. It was still up

Table 9.4

Web Sites for State Speech-Language-Hearing Associations

State	Association		Web Site (if available)
Alabama	Speech and Hearing Association of Alabama	(SHAA)	
Alaska	Alaska Speech-Language-Hearing Association	(ALSHA)	
Arizona	Arizona Speech-Language-Hearing Association	(ArSHA)	*www.healthcaresource.com/arsha*
Arkansas	Arkansas Speech-Language-Hearing Association	(ArkSHA)	*www.byers-soft.com/arksha*
California	California Speech-Language-Hearing Association	(CSHA)	*www.csha.org*
Colorado	Colorado Speech-Language-Hearing Association	(CSHA)	*www.cshassoc.org*
Connecticut	Connecticut Speech-Language-Hearing Association	(CSHA)	
Delaware	Delaware Speech-Language-Hearing Association	(DSHA)	
DC	District of Columbia Speech-Language-Hearing Assoc.	(DCSHA)	
Florida	Florida Association of Speech-Language Pathologists & Audiologists	(FLASHA)	*www.flasha.org*
Georgia	Georgia Speech-Language-Hearing Association	(GSHA)	*www.gsha.org*
Hawaii	Hawaii Speech-Language-Hearing Association	(HSHA)	*www.hsha.org*
Idaho	Idaho Speech-Language-Hearing Association	(ISHA)	*www.idahosha.org*
Illinois	Illinois Speech-Language-Hearing Association	(ISHA)	*www.ishail.org*
Indiana	Indiana Speech-Language-Hearing Association	(ISHA)	*www.islha.org*
Iowa	Iowa Speech-Language-Hearing Association	(ISHA)	*www.isha.org*
Kansas	Kansas Speech-Language-Hearing Association	(KSHA)	*www.ksha.org*
Kentucky	Kentucky Speech-Language-Hearing Association	(KSHA)	*http://msumusik.mursuky.edu/ksha*
Louisiana	Louisiana Speech-Language-Hearing Association	(LSHA)	*www.softdisk.com/comp/lsha*
Maine	Maine Speech-Language-Hearing Association	(MSLHA)	
Maryland	Maryland Speech-Language-Hearing Association	(MSHA)	*www.mdslha.org*
Massachusetts	Massachusetts Speech-Language-Hearing Association	(MSHA)	*www.healthcaresource.com/msha*
Michigan	Michigan Speech-Language-Hearing Association	(MSHA)	*www.michiganspeechhearing.org*
Minnesota	Minnesota Speech-Language-Hearing Association	(MSHA)	*www.msha.net*

Table 9.4—*Continued*

State	Association	Abbreviation	Website
Mississippi	Mississippi Speech-Language-Hearing Association	(MSHA)	*www.mshausa.org*
Missouri	Missouri Speech-Language-Hearing Association	(MSHA)	*www.showmemsha.org*
Montana	Montana Speech-Language-Hearing Association	(MSHA)	*www.mtspeechhearing.org*
Nebraska	Nebraska Speech-Language-Hearing Association	(NSLHA)	
Nevada	Nevada Speech-Language-Hearing Association	(NSHA)	
New Hampshire	New Hampshire Speech-Language-Hearing Association	(NHSLHA)	*http://nhslha.org*
New Jersey	New Jersey Speech-Language-Hearing Association	(NJSHA)	*www.njsha.org*
New Mexico	New Mexico Speech-Language-Hearing Association	(NMSHA)	*www.healthcaresource.com/nmsha*
New York	New York State Speech-Language-Hearing Association	(NYSSLH)	*www.healthcaresource.com/nysslha*
North Carolina	North Carolina Speech, Hearing and Language Association	(NCSHLA)	*www.geocities.com/~ncshla*
North Dakota	North Dakota Speech-Language-Hearing Association	(NSDLHA)	
Ohio	Ohio Speech and Hearing Association	(OSHA)	*www.osha.org*
Oklahoma	Oklahoma Speech-Language-Hearing Association	(OSHA)	*www.oslha.org*
Oregon	Oregon Speech-Language-Hearing Association	(OSHA)	*www.healthcaresource.com/osha*
Overseas	Overseas Association of Communication Sciences	(OSACS)	
Pennsylvania	Pennsylvania Speech-Language-Hearing Association	(PSHA)	*www.healthcaresource.com/psha*
Rhode Island	Rhode Island Speech-Language-Hearing Association	(RISHA)	
South Carolina	South Carolina Speech-Language-Hearing Association	(SCSHA)	*www.midnet.sc.edu/scsha*
South Dakota	South Dakota Speech-Language-Hearing Association	(SDSLHA)	
Tennessee	Tennessee Assoc. of Audiologists and Speech/Language Pathologists	(TAASLP)	*www.taaslp.org*
Texas	Texas Speech-Language-Hearing Association	(TSHA)	*www.txsha.org*
Utah	Utah Speech-Language-Hearing Association	(USHA)	*www.healthcaresource.com/usha*
Vermont	Vermont Speech-Language-Hearing Association	(VSHA)	
Virginia	Speech-Language-Hearing Association of Virginia	(SHAV)	*www.healthcaresource.com/shav*
Washington	Washington Speech and Hearing Association	(WSHA)	*www.wslha.org*
West Virginia	West Virginia Speech-Language-Hearing Association	(WVSHA)	
Wisconsin	Wisconsin Speech-Language Pathology and Audiology Assoc.	(WSHA)	*www.wisha.org*
Wyoming	Wyoming Speech-Language-Hearing Association	(WSHA)	*www.healthcaresource.com/wsha*

Professional Organizations Useful to Speech-Language Pathologists in Schools

Examples of valuable specialization organizations outside ASHA are listed below. The ones marked with an asterisk (*) include consumers as well as professionals, an authenticity that is missing in professionals-only groups. Others are particularly valuable because they are international and bring speech-language pathologists into contact with professionals from school systems beyond the United States. International organizations can often be recognized by their titles.

- Alexander Graham Bell Association for the Deaf and Hard of Hearing* *(www.agbell.org/)*
- American Academy of Audiology *(www.audiology.org/)*
- American Council on Learning Disabilities
- Association for Supervision and Curriculum Development *(www.ascd.org/)*
- Auditory-Verbal International* *(www.auditory-verbal.org/)*
- Autism Society of America* *(www.autism-society.org)*
- Council for Exceptional Children *(www.cec.sped.org)*
  - Council of Administrators in Special Education *(members.aol.com/casecec/)*
  - Division for Children's Communicative Development
  - Division for Early Childhood
- Council for Learning Disabilities (International) *(www.cldinternational.org/)*
- International Association of Logopedics and Phoniatrics *(www1.ldc.lu.se/logopedi/IALP/)*
- International Reading Association *(www.reading.org)*
- International Society for Augmentative and Alternative Communication* *(www.isaac-online.org)*
- National Association for the Education of Young Children *(www.naeyc.org/)*
- National Cued Speech Association* *(web7.mit.edu/CuedSpeech/ncsainfo.html)*
- National Down Syndrome Congress* *(www.ndsccenter.org)*
- Rehabilitation Engineers of North America*
- United States Society for Augmentative and Alternative Communication*

to me if I wanted to get on it, but at least I knew where it was" (Leubetken, M., personal communication, May 1, 1998). One of the authors of this book found that joining the National Association for the Education of Young Children (NAEYC) was like looking up from the microscope and seeing a whole laboratory for first time. These organizations are national, however, states and regions have similar organizations on smaller scales that focus on state issues. Again, these groups have great value for speech-language pathologists because education is a state issue, and the decisions about education are made by local legislatures and school boards who listen to their constituents, not to a group that represents other states. Bigger is not necessarily better when it comes to influencing opinion makers about their personal ideas of quality.

It is important to recognize the key organizations for other school professionals even if you cannot or do not join them. A few national organizations focused on the broader view of general or special education include National Association of Secondary Schools Principals (NASSP), National Association of Elementary Schools Principals (NAESP), and National Association of School Psychologists.

As noted earlier, some speech-language pathologists find it advantageous to join an organization that specializes in a particular disorder, approach, philosophy, or subgroup. Although special interest groups in both ASHA and state associations may have similar subgroups, these are still managed by the parent organization and have the same basic orientation and resources.

Professional organizations play an important part in the school-based speech-language pathologist becoming someone who knows the discipline within the larger context of education, plus one or two specialty areas in great depth. Membership in more than one organization allows speech-language pathologists to hone skills in one activity and use them with another

related group. The new energy that professional organizations add to the practice of speech-language pathology in schools is a great reason to join them.

Teacher Unions

Having a professional career as a speech-language pathologist in the schools means working in a specialized environment. The speech-language pathologist is an employee of the school district but is not a teacher in the sense of CLASSROOM INSTRUCTION. The speech-language pathologist is a service provider who selects which students will receive speech-language services and to what extent but typically is not an administrator. The speech-language pathologist's position exists to provide supports to students who require specialized assistance in order for them to be successful in the classroom and curriculum.

In some states, speech-language pathologists are viewed as teachers for purposes of credentialing, union membership, and salary placements. In other states, they have all of the above-named teacher rights but are considered nonteaching employees when they apply for related credentials or mentor teacher pay. Within states, some districts will place their speech-language pathologists on the management or support services track (i.e., nonunion) to receive additional pay but not management responsibilities.

Unions are prevalent for educators in some states and nonexistent in others. Table 9.5 lists states that have unions and specifies if speech-language pathologists are members. Teacher union employee groups are organized for the purpose of collective bargaining and are considered to be a "community of interest" (Webb, Greer, Montello, and Norton, 1987). Unions seek to cover fragmentation groups such as nonmanagement employees, but may not always do so. Unions may have local chapters and most are aligned nationally with either the National Education Association (NEA) or the American Federation of Teachers (AFT).

Table 9.5

Does Your State Have Unions/Collective Bargaining Units?

Responses of Council of State Association Presidents to November 1999 Survey for 28 States

Have Bargaining Units	Bargaining Units Include SLP Membership	Do Not Have Bargaining Units
California	Yes	Florida
District of Columbia	Yes	Georgia
Delaware	Yes	Hawaii
Indiana	Yes	Louisiana
Iowa	Yes	Maine
Kansas	Yes	Mississippi
Kentucky	Yes	North Carolina
Missouri	Yes	South Carolina
Montana	Yes	Vermont
Nebraska	Yes	
New Mexico	Yes	
New York	Yes	
North Dakota	Yes	
Ohio	Yes	
Oregon	Yes	
Pennsylvania	Yes	
Rhode Island	Yes	
South Dakota	Yes	
Utah	Yes	

Source: Moore-Brown and Montgomery (1999)

When a speech-language pathologist is hired by a school district, county agency, or regional special education unit, the local leader of the teachers' bargaining unit usually contacts the new employee to provide information on the union. If the union is a closed shop, all teaching employees—which may or may not include speech-language pathologists—must pay dues to that union. If it is an open shop, the speech-language pathologist may choose whether or not to join the union which bargains on behalf of the members, but can only select the currently situated union.

Advantages of union membership are hotly debated, though the issue of joining is often moot if the speech-language pathologist is employed in a district with a closed shop union. Speech-language pathologists are typically well represented by unions, if they bring their issues to the attention of the union's leadership.

At times, speech-language pathologists will bring concerns about employment conditions to the attention of ASHA or a state association and seek intervention from the professional association. Often these are not professional issues but rather bargaining issues that must be worked out between the parties in the employment contract (i.e., the school district and its employees). ASHA has developed a document (ASHA, 2000f) to assist speech-language pathologists and unions in their joint work. Speech-language pathologists from one district can also assist colleagues in a neighboring district with contract wording or work conditions that have been successfully resolved.

Liability and Insurance

General and special educators currently find they work within a highly litigious environment at times. While most professionals do not expect to be involved in litigation or to have their ethics or professional behavior questioned, in fact this does happen. Occasionally, spurious accusations are made or, unfortunately, unprofessional conduct occurs. The vast majority of the time, if professionals conduct themselves in a professional manner, their work behavior will not be challenged. The realities of a modern society dictate, however, that speech-language pathologists in public schools be informed and take adequate precautions regarding their own professional liability. Throughout this book, the importance of documentation and using research-based practice patterns has been emphasized. These habits will serve a speech-language pathologist well should he or she become involved in litigation. In addition, speech-language pathologists should take the steps that professionals in related fields take and carry professional liability insurance.

Professional liability and related insurance has several applications in the public school setting. There are basically three aspects to the liability issue:

- Liability for one's professional conduct in assessment and treatment of students with communication disabilities

- Liability for working as an educator of children to carry out the school district's curriculum, policies, procedures, and expectancies

- Liability as a citizen to abide by the civil laws and regulations of the city, state, and country (including laws that protect against discrimination toward persons with disabilities)

In the first case, to protect oneself from a claim regarding the conduct of professional practice, the speech-language pathologist needs to purchase professional liability insurance through an ASHA-approved agency or a similar service. Union membership sometimes provides this coverage. In the second case, the school district's insurance will cover an employee who is accused of negligence or incompetence if the person has operated under the district's policies and guidelines. In the third case, the person is liable for her own conduct as a law-abiding citizen.

After investigation, if the speech-language pathologist is found responsible for inappropriate action, reprimands can take many forms. One's certification and/or state license could be forfeited if found guilty of a violation of professional practice. One's job, credentials, or both could be forfeited for not properly carrying out district procedures, and one could face civil action for a violation of civil rights laws.

Because school district policies are understandably silent on many aspects of a communication intervention program and permit speech-language pathologists to make their own judgments for assessment and intervention, the wise professional should carry professional liability insurance in addition to the coverage the school district provides. The scope of practice of the speech-language pathologist is an ever-changing landscape. For example, engaging in an evolving practice such as dysphagia treatment with children in a school setting is exciting but has greater liability for the speech-language pathologist (O'Toole, 2000; Homer, 2000a). Speech-language pathologists who are covered by liability insurance can be reassured that they are protected when engaging in appropriate practice, in the event that their practices are challenged.

Teacher associations and unions are also very helpful with insurance arrangements or immediate assistance if allegations of wrongdoing are brought against a speech-language pathologist. Assistance with insurance and liability issues may also be available from school-based colleagues, ASHA, state associations, unions, and insurance brokers. All professions have well-structured insurance plans to protect clients against workplace hazards, such as false claims against the insured, unsubstantiated terminations, costly defense actions, and unfair treatment.

Who to Ask When You Have a Question on the Job

No matter how long someone works in the schools, questions about situations that are new and novel come up frequently. The first rule of working in public schools is "Don't be afraid to ask for help!" Where to go for that help may vary depending on the nature of the question. One thing to remember is that public school staff members are generally thoughtful and helpful, since this is the nature of people drawn to working with children. As a new person, though, seek advice from someone who has the knowledge to answer your question and has the experience to help you learn the expected methods of working within your school culture.

Support Networks

Speech-language pathologists need to develop several networks to acquire the types of information they need. Table 9.6 (pages 310–311) illustrates who and what might be helpful for speech-language pathologists to know when working in public schools.

There are other important people who can be a resource to beginning speech-language pathologists. Such people might include:

- Other speech-language pathologists in schools

- Speech-language pathologists in health care

- District or regional resource support staff for technology, staff development, categorical programs (e.g., Title I, bilingual education, American Indian education, or school-to-work), child welfare and attendance, and research and evaluation

- Directors of curriculum and instruction

- Assistant superintendents

- Business managers

- Superintendents (depending on the issue and size of the district)

- Parent groups

- Advisory groups

When seeking information, speech-language pathologists should know the culture of the district and understand the hierarchy for gaining information or obtaining resources. While most people will be relatively friendly, some school districts are very sensitive about the ways that employees go about getting what they need. While a new person should feel comfortable asking questions, be sensitive in terms of from whom and where the information is sought. Sometimes an employee may be told they "do not need to know about that." In such a circumstance, speech-language pathologists should simply ask who handles the matter and find out how to work with that person.

Existing structures for problem solving will also likely be in place. Examples would be department, job-alike (i.e., people with the same job titles), regional, or school site meetings. Another example of problem solving systems is to hold lunch meetings to discuss cases, which the authors have found to be a most successful learning and team-building experience. If such a system does not exist where you work, you might set it up!

Speech-language pathologists should also go to their state and national associations for guidance on specific issues. Such organizations often have policy and practice statements that may be useful to the speech-language pathologist in making decisions or communicating a position to administrators, parents, or teachers. Many helpful ASHA documents are available on the ASHA Web site *(www.asha.org),* including:

Table 9.6

People and Places for Finding Assistance

Level	Person	Nature of Information	Type of Question
Site	Secretary	Supplies, equipment, meetings, schedules, absences	Where do I get pencils and other supplies? Can I use the copier at the school site? Where do I report my absences? Who do I report to regarding changes in my schedule? Where do I get a key for my room?
	Custodian	Furniture, cleaning, supplies	How often is my room cleaned? Could I get another chair for this room?
	Principal	Schedules, meetings, resources, books and materials, funds, families, curriculum trends	Where is my room? Where can I obtain curriculum material? Who will chair IEP meetings? When do you want those meetings scheduled? What schoolwide and district meetings should I attend? What are the special programs that I should know about?
	Special Education Teacher	Policies and procedures for special education, service delivery models used at the site, student data, strategies for instruction	Which students receive duplicated services? How can we work together to provide services?
	General Education Teacher	General education curriculum, Student Study Team (SST) practices, student performance information, current instructional methodology	How is a particular student doing in class? What modifications/accommodations are being used? What is the program/curricular emphasis in the classroom?

Table 9.6—*Continued*

Level	Person	Nature of Information	Type of Question
District/ Region	Secretary (Special Education)	Student database, forms, ordering/budget	Who sets up IEP meetings? What is the process for turning in paperwork? What data am I required to keep? How do I order supplies?
	Psychologist	Behavior/social issues, testing, program issues, eligibility questions	Are there characteristics being demonstrated that might be considered emotional disturbance? What is the student's performance on processing tests? What programmatic considerations should we be making? What if the student does not qualify?
	Program Specialist/ Manager	Assistance with student issues, referral to more restrictive environments, assistance with referrals to outside agencies, assistance with issues involving advocates or attorneys	Please come and observe this student. This student is not being successful. What should we consider? Parents say they will bring an advocate to the meeting. What should I do?
	Program Administrator (Coordinator; Director)	Allocations of funds and resources, assignments, assistance with student issues, due process issues, hiring, supervision, program coordination	What is my assignment? What is my budget? Can I discuss suggestions for program changes with you? Who is conducting my performance evaluation?
	Regional Administrator	Legal assistance, allocations of funds, assignments (in some organizations)	(Same as those for the Program Administrator, depending on the organizational structure.)

- Scope of Practice Statements: A list of professional activities that define the range of services offered within the professions of speech-language pathology

- PREFERRED PRACTICE PATTERNS: Statements that define universally applicable characteristics of activities directed toward individual patients/clients, and that address structural requisites of the practice, processes to be carried out, and expected outcomes

- Position Statements: Statements that specify ASHA's policy and stance on a matter that is important not only to the membership but also to other outside agencies or groups

- Practice Guidelines: A recommended set of procedures for a specific area of practice, based on research findings and current practice, that details the knowledge, skills, and/or competencies needed to perform the procedures effectively

The sidebar provides activities for the aspiring speech-language pathologist to begin engaging in professional activities common to the work world of school-based speech-language pathologists.

Activities for Aspiring Speech-Language Pathologists

Invite an officer of your state association to class, or interview him or her on your own. Prepare questions about the role that your association plays in legislation, recruitment, and retention of school-based speech-language pathologists. Inquire whether there is a committee or a board position to represent school issues. Inquire whether there is a student chapter or reduced student membership fee, and how you can get involved.

Plan to attend the next state or national conference for speech-language and hearing professionals that is held in your geographic area, or plan to travel to one. Register in advance so you receive a copy of the program and note how many topics are on school-based issues. Plan to attend those sessions, especially any committee meetings or task force meetings that are open to you. Ask questions and get to know the professionals involved in these issues in your state.

Join or become more active in your campus NSSLHA chapter. Bring issues from this class or this book for discussion at the next meeting. Record the responses and keep track of the certifications, regulations, and procedures in your state for the topics discussed in this chapter.

Create a personal portfolio of your continuing education and professional development activities thus far. Begin to collect documentation of conference and course attendance that is necessary to maintain your state and national certifications. Record activities that have developed your professional skills even if they are not immediately needed for minimum requirements. List professional organizations, volunteer activities with children, leadership tasks in your school, and extra curricular activities that demonstrate your knowledge and commitment to public education.

Local and Regional Supervisors

Speech-language pathologists in public schools will work with a variety of individuals who will serve in different supervisory positions. The person who writes the speech-language pathologist's evaluations may or may not have a background in speech-language pathology, or even special education. Speech-language pathologists, as much as any other professional in the system, may be promoted into general or special education administration.

Building-level staff, including speech-language pathologists, are likely to report to a principal. In some systems, the supervisor is from the special education department and may have a background from either general or special education. There is not one particular career track for general or special education administrators.

Many special education systems have a middle management person called a program specialist or program manager. These individuals may or may not be administrators, but they have significant involvement in program development, program placement decisions, and staff development. Some also are involved in employment decisions, such as making recommendations for hiring and termination. Job performance evaluations are typically conducted by individuals who are administrators, which is why a principal often performs that function for the specialist staff.

Depending on the size of the district, the special education department may also have a director or coordinator who oversees the entire operation of special education in the district. This person may also have job responsibilities other than special education, such as other pupil services functions (e.g., health, psychological, counseling, discipline, home study, or other services). The speech-language pathologist may or may not interact on a regular basis with the district-level special education administrator. If the district is large, program support persons will provide guidance. A large district or consortium of smaller districts may even have one individual who oversees only the speech-language programs. In a midsize or smaller school district, the speech-language pathologist may have regular contact with the district-level administrator.

Speech-language pathologists who have moved into supervisory and administrative roles in public schools have access to groups such as the ASHA special interest division in administration (number 11) and the Council for Administrators and Supervisors of Speech, Language, and Hearing Programs (CASSLHP) to provide support and collegial interaction. Supervisors who are not speech-language pathologists, may need input regarding program goals, the speech-language pathologist's role, and the work of the field. When sharing information with a supervisor, it is usually helpful to recognize that person's perspective and what is important to him or her. Speech-language pathologists may find that discussing how their activities promote improved reading ability may be of greater interest to a principal than information about oral motor exercises, for example. Certainly, once the principal learns the extent of skills and abilities of the speech-language pathologist, a great partnership can occur.

State Consultants

In the early days of special education, most SEAs had consultant positions for all specialty areas (e.g., visual impairments, deaf/hard of hearing, preschool, and speech-language). By the end of the 1990s, several states still had consultants with a speech-language background, but these individuals had job responsibilities that extended far beyond the field of speech-language. Such responsibilities included working with the complaints and monitoring division of the SEA, working with school reform issues, and working with Medicaid billing. Despite these other job responsibilities, today's SEA consultants connect to speech-language pathologists in the field in a variety ways. They also connect with each other through an ASHA-related organization called the Council of Language, Speech, and Hearing Consultants in State Education Agencies (CLSHCSEA). CLSHCSEA members:

- ADVISE AND CONSULT with appropriate federal agencies, state agencies, and other public and private organizations and committees on philosophies, principles, practices, and needs in all areas relating to services for individuals who have language, speech, or hearing disabilities

- FORMULATE AND RECOMMEND policies and procedures in the field of language, speech and hearing, and disseminate them to appropriate agencies and organizations.

- ESTABLISH liaisons with other organizations and associations whose primary purpose is to promote the pro-

vision of appropriate speech, language, and hearing services to children from birth through twenty-one.

- NETWORK AND SHARE information, ideas, solutions, guidelines, innovative programs and practices, etc. with other CLSHCSEA members (CLSHCSEA, 1999, p. 1).

In their daily work, state consultants focus their energies in the following areas:

- Consult with university training programs, especially in the area of speech and language

- Assist noncertified people who are working in the field

- Assist certified speech-language pathologists who have questions about issues, and need an outside recommendation

- Provide recruitment connections between graduates and school systems

- Conduct trainings

- Serve as a liaison between county level systems and the state

- Maintain a library of resources

- Serve as the connection between general education and speech-language pathologists in early literacy trainings (especially in the area of PHONEMIC AWARENESS)

- Work closely with state associations, and possibly conduct round table discussions or update sessions at the annual state conference (K. Knighton, personal communication, December 28, 1999).

As of November 1999, the following states had representatives to the CLSHCSEA group: Alabama, California, Colorado, Connecticut, District of Columbia, Florida (2), Illinois, Louisiana, Maryland, Minnesota, Mississippi, Montana, Nebraska, Nevada, Oklahoma, Pennsylvania, Texas, Utah, West Virginia, Wisconsin (CLSHCSEA, 1998).

Speech-language pathologists in public schools are encouraged to contact their SEA and ask who is the consultant responsible for speech-language and hearing programs in the state. This person can be one more valuable resource for answers and ideas.

Continuing Education

School-based speech-language pathologists have a professional responsibility to maintain and update their clinical skills to meet the needs of myriad developmental levels and ever-expanding range of disabilities presented by students. When assignments change, new skills often are needed or previously learned skills need to be updated. This might be particularly true when speech-language pathologists encounter students in secondary school for the first time or students with specialized needs such as autism, cerebral palsy, augmentative communication, or perhaps a cochlear implant. In most schools, the speech-language pathologist is the only professional who can assess and implement a plan for these students' communication needs. Much of one's graduate program in communication sciences and disorders is devoted to recognizing and serving students with these disorders, as well as identifying sources of information that the speech-language

pathologist can access later to stay current with the field. Part of the allure of this profession is the steady stream of new developments in so many areas and continued expansion into new areas. School-based speech-language pathologists also play expanding roles in reading instruction and classroom-based services, so continuing education in these areas is essential.

Continuing education is the vehicle to assure parents and other team members that qualified providers with state or national licensure and certification remain knowledgeable and qualified. In some states, a certain number of continuing education units (CEUs) is mandatory for renewing credentials, while others rely on professional integrity. The Continuing Education section of ASHA's Web site (*www.asha.org/continuing_ed/continuing_ed.htm*) maintains a list of each state's requirements for licensure and the contact agencies for speech-language licensure and teacher certification. ASHA has been discussing the possibility of mandatory CEUs to maintain the CCC in speech-language pathology, but no change in policy is pending.

State organizations for speech-language pathologists are excellent sources of continuing education through their conferences, workshops, and professional study groups. ASHA offers the broadest array of continuing education formats, including conferences, workshops, seminars, audiotapes, video conferences, journal and newsletter read-and-test situations, study groups, special interest divisions, and refereed scholarly journals. Universities offer classes and courses, but enrolling may be difficult if one is not pursuing a degree. University courses can be more expensive and time-consuming than training offered by professional organizations and may not have the advanced level of information the experienced professional is seeking. Continuing education offerings by school districts, state educational agencies (SEAs), and extended adult education programs, which are often free or low cost, can be problematic in other ways. While these offerings can provide valuable information on general education curriculum and instruction, they have less direct application to the field of speech-language pathology. These courses may suffice for school district salary schedule advancement (a local union or school district decision in most areas), but they may not be acceptable for state licensure or the future renewal of CCC if that becomes a requirement.

CEUs must be approved by the certificate-granting body in order to be counted as professional growth hours. This circumstance could require the speech-language pathologist to take multiple classes to accommodate what several boards, panels, and certification agencies require. Some states have developed arrangements that assist in coordinating these requirements. The speech-language pathologist should keep in mind that school districts, university curriculum and instruction departments, and SEAs are the only agencies likely to offer courses that help speech-language pathologists understand general education curriculum and instruction, a requirement of IDEA (1997). Learning the state and district curriculum frameworks and standards is a responsibility of the speech-language pathologist in schools and can be met with teacher education CEUs. Participating and learning alongside teachers also gives insight into the expectations for teachers and helps to create partnerships.

The important factors to keep in mind regarding continuing education are:

- Maintain your CCC yearly.

- Choose your professional development training options carefully.

- Know what your state requires to maintain your credential.

- Know what your state requires to maintain your speech-language pathology license.

- Know what you need to extend your clinical skills in schools.

- Know what you want to add to your repertoire.

- Know what to add to your professional portfolio to help you stay viable in the job market.

- Look for continuing education providers who have received endorsement by all the certifying agencies to which you must report, to keep it affordable for you.

- Join other school-based speech-language pathologists and work with your state organization to streamline an unwieldy state continuing education process.

- Remember all continuing education brings added value to your knowledge and skills; some is just more immediately evident than others.

Finally, IDEA (1997) stipulates that if the speech-language pathologist or any other member of the student's educational team needs specific training to be effective with that student, the training can be written into the student's IEP (34 CODE OF FEDERAL REGULATIONS [C.F.R.] § 300.346 [d]). This is referred to as "supplementary aids and services, program modifications, or supports for school personnel." If a team member needs specific training to help the child with a communication disorder (e.g., sign language, DISCRETE TRIAL TRAINING, or augmentative or alternative communication) this training can be listed as a supplementary support for school personnel in the IEP. This could provide specific training for the speech-language pathologist or might enable a paraprofessional or another team member to learn a supporting skill for the classroom. The LEA representative is present on the IEP in order to authorize this type of commitment of LEA resources.

Continuing education can take many forms, but it is always an important component of the school-based professional's role. Even if continuing education is not mandated, it is a professional responsibility as is keeping track of one's continuing education growth activities each year. Table 9.7 is an example of one school based speech-language pathologist's continuing education activities for two years that enabled her to maintain all of her credentials and keep her skills sharp.

Table 9.7

One Speech-Language Pathologist's Continuing Education Log

(The Personal Portfolio contains notes and registration from each activity.)

Year	Action	Hours
1	Attended ASHA convention in home state	8*
	Attended one day of state SLP convention	5*
	Attended two days of school district reading curriculum workshops (stipend)	8
	Read journals with Journal Group from the district for ASHA CEUs	10*
2	Attended three days of state convention	16*
	Took a three-day summer workshop on bilingual assessment from the SEA	18
	Completed two-day fluency seminar for school practitioners	10*
	Read the Special Interest Division newsletters and took the quizzes	6
	Responded on Special Interest Division listserv at least once a week	24
	Organized and attended the May Is Better Hearing and Speech Month all-day speaker on functional outcomes in the schools	13 (5*)

*These hours convert to CEUs and each activity was registered with an approved CE sponsor for that credential.

CHAPTER 10

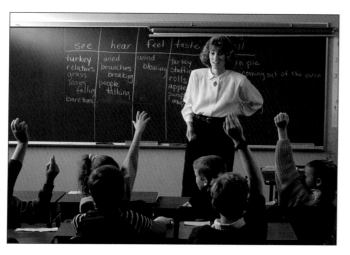

A Promising Future for School-Based Speech-Language Pathologists

IN THIS CHAPTER

Three national reports that focus on future issues in education and in speech-language pathology introduce this chapter. The concept of future study is explored as a way of anticipating and shaping the future. Social and educational trends that will likely affect the field of speech-language pathology are examined to prepare for the ongoing changes in the profession. Interpersonal competencies will be just as important as technical competencies for speech-language pathologists working in a climate of collaboration, reform, technological change, and community diversity.

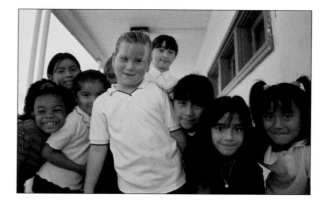

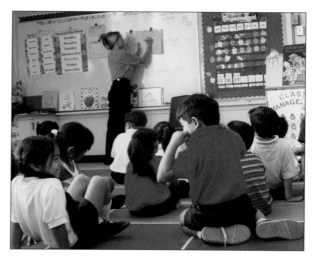

1. The National Education Goals were not met after 10 years of effort. What would be the advantages and disadvantages of continuing to have a national focus on these goals for another decade?

2. The need to attract, educate, recruit, and retain bilingual and bicultural speech-language pathologists continues. What efforts could university departments and their students make to address this need?

3. Select one of the trends listed in the sidebar beginning on page 324 and describe the effects you project this trend will have on schools and speech-language pathologists.

4. What knowledge and skills would be needed by a speech-language pathologist who wishes to become a curriculum consultant and be knowledgeable about methods for delivering large group instruction to diverse learners? How would a school-based speech-language pathologist go about developing these skills and knowledge?

5. Ask a school-based speech-language pathologist about the issues listed in the sidebar on page 332, and determine which are the most critical to that professional. Compare your results with those of other class members and look for trends.

Foundations for Envisioning the Future

Three reports from the 1990s might be considered foundational for our leap into the future of school-based speech-language pathologists. One report, the *National Education Goals Report* (National Education Goals Panel [NEGP], 1999), was established as the national focus for all public schools, and the other two reports—"Future Watch: Our Schools in the 21st Century" (Montgomery and Herer, 1994) and "Partnerships in Education: Toward a Literate America" (ASHA, 1989b), which was the seminal document that evolved into "Trends and Issues in School Reform and Their Effects on Speech-Language Pathologists, Audiologists, and Students with Communication Disorders" (ASHA, 1997d)—were created directly by and for professionals involved in school speech-language services.

The National Education Goals

In 1989, an educational summit held at the University of Virginia produced six National Education Goals. The goals were formally announced by President George Bush in his 1990 State of the Union address. They were ratified by the National Governors Association a month later, and Congress added two more goals in 1994 (NEGP], 1999). The eight goals from this unprecedented state and national government partnership were presented in Chapter 1. (See page 6 for the National Education Goals.)

In December 1999, a rather subdued news conference was held in Washington, DC, by the NEGP to announce disappointing results of the 10-year effort. The nation had not fully met any of the eight goals. The NEGP reported that measurable progress had been made in the goals pertaining to preschoolers and student achievement in math and reading (Cooper, 1999). Overall, there was general improvement in 12 of the 27 statistical indicators used to measure the goals and a decline in 5 others. In many cases, insufficient information did not allow for accurate judgments to be made, reflecting problems with data gathering and reporting. Five states—Colorado, Connecticut, Kentucky, North Carolina, and South Carolina—improved on nearly half of the indicators. Maryland was recognized for having 95 percent of its students finish high school—the highest percentage in the country. Forty-nine states did have increases in the proportion of students with disabilities participating in preschool. While 12 states reduced their high school dropout rate, 11 states reported increases. Unfortunately, more states reported that teachers were not holding a college degree in the area in which they were actually teaching. More states also reported issues of safety and disruptions.

Education Secretary Richard W. Riley shared the opinion of many educators when he commented, "We're not where we want to be—by a long shot—and we have to pick up the pace.... The goals we have set are like a North Star. They give a sense of direction" (as quoted in Cooper, 1999, p. A2). Americans now question if the goals will simply be extended for 10 more years. Wisconsin's Governor, Tommy Thompson, the only remaining member from the original 1989 NEGP, suggested that every school district be responsible to meet the goals by 2010 (Cooper, 1999).

Judging by the coverage in professional newsletters, journal articles, and AMERICAN SPEECH-LANGUAGE-HEARING ASSOCIATION (ASHA) Executive Board initiatives, speech-language pathologists first turned their attention to these National Education Goals in 1994 (ASHA, 1999a; S. Karr, personal communication, November 19, 1999; Montgomery, 1995). Halfway through the 1990s, school districts began to realize that their special education personnel needed to support these general education goals. In 1995, as Congress began to review the wording in IDEA for impending reauthorization, the National Education Goals served as one of their sources of information on public policy. FUNCTIONAL OUTCOMES in health care focused on effectiveness indicators that also showed utility as accountability tools in measuring progress for individual students and National Education Goals. Striving for National Education Goals will likely remain an important part of speech-language pathologists' work ethic in schools and a signal of the ongoing partnership with general education.

A National Forum on Schools

The same year that the Governors Summit produced the National Education Goals, a first-ever National Forum on Schools was held by ASHA in Washington, DC. This forum featured nationally known speakers in three areas: young children at risk, language and LITERACY in an information age, and education in a multi-cultural society. Three of the 12 speakers were from the field of speech-language pathology, but the majority of speakers invited to discuss these three critical areas represented the fields of education, developmental psychology, reading research, human development, journalism, government, and public policy. For ASHA, it was time to learn from colleagues outside the profession and announce our intention to stand ready to pledge our support for the National Education Goals rumored to be on the horizon (Herer, 1989).

Describing the current situation in their discipline, each speaker proposed how speech-language pathologists and others in schools could and should make a difference for students in the next decade. The final discussant, Shirley Jones Daniels, formerly of the U.S. Office of Special Education and Rehabilitation Services, outlined seven recommendations that reflected the specific roles that speech-language pathologists in public schools should play as partners with educators in schools (ASHA, 1989):

1. ASHA, with public and private agencies, should jointly develop documents on the nature of, and SERVICE DELIVERY to, the population embraced by the term *at-risk*.

2. ASHA and individual states must decide how best to identify at-risk children, whether they are eligible for federal special education funds, and decide what role speech-language pathologists will have with underachieving children in our schools.

3. Speech-language professionals need to forge relationships and partnerships with learners to help them achieve, and with related fields of education, human development, and reading/literacy research to help us to achieve the knowledge we need to be more effective in literacy, reading, and language.

4. Speech-language pathologists need to learn the research on competencies in COLLABORATION and prepare to engage ourselves in the educational partnership.

5. The profession needs to help determine which limited English proficient children need what kind of instruction, while remaining wary of the known flaws in bilingual evaluation research.

6. Speech-language pathologists must recognize that the ability to communicate is the link among the topics of at-risk and marginalized children, literacy acquisition, and serving culturally and linguistically diverse populations.

7. We need to make a dramatic effort to attract, educate, recruit, and retain bilingual and bicultural speech-language pathologists to work in our schools in every state.

So what happened 10 years later when these recommendations were reassessed? It is safe to say that, like the National Education Goals, these seven goals have become ongoing "North Star" efforts. The three themes of the recommendations—young children at risk, language and literacy in an information age, and education in a multicultural society—are of vital importance, are not easily vanquished in a decade, and remain in the forefront of speech-language intervention today. Specific indicators, such as how to measure a partnership or how many new bilingual professionals joined ASHA, were not attached to these goals at the time they were developed. It is likely we have become better goal setters today. By adding objective statements to our professional goals, we will be able to more clearly identify how we expect the future to look.

In the early 1990s, speech-language pathologists felt the urging to partner with their general education colleagues change from gentle nudges to strongly worded regulations found in IDEA (1997) to address curricular areas and academics. We are highly cognizant of the hand held out by reading teachers in both elementary and secondary schools. They want help with their struggling readers, and a speech-language pathology background intersects with reading development in many ways (see ASHA, 2000d).

We have made some significant strides in this country to become culturally competent practitioners. We have recognized the value and richness of second-language learners' experiences and no longer label them with limited proficiency. Sadly, only very small numbers of bilingual individuals are attracted into our profession, and we graduate even smaller percentages (ASHA, 1999d). Certainly, the three themes of young children at risk, language and literacy in an information age, and education in a multicultural society are reflected everywhere in our professional literature, in our discussions, and in this textbook. The authors are convinced that the ability to communicate is the link between and among these three issues for school-based speech-language pathologists.

Future Watch

Future studies is a discipline that involves a systematic way of examining factors that can influence the future, then projecting possible futures on the basis of their interaction and trends (Montgomery and Herer, 1994). In fact, the word *futures,* often used in these studies,

refers to more than one future or multiple directions that trends will take us. Some are more preferable than others, and the persons who track and thereby influence these trends are also the ones who have the greatest impact on which future actually occurs according to Whaley and Whaley (1986). Speech-language pathologists want to track and influence as many trends as possible in the school environment. John Goodlad (1984) reported in a landmark book, *A Place Called School,* that the future should be viewed as a "succession of days and years between now and then that will determine what life will be like. Decisions made and not made will shape the schools of tomorrow" (p. 7).

A 1994 article "Future Watch: Our Schools in the 21st Century" (Montgomery and Herer) used the social trends identified by Cetron and Gayle (1990) to identify 19 forecasts judged most likely to affect speech-language pathologists by the year 2000. These forecasts are presented in the sidebar.

Examined in hindsight, the first eight projections are easily recognizable in the current

**Social Trends Likely to Impact
Speech-Language Pathologists by the Year 2000**

1. Education will be the major public agenda item and will be viewed as key to our economic growth.

2. There is growing mismatch between the vocabulary, reading and writing skills of our workforce and the competencies required on the job. This involves entry-level workers, as well as those on the job who are not adapting to new technology.

3. Public school enrollment will increase to 43.8 million in the year 2000, up from slightly below 40 million in the 1980s.

Continued

4. One million will drop out of school yearly due to increased academic standards, drug abuse, and teen pregnancy (to cite only a few key reasons) costing an estimated loss in earnings and taxes of $240 billion over a lifetime.

5. The supply of newly graduated teachers will meet only 60% of the new hire demands of public schools during this decade. We will need a million more than available due to retirement, class size requirements, and enrollment projections.

6. Minorities among students will grow, as they will in the general population, but this increase will not be reflected in the ranks of teachers. The pool of minority teachers in training is small.

7. Lifelong learning will be reflected in education delivery systems.

8. A core curriculum will emerge from a debate of teaching basic skills versus arts, and vocational education versus critical thinking.

9. Foreign language/bilingual instruction will be necessary for all students as states prepare them for a worldwide marketplace.

10. Vocational education emphasizing technical literacy will be demanded by and required of an increasing number of students, and it will be integrated with academics in a re-structured curriculum.

11. Although valued in principle, a liberal arts college education will not be valued in pay or competitiveness for jobs requiring special skills.

12. More than half of all jobs will require postsecondary education and training, but only 15% will require a college degree. Technical institutes and community colleges will supply the former.

13. The ingredients of school reform will continue to be debated in the 1990s (e.g. merit pay, longer school year, local control, accountability measures, curriculum design, etc.) with improvements occurring in some areas but not in national averages on standardized tests. A national consensus on reform will be necessary to achieve the latter and to reassert the supremacy of U.S. education versus that of other industrialized nations.

14. A futures perspective of basics in education will occur, using telecommunications technologies, advanced science knowledge, and technical skills to achieve problem solving.

Continued on next page

Making a Difference
for America's Children

Continued

15. Educational bureaucracies at all levels of government will lose power as reforms occur in the 1990s. Parents, teachers, students and business leaders will demand more involvement in decisions, have little knowledge of how to restructure, and move forward with little research.

    Speech-language pathologists will see county and regional special education agencies weaken in power and control less and less of the programming for children with communication disorders. State credentials and licenses will undergo significant changes, including speech-language pathologists and audiologists in one place and completely overlooking them in others. Speech-language pathologists will find it necessary to define themselves as teachers or specialists, but not both. The audiologists will be aligned with medical personnel and collaborate with educators.

16. Curriculum, teacher training, and achievement standards will be controlled centrally, but decentralization of school and classroom management will occur.

    Curriculum will be characterized by large loose state frameworks and specific local requirements. Literacy will become the hallmark of all special education, and speech-language pathologists will be helping to write the metacognitive and metalinguistic components of local curriculum.

    As IQ tests fall out of favor, the functional and authentic assessments used by speech-language pathologists will be in great demand. They will need to be computerized, administered, and scored holistically to be useful for schools.

17. Principals will be the leaders of change in schools and will share responsibility for school-based management with staff. This will require high-quality professionals during a time (the 1990s) of shortages for qualified school administrators.

    Many speech-language pathologists will be moving into administrative posts in schools, particularly positions in managing special education, preschool, Head Start, and at-risk students.

18. Numerous school alternatives will fragment the traditional education system. Initiatives will range from extreme centralization/financial control to vouchers used by parents selecting private schools.

    Although traditional public school programs will persist, many will have increased private sector partnerships.

19. Parents and special interest groups will raise legal challenges to issues such as curriculum, expenditures, and access, especially as they pertain to minorities and those with low incomes. Educational equity issues will be redefined in terms of expenditures and not access.

From "Future Watch: Our Schools in the 21st Century" by J. Montgomery and G. Herer, 1994, *Language, Speech, and Hearing Services in Schools, 25,* pp. 134–135. © 1994 by the American Speech-Language-Hearing Association. Reprinted with permission.

state of affairs. Forecasts 11–13 are also acknowledged today. Forecast 15 can be found in more than half the states today. Forecast 16 can be found in all the field's current professional conferences and journals. Forecasts 17–19 describe a future that has arrived in many ways in our schools, including speech-language pathologists in administrative roles, special and alternative education joining forces, and more legal challenges to our delivery of services. Forecasts 9, 10, and 14 remain issues that have changed very little.

This review of forecasts speaks directly to the importance of the individual speech-language pathologist in public schools. Knowing trends and influencing them does appear to have an impact on the future. Did a projected trend happen because we said it would, or did the series of events occur because we recognized and reported on the trends that were shaping it? We are always in a position to shape the future by being aware of what is shaping the present. Speech-language pathologists have a responsibility to know the current expectations and trends for their profession, share them with others, and respond to them to craft our preferable futures.

Educational Services in the Twenty-First Century

That speech-language pathologists in public schools serve as partners with others to realize the *transformation* of educational systems is evident. *Transformation* means the "inventing of a different kind of educational system for tomorrow" (Paul, Yang, Adiegbola, and Morse, 1995, p. 11). These partnerships necessitate the extension of our scope of practice, thereby expanding our roles and responsibilities (see sidebar in Chapter 9 on pages 286–287). As the educational system is transformed, speech-language pathologists are also called on to develop methods of service delivery designed to meet the needs of an ever-changing student population.

School-based speech-language pathologists are part of an educational system that, itself, is in a constant state of flux. As we consider the future for speech-language pathologists in schools, we must again step out of our profession and consider the thoughts, ideas, and predictions of our partners, our education colleagues. As we return to Chapter 1's predictions for the future by O'Shea and O'Shea (1997), we will also consider what others think about education's future in the twenty-first century.

General Education: Areas in Need of Change

Researchers recognize that the future of educational practice is complex and multidimensional. Luke and Elkins (2000b) described how the science of education has moved from looking for simple answers to recognizing the uncertainty of working in dynamic systems:

> As teachers and as learners, we are on new, tricky, and shifting ground. The notion that our work as literacy educators

is about the development of scientific "methods" can be traced back to the last turn of the century, when it was assumed that all educational problems could be solved with efficiency and precision. At this turn of the century, our position is different. Where once scientific certainty appeared to provide answers, we are now living in the midst of unprecedented diversity and complexity, dynamic change, and, often chaos. Whether we are biologists, social planners, or educators, New Times are requiring sensitive, contextual, and flexible blends of cultural and scientific analysis. (p. 396)

The influence of cognitive psychology and insights from brain research are identified by Marzano (2000) as being foundations of twentieth-century pedagogy that will strongly influence general education's instructional models in the future. He makes two simple, "safe" (p. 84) predictions for instructional models:

> **Prediction 1:** Instruction will become more of a science (p. 84).

> **Prediction 2:** Instructional models will become more comprehensive (p. 85).

To realize such predictions, professionals must develop expertise and be provided the requisite tools and an appropriate environment. Additionally, six areas of educational practice (described in the following sections) need to change, according to Allington and McGill-Franzen (2000). These areas are of interest to special educators, as they speak to areas that

students with special learning needs find challenging in schools. Consider how these six areas might apply and extend to the work of speech-language pathologists in public schools.

Discourse of the Classroom

A criticism of classroom instructional practices at the end of the twentieth century was that the discourse pattern of I-R-E (Initiate-Reply-Evaluate) continued to be the predominant mode of instructional delivery in most classrooms. In order for all learners, especially those with specialized learning needs, to be engaged in the learning of the classroom, this discourse pattern needs to change.

Who better than the speech-language pathologist—with our extensive knowledge in discourse, communication, and learning—to work with classroom teachers to identify models of teaching that will expand learning and interaction in the classroom? Speech-language pathologists then become not only curriculum consultants to classroom teachers, but also extend the methodologies of delivering instruction to large groups of diverse learners.

Standards and Educationally Challenged Students

Throughout several chapters, this book has referred to the requirements of standards-based reform and their impact on service delivery by speech-language pathologists and all educators when working with students who are educationally challenged. Allington and McGill-Franzen (2000) essentially addressed the same issues that were identified in Chapter 1 as the complicators of Wave Three reform (see "Three Waves of Educational Reforms"). The challenge involved in including all students in expectations for high performance and accountability for all learners require new methods of curriculum and instruction. This evolving future may be achieved through the concept of UNIVERSAL DESIGN, described in "Development of Goals and Short-Term Objectives or Benchmarks" in Chapter 4. Special educators typically have not been involved in curriculum choices or development, but must increase their involvement to realize the goals set forth in legislation and by society.

Expert Teachers Are the Key

This area of need appears self-evident and is closely tied to the next area. Professional expertise has become a necessity in the twenty-first century. Speech-language pathologists, teachers, psychologists, counselors, administrators, and others working with children must possess a current knowledge base in their own and in related fields. Most professionals are inundated with the resources available in our information society. IDEA (1997) and standards-based reform moved educators in the direction of making instructional decisions based on research-proven methods. The school-based speech-language pathologist will need to be a continuous learner to remain on the cutting edge of professional expertise.

> Access...deals not only with the issues of access to equipment, but also access to teachers who are knowledgeable in the use of technology.

Professional Development

Teachers and specialists must be well trained and expert in their choices and execution of their responsibilities in the classroom. Personal responsibility for professional development was addressed in Chapter 9 (see "Continuing Education"). School districts and state educational agencies will also need to continue to expand their provision of learning opportunities for teachers to align their teaching with the standards.

Technology

The need to support the evolving use of technology within curriculum and instruction may seem obvious. Allington and McGill-Franzen (2000) draw attention to concerns regarding access. Children from low socioeconomic status homes typically do not have the out-of-school access to computers that their more economically advantaged peers have. President Bill Clinton addressed concerns about the Digital Divide in his State of the Union address in January 2000, followed by initiatives from his administration to move "from Digital Divide to Digital Opportunity" (The White House, 2000). Education seeks to bridge the Digital Divide through building a "digital curriculum" (Technology Counts '99, 1999). Access, in the context of these discussions, deals not only with the issues of access to equipment, but also access to teachers who are knowledgeable in the use of technology. (See more on technology on page 334.)

Common School Experience/School Choice

Allington and McGill-Franzen (2000) express great concern over the impact of choice or charter schools on disadvantaged children when addressing the ongoing movement toward privatization of public education. This movement has implications not only for children with special needs, but for the whole of the public education system. It seems somewhat ironic that IDEA (1997) indicated that access had seemingly been achieved for children with disabilities, yet now that home school and general education classroom PLACEMENTS are no longer the major concern of SPECIAL EDUCATION, an entire movement is afoot to change the reality of the neighborhood school itself.

> The expanded definition of literacy will include the need for competence in several genres, including print text of various modes, texts of the Internet, and multimedia texts.

Expanded Definition of Literacy

This book has made significant reference to the emerging role of speech-language pathologists in working with literacy. The expanded definition of literacy will include the need for competence in several genres, including print text of various modes, texts of the Internet, and multimedia texts. Students and workers in the digital age must be able to process massive amounts of information presented in all of these new areas of literacy (Helfand, 2000; Kist, 2000; Luke and Elkins, 2000a, 2000b; Moje, Young, Readence, and Moore, 2000; Neuman, Smagorinsky, Enciso, Baldwin, and Hartman, 2000; Tierney, Johnston, Moore, and Valencia, 2000).

An ASHA document (2000d) on the roles and responsibilities of speech-language pathologists clearly defines why and where speech-language pathologists should be involved in reading and writing. The role of speech-language pathologists in literacy activities in schools remains inconsistent with variability between practitioners in terms of their chosen level of involvement. Speech-language pathologists of the future must be connected in a meaningful way to literacy activities in the school and district. The education and research base in our field have provided expertise in this area. Practice patterns must expand so that speech-language pathologists can use their expertise to benefit an entire school program. We must also extend our study to allied and related fields, such as teacher education, linguistics, reading, counseling, psychology, child health, and sociology. The new literacies will provide new challenges for individuals with COMMUNICATION DISORDERS, and new opportunities for extension of practice and novel interventions for speech-language pathologists.

Speech-language pathologists must attend to the implications of this trend. Moje et al. (2000) predict, "If we cannot address these new literacies and the increasing diversity that we encounter, then we may find that more and more students will struggle to be successful in school" (p. 405). If this is a concern for the typical learner, certainly students with communication disorders—who already have difficulties processing and retaining text information—are likely to be further challenged. Perhaps, however, speech-language pathologists will find that these new modes of literacy will also provide new areas of assessment (Tierney et al., 2000) and intervention, which may assist students in "re/mediating" (Luke and Elkins, 2000b, p. 396) their communication disorders.

Our Predicted Future: Speech-Language Pathologists in Public Schools

In 1996, an *Asha* magazine article peered into the future of the professions and identified the forces of technology, decentralization, and cost containment as revolutionizing both education and health care (Goldberg, 1996). Special education researchers identified the late 1990s trends of "integration and inclusion, collaboration and teaming, acceptance of diversity, and use of advanced technology" as shaping the future of special education (Lombardi and Ludlow, 1996, pp. 7–8). Presidents of state speech-language and hearing associations from all over the country were surveyed in 1999 as to

the critical issues facing school-based speech-language pathologists in schools. The results of this survey, presented in the sidebar on page 332, reveal commonalities across the country (Moore-Brown and Montgomery, 1999).

Beyond technical competencies, speech-language pathologists in the twenty-first century will also need to be adept at interpersonal skills. When considering workplace success skills that graduate students need to learn, ASHA (2000c) identified the following as critical for success in the work environment, in addition to technical expertise:

- Planning and priority setting
- Organizing and time management
- Managing diversity
- Team building
- Interpersonal savvy and peer relationships
- Organizational agility
- Conflict management
- Problem solving, perspective, and creativity
- Dealing with paradox and learning on the fly

It was interpersonal skills, a method of thinking, and a service delivery model that O'Shea and O'Shea (1997) identified as being critical to insuring the success of school reform when they wrote: "Regardless of the impediments that currently block forward thinking, local collaboration is a cornerstone of effective school reform" (p. 454). Speech-language pathologists must possess both technical competence and interpersonal skills in a digital society to better meet the needs of all children.

Critical Issues Facing Speech-Language Pathologists in Public Schools

Responses to Survey of Council of State Association Presidents (CSAP) in November 1999

Please identify what you see as the most critical issue(s) facing school-based practitioners in your state.

Caseload size/Management (14 responses)

Compliance/Procedural paperwork (7 responses)

Highest state standard (B.A. v. M.A. entry level) (4 responses)

Compensation (3 responses)

Speech-language pathology assistants (SLPAs) (3 responses)

Providing services to multicultural populations (2 responses)

Speech-language pathologist staffing (2 responses)

Supervision of programs by qualified administrators (2 responses)

Third-party billing/Medicaid regulations (2 responses)

Dual certification as teacher/speech-language pathologist

Implications for students with communication disorders passing high school exit exam

Preschool issues: Increasing numbers and complexity of needs

Licensure/Credentialing

Increasing litigation

Assuming new roles that are teacherlike

Expanding services through new models

Change

Supervision of SLPAs—state code conflicts with ASHA

Documentation

Benchmarks

Behavior/Communication Intervention

Autism—matching goals with standards

Matching speech-language goals and outcomes to state curriculum standards

Eligibility/Exit criteria

Continuing education

Funding of services

Role of the speech-language pathologist in literacy development

National certification bonus for teachers but not for speech-language pathologists

Increase in medically fragile students needing diagnosis and treatment

Source: Moore-Brown and Montgomery (1999)

In "Predictions for the Future" in Chapter 1, we invited readers to consider 10 predictions for education (O'Shea and O'Shea, 1997) in the context of the educational system as a whole and to consider how the evolving roles for speech-language pathologists in schools embraced system change. The "safe" predictions of Marzano (2000) have been presented, as well as recommendations for change in general education by Allington and McGill-Franzen (2000) and how these changes will affect children with special needs. We ask that you consider once again the 10 predictions of O'Shea and O'Shea (1997) to understand the forces that will affect speech-language pathologists in the future.

1. **Interagency Processes Will Become More Prominent (p. 454).**

   Education has formed new partnerships with external agencies. Speech-language pathologists in schools will work within departments of the building, district, and region, but will also collaborate with mental health agencies, health services agencies, private practitioners, hospitals, and other organizations that provide services to children with disabilities. Extending beyond our traditional scope of partnerships will be a greater part of the future.

2. **Despite New Collaborative and Collective Visions, Legal and Ethical Issues, Political Issues, Administrative Structures, and Educational Practices Will Continue to Shape Assessment and Programming in Learning Support (p. 455).**

The presentation of legal, ethical, and political issues throughout this book has been designed to help speech-language pathologists understand the forces that affect how student learning is evaluated, as well as how resources are allocated to support programs.

3. **Preservice Training Agendas Will Change in Order to Address School Restructuring and Service Delivery Systems (p. 455).**

   School reform is impacting pre-service training. Change in the university instructional delivery system is necessitated by the changes in public education discussed throughout this book. Universities are also being held to the state educational standards and the outcomes of their graduates.

4. **School Reform Will Affect Experienced Teachers (p. 457).**

   With all the changes in educational systems, especially in terms of instructional practices and accountability for all learners, experienced speech-language pathologists will need to be as much a part of ongoing staff development as any other educators in the school. Opting out of reform or working with certain student populations will not be possible for anyone in the system. Being an educator in any capacity will require lifelong learning.

5. **Learning Settings Will Expand (p. 458).**

   Students with communication disorders will receive their education in all possible settings within a school environment.

This is one of the reasons why this book has covered the topic of service delivery in such depth. The ways and places that speech-language pathologists will deliver services will continue to expand. Besides assisting students with communication disorders, speech-language pathologists will also find themselves central to enhancing the communication skills of all students in the educational environment through an extension of their role in serving a school or a community.

6. Technology Will Shape the Collaboration Format (p. 458).

Speech-language pathologists have a long history of using technology as a communication tool. The expanded areas of AUGMENTATIVE AND ALTERNATIVE COMMUNICATION (AAC) and ASSISTIVE TECHNOLOGY (AT) were discussed in Chapter 7. As classroom teachers become more experienced with using technology as a teaching tool, speech-language pathologists will be able to partner with them, to the benefit of students. As a result of technology, speech-language pathologists will also form new types of collaborative relationships, including designing intervention that uses and addresses the literacies presented with technology. As technology improves, educators and medical personnel will also learn more about the specifics of learning and attention deficit/hyperactivity disorder (ADHD), LEARNING DISABILITIES, AUTISM SPECTRUM DISORDER, and fluency, among others. Speech-language pathologists will collaborate with nurses, physicians, and parents

regarding services for children who have survived medical traumas or who are experiencing high-tech medical intervention. Continued research in genetics, such as the Human Genome Project, will likely have profound implications for children with communication disorders. As a result of such medical advancements, speech-language pathologists will continue to adjust and adapt to the ever-changing needs of the student population.

7. The Effects of Parent and Community Advocacy Groups Will Increase in Prominence (p. 459).

Involving parents in their child's education has been described as critical and therefore mandated. Increasingly, parents and parent advocacy groups are bringing to the IEP table requests for specific types of diagnostic and treatment protocols,

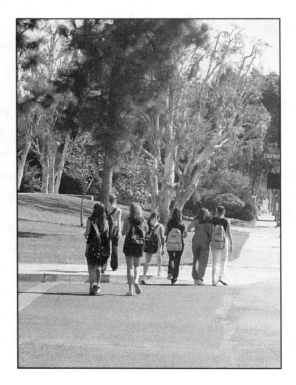

including specific service providers. In the future, the role of new partnerships with parents must be realized. Parents will be both implementers of services to their children and positive partners in the decision making. Additionally, speech-language pathologists and all educators will form new relationships with advocates and advocacy groups to assist parents in making decisions about their child's education.

8. **Family Diversity Will Change Professionals' Roles (p. 459).**
Chapter 1 presented information about children and families. The role of all educators is to work with the family structure in ways that support a student. This may mean that the speech-language pathologist will be working with a child's extended family who take part in raising the child, some of whom may not be blood relatives. Speech-language pathologists may find themselves in situations where complex family structures are involved in the decision-making about a child's program. This means that speech-language pathologists will need skills in how to work with possible opposing opinions. They may also need to extend into the community and work with supportive structures within a particular cultural or linguistic community to achieve good working relationships with families.

9. **Student Diversity Will Affect Professionals' Roles (p. 459).**
This topic has been discussed throughout this book and is evident in the trends identified by Lomardi and Ludlow (1996). Student diversity will continue to evolve,

including not only social, economic, and learning capacities, but also lifestyle choices and technological and linguistic skills. One example of how student need will expand professional roles is the addition of swallowing and dysphagia programs, which were introduced in some districts in the year 2000, but are expected to grow.

10. **Local Groups Will Shape Local School Structures (p. 460).**
Speech-language pathologists will find that they may become actively involved in parent councils, specialist groups (e.g., disability support groups), activity groups (e.g., reading councils), school site councils, or district advisory committees, which influence both the educational directions and the financial decisions made in a school or district. Increasing calls for accountability are mandating public reports of service delivery options and financial expenditures. The speech-language pathologist may find that local involvement is a positive way to influence the decisions made for children and school employees.

In the spirit of promoting a unified system between general education and special education, we have examined the future of school-based speech-language pathologists in public schools, through the lens of general education. We believe that this provides meaningful perspective for those who will be working in and creating this future. The predictions presented here clearly have implications for all educators, and all of those who are concerned with children. Understanding these forces and how to be a part of the solution will enhance the work of school-based speech-language pathologists.

Speech-Language Pathologists' Future Watch: Expanded Practice and Professionalism

The influence of the forces of general and special education leads to a vision of expanded practice and professionalism for speech-language pathologists in the schools. The following areas seem to be among those that will pose the most immediate challenges.

- The recruitment and retention of well-trained, competent, fully certified speech-language pathologists in the workplace

- The need for speech-language pathologists who are culturally competent to serve a diverse population in an environment of school reform

- The need for speech-language pathologists to possess traditional and expanded technical skills for diagnostics and intervention in a broad arena, including with specialized populations and specialty areas. Application of these skills to the curricular program will be required

- The evolution of the paraprofessional position and the evolution of the speech-language pathologist's skills in the supervisory/advisory capacity

- Service delivery models that are expanded and flexible, providing speech-language pathologists with a greater ability to address student needs

- The use of outcome data to expand clinical decision-making abilities

- The expansion of the role of speech-language professionals in literacy and curriculum, which will create an opportunity to take a leading role in literacy and reading instruction

- The need for speech-language pathologists to advocate for students and the professions

- The expansion or redefinition of the scope of practice of speech-language pathologists, creating a greater need to work with allied disciplines assisting children and families in settings that extend beyond the school building. Speech-language pathologists will spend time teaching other team members how to intervene with or prevent communication disorders.

- Significant impact of technology on diagnostic, therapeutic, and student needs

- Learning how to engage and support parents in ways beyond goal CONSULTATION

- The expansion of service delivery to address students' communication skills in areas such as violence prevention/intervention and self-determination. In doing so, speech-language pathologists will find themselves teaming with counselors, psychologists, and classroom educators in new and novel ways

- Increasing involvement in early intervention related to improvements in technology (i.e., universal newborn hearing SCREENING, genetic counseling, and so on), which allow for earlier identification of possible communication challenges

The skills and talents of others will extend services as speech-language pathologists train parents and other multidisciplinary team members to provide intervention and prevention services, and with the expanded use of SPEECH-LANGUAGE PATHOLOGY ASSISTANTS. Although it may be difficult to "let go" of direct service delivery to all children with communication needs, speech-language pathologists must examine the best use of time as the number of children served increases.

In the future, speech-language pathologists will have newly defined and expanded roles, including consultant, diagnostician, supervisor, curriculum/literacy advisor, and more. CASELOAD size will be adjusted to accommodate expanded roles and schoolwide responsibilities. For a more comprehensive listing of the skills and competencies needed by school-based speech-language pathologists, see Appendix G.

Closing Thoughts

Being a speech-language pathologist in public schools will be exciting, energizing, and rewarding. Educational reforms will continue, enabling speech-language pathologists and those concerned about children—*all* children—to be dramatically involved in creating a system that works for children with communication disorders. Allington and McGill-Franzen (2000) commented:

> So I guess the answer to what sort of schools will we have in the 21st century can be best stated as "It will depend." It will depend on the decisions we as a society make about what it means to teach and what it means to learn and to be literate, and whether schools are seen as important in achieving the ideals of a just, democratic society. (p. 151)

And it will depend on the work of speech-language pathologists, who do, indeed, make a difference for America's children.

Appendixes

ASHA's Preferred Practice Patterns in Assessment

Guiding Principles

The following guiding principles formed the basis of the Preferred Practice Patterns.

The practice patterns—

1. Keep paramount the welfare of patients/clients served in all practice decisions and actions.

2. Acknowledge that a primary purpose for addressing communication and related disorders is to effect measurable and functional change(s) in an individual's communication status in order that he or she may participate as fully as possible in all aspects of life — social, educational, and vocational.

3. Recognize that communication is always an interactive process, and that the focus of intervention may include training of communication partners (e.g., caregivers, family members, peers, educators, etc.).

4. Identify the professionals and support personnel within the discipline of human communication sciences and disorders who may perform any given procedure.

5. Address the clinical indications for performing any given procedure; treatment plans should be predicated on assessment/reassessment findings and consistent with current practice.

6. Define appropriate environmental factors related to procedures (e.g., setting, equipment, and materials).

7. Address demographic factors pertinent to the individual (e.g., age, developmental level, education), as well as cultural, ethnic, linguistic, social, and vocational factors.

8. Consider risk as it relates to the health, safety, and welfare of patients/clients and practitioners; severity of illness or disability, severity of communication, swallowing, or other related disorder(s); premorbid health and cognitive status; related conditions and complications; effects of medications, surgery, and other interventions; special needs (e.g., glasses, hearing aid, wheelchair); social needs/support system; and other services needed.

9. Consider outcomes including prevention of communication, swallowing, and other related disorders; improvement and/or maintenance of functional communication; and enhancement of the quality of life.

10. Consider intradisciplinary (speech-language pathology and audiology) and interdisciplinary approaches to service delivery.

11. Recognize the dignity and privacy of individuals and consider patient/client rights, expectations, needs, and preferences.

12. Recognize the value and importance of obtaining fully informed consent for procedures that may present risk or are part of a research protocol, and appropriate releases of information prior to sharing any in-formation about patients/clients with others.

13. Recognize the importance of documentation.

14. Recognize a variety of appropriate service delivery models and procedures (e.g., collaborative consultation, participation in multi-, inter-, and transdisciplinary teams, use of support personnel, and new and advanced technologies).

15. Adhere to the specifications and intent of the current Code of Ethics.

Fundamental Components of Preferred Practice Patterns

Professionals Who Perform the Procedure(s)

- Only those professionals who hold the appropriate credentials in speech-language pathology and who have pertinent training and experience may provide specific procedures.

Support Personnel Who Perform the Procedure(s)

- Speech-language pathology assistants who provide services must do so under the supervision of a certified speech-language pathologist (in accordance with the current ASHA Guidelines for the Training, Credentialing, Use, and Supervision of Speech-Language Pathology Assistants). The speech-language pathologist who supervises speech-language pathology assistants maintains full responsibility for the quality and appropriateness of services provided to the patient/client.

Expected Outcome(s)

- Although the outcome of any specific procedure may not be guaranteed, a reasonable statement of prognosis may be made to referral sources, clients/patients, and families/caregivers.

- Outcomes of services should be monitored and measured in order to ensure the quality of services pro-vided and to improve the quality of those services.

- Appropriate follow-up services are provided to determine functional outcomes and the need for further services after discharge.

Clinical Indications

- Screening procedures may be used for identification of those individuals who may be at risk for communication disorders or differences and who may benefit from evaluation or treatment services.

- Services are provided when there is a reasonable expectation of benefit to the patient/client or in order to rule in or out a specific disabling condition.

Clinical Process

- Procedures are conducted in the patient's/client's chosen communication mode and linguistic system and in consideration of his or her cultural background and community.

- An essential component of each procedure is patient/client and family counseling, which may address the nature of the communication or related disorder or difference and its impact, and outcomes of the procedure.

- Speech-language pathologists work in collaboration with other professionals, the patient/client, and family/ caregivers.

- Procedures address patient/client and family preferences, goals, and special needs. Materials and approaches used and products dispensed are appropriate to the patient's/client's chronological and developmental age, medical status, physical and sensory abilities, education, vocation, cognitive status, and cultural/ethnic, social, and linguistic background.

Setting/Equipment Specifications

- Equipment is maintained according to manufacturer's specifications and recommendations. Instruments are properly calibrated and calibration records are maintained.

Safety and Health Precautions

- All procedures ensure the safety of the patient/client and clinician and adhere to universal health pre-cautions (e.g., prevention of bodily injury and transmission of infectious disease).

- Decontamination, cleaning, disinfection, and sterilization of multiple-use equipment before reuse are carried out according to facility-specific infection control policies and procedures and according to manufacturer's instructions.

Documentation

- Speech-language pathologists prepare, sign, and maintain, within an established time frame, documentation that reflects the nature of the professional service. When appropriate and with written consent, reports are distributed.

- Except for screenings, documentation addresses the type and severity of the communication or related disorder or difference and associated conditions (e.g., medical diagnoses, disability).

- Documentation includes results of previous related screening, assessment, and treatment procedures, if available.

- Results of assessment and treatment are reported to the patient/client and family/caregivers.

02.0 Speech Screening—SLP

(as performed by Speech-Language Pathologists)

A pass/fail procedure to identify individuals who require further speech (articulation, voice, resonance, fluency), and/or orofacial myofunctional assessment.

Speech screening is conducted according to the Guiding Principles and the Fundamental Components of Preferred Practice Patterns.

Professionals Who Perform the Procedure(s)

- Speech-language pathologists

Support Personnel Who Perform the Procedure(s)

- Speech-language pathology assistants under the supervision of a certified speech-language pathologist (in accordance with the ASHA Guidelines for the Training, Credentialing, Use, and Supervision of Speech-Language Pathology Assistants, performed without interpretation, recommendations, or documentation).

Expected Outcome(s)

- Speech screening identifies those persons most likely to have speech and/or orofacial myofunctional disorders that may interfere with education, health, development, or communication.

- Screening may result in recommendations for rescreening or comprehensive assessment, or in referral for other examinations or services.

Clinical Indications

- Individuals of all ages are screened as needed, requested, or mandated, or when they have conditions that place them at risk.

Clinical Process

- Standardized and nonstandardized methods are used to screen oral motor function and speech production skills: articulatory, fluency, resonance, and voice characteristics.

- Patients/clients who fail the screening are referred to a speech-language pathologist for further assessment.

Setting/Equipment Specifications

- Speech screening is conducted in a clinical or natural environment conducive to eliciting a representative sample of the patient's/client's speech.

Safety and Health Precautions

- All procedures ensure the safety of the patient/client and clinician and adhere to universal health precautions (e.g., prevention of bodily injury and transmission of infectious disease).

- Decontamination, cleaning, disinfection, and sterilization of multiple-use equipment before reuse are carried out according to facility-specific infection control policies and procedures and according to manufacturer's instructions.

Documentation

- Documentation includes a statement of identifying information, results, and recommendations, including the need for rescreening, assessment, or referral.

ASHA Policy and Related References *[sic]*

In addition to the references on p. I-50 [page number refers to original ASHA (1997c) document. Available: http://www.asha.org/library/images/pppslp.pdf.], the following references apply specifically to these procedures:

American Speech-Language-Hearing Association. (1993). Definitions of communication disorders and variations. *Asha, 35* (Suppl. 10), 40–41.

03.0 Language Screening—SLP

(as performed by Speech-Language Pathologists)

> *A pass/fail procedure to identify individuals who require further language assessment.*
>
> Language screening is conducted according to the Guiding Principles and the Fundamental Components of Preferred Practice Patterns.

Professionals Who Perform the Procedure(s)

- Speech-language pathologists

Support Personnel Who Perform the Procedure(s)

- Speech-language pathology assistants under the supervision of a certified speech-language pathologist (in accordance with the ASHA Guidelines for the Training, Credentialing, Use, and Supervision of Speech-Language Pathology Assistants, performed without interpretation, recommendations, or documentation).

Expected Outcome(s)

- Language screening identifies those persons most likely to have language and/or cognitive communication disorders that may interfere with education, health, development, or communication.

- Screening may result in recommendations for rescreening or comprehensive assessment, or in referral for other examinations or services.

Clinical Indications

- Individuals of all ages are screened as needed, requested, or mandated, or when they have conditions that place them at risk.

Clinical Process

- Standardized and/or nonstandardized methods are used to screen comprehension and production of language (including phonological processes) and cognitive aspects of communication.

- Patients/clients who fail the screening are referred to a speech-language pathologist for further assessment.

Setting/Equipment Specifications

- Language screening is conducted in a clinical or natural environment conducive to eliciting a representative sample of the patient's/client's language.

Safety and Health Precautions

- All procedures ensure the safety of the patient/client and clinician and adhere to universal health precautions (e.g., prevention of bodily injury and transmission of infectious disease).

- Decontamination, cleaning, disinfection, and sterilization of multiple-use equipment before reuse are carried out according to facility-specific infection control policies and procedures and according to manufacturer's instructions.

Documentation

- Documentation includes a statement of identifying information, results, and recommendations, including the need for rescreening, assessment, or referral.

ASHA Policy and Related References

In addition to the references on p. I-50 [page number refers to original ASHA (1997c) document. Available: http://www.asha.org/library/images/pppslp.pdf.], the following references apply specifically to these procedures:

American Speech-Language-Hearing Association. (1982). Definitions of language. *Asha, 24*(6), 44.

American Speech-Language-Hearing Association. (1989). Issues in determining eligibility for language intervention. *Asha, 31*(3), 113–118.

American Speech-Language-Hearing Association. (1993). Definitions of communication disorders and variations. *Asha, 35* (Suppl. 10), 40–41.

12.0 Prespeech, Prelanguage, and Language Assessment for Infants and Toddlers

Procedures to assess prelanguage and language systems in infancy and early childhood, delineating strengths, deficits, contributing factors, and family needs for fostering functional communication development.

Prespeech, prelanguage and language assessment for infants and toddlers is conducted according to the Guiding Principles and the Fundamental Components of Preferred Practice Patterns.

Professionals Who Perform the Procedure(s)

- Speech-language pathologists.

Expected Outcome(s)

- Assessment is conducted to identify and describe the infant's or toddler's existing prespeech abilities and prelanguage or language interactions, and primary caregivers' support for these, preferably in the infant's or toddler's primary or home language. Prespeech, prelanguage, and language assessment contributes to the diagnosis of a communication disorder.

- Assessment may result in a diagnosis and clinical description of a disorder, recommendations for treatment or follow-up, confirmation that an infant or toddler is at risk for communication disorder even if a disorder is not currently diagnosed, recommendations for fostering communication and language development, and/or referral for other examinations and services.

Clinical/Early Educational Indications

- Infants and toddlers are assessed as needed, requested, or mandated, or when infants and toddlers have confirmed or suspected risks for developmental or acquired speech-language disorders.

- Assessment is prompted by referral, by the infant's or toddler's medical status, or by failure of a developmental screening.

Clinical Process

- Review of auditory, visual, motoric, and cognitive status.

- Assessment includes:

— Case history

— Determination of family/caregiver capacity for supporting the child's development

— Standardized and/or nonstandardized methods to observe and describe gestural communication, interactive play (including interaction with toys and people), babbling, spoken language comprehension, and spoken language expression, as well as sign language comprehension and expression (if applicable)

— If indicated, standardized and/or nonstandardized methods to assess the infant's or toddler's oral-motor skills

— Standardized and/or nonstandardized methods to gather systematic parental or caregiver report of communication and language behaviors that appear regularly but not within the assessment activities

— Standardized and/or nonstandardized methods to observe and describe parental or caregiver support of infant's or toddler's communication attempts

— Integration of information from other disciplines (e.g., early interventionists, developmental pediatricians, pediatric physical therapists) about such issues as social interactions, play, and feeding

Setting/Equipment Specifications

• Assessment is conducted in a clinical, home, community-based service, or educational environment conducive to eliciting a representative sample of the infant's or toddler's prelanguage and language abilities. Samples may be videotaped to document nonverbal, as well as verbal, communication attempts.

• Parental report is used to augment, but not replace, actual observations of the infant or toddler interacting with a familiar partner.

Safety and Health Precautions

• All procedures ensure the safety of the patient/client and clinician and adhere to universal health precautions (e.g., prevention of bodily injury and transmission of infectious disease).

- Decontamination, cleaning, disinfection, and sterilization of multiple-use equipment before reuse are carried out according to facility-specific infection control policies and procedures and according to manufacturer's instructions.

Documentation

- Documentation may include pertinent background information, assessment results and interpretation, prognosis, and recommendations. Recommendations may include the need for further assessment, follow-up, or referral. When treatment is recommended, information is provided concerning frequency, estimated duration, type of service (e.g., home-based, center-based, clinic-based, consultative, care-coordination), and family involvement.

- Documentation of hearing status is a critical element.

- Documentation may include videotaped samples and descriptions of the infant's or toddler's communication interactions with a caregiver or other familiar adult.

ASHA Policy and Related References

In addition to the references on p. I-50 [page number refers to original ASHA (1997c) document. Available: http://www.asha.org/library/images/pppslp.pdf.], the following references apply specifically to these procedures:

American Speech-Language-Hearing Association. (1982). Definitions of language. *Asha, 24*(6), 44.

American Speech-Language-Hearing Association. (1990). The roles of speech-language pathologists in service delivery to infants, toddlers, and their families. *Asha, 32* (Suppl. 2), 4.

American Speech-Language-Hearing Association. (1991). The prevention of communication disorders tutorial. *Asha, 33* (Suppl. 6), 15–41.

12.1 Language Assessment for Children and Adolescents

Procedures to assess the developing language systems of children and adolescents, delineating strengths, deficits, contributing factors, and social, academic, and vocational (including prevocational) needs for using language functionally to listen, speak (or sign), read and write; and related cognitive-communication processes.

Language assessment for children and adolescents is conducted according to the Guiding Principles and the Fundamental Components of Preferred Practice Patterns.

Professionals Who Perform the Procedure(s)

Speech-language pathologists.

Expected Outcome(s)

- Assessment is conducted to identify and describe the child's or adolescent's language knowledge and skills, preferably in the child's primary or home language, in areas of concern raised by the parents or school. Language is described in the areas of spoken language comprehension and expression, and in the areas of reading and writing if identified as areas of concern.

- Assessment may result in a diagnosis and clinical description of a disorder, recommendations for treatment or follow-up, and/or referral for other examinations and services.

Clinical/Educational Indications

- Children or adolescents are assessed as needed, requested, or mandated, or when they have communication, educational, vocational, social, behavioral, and health needs due to their language status.

- Assessment is prompted by referral, by the child's or adolescent's medical status, or by failure of a speech and language screening (see Procedures 02.0 and 03.0).

Clinical Process

- Review of auditory, visual, motoric, and cognitive status.

- Assessment includes:

  — Case history

  — Parental, school, and child or adolescent report of areas of concern (listening, speaking, reading, writing, or cognitive-communication) and contexts of concern (e.g., social interactions, academic subject areas, vocational interactions)

— Standardized and nonstandardized methods to observe and describe the child's or adolescent's comprehension and production of spoken language form (phonology, morphology, and syntax), content (semantics), and use (pragmatics) in varied communication events (formal tests and natural communication samples) and contexts of concern

— Oral motor/motor speech function

— If indicated, standardized and/or nonstandardized methods to observe and describe the child's or adolescent's comprehension (reading) and production (writing) of written language form (phonology, morphology, and syntax), content (semantics), and social use of language in multiple discourse contexts (pragmatics)

— If indicated, standardized and/or nonstandardized methods to observe and describe the child's or adolescent's phonological awareness, reading decoding, and comprehension processes (or evidence of emergent literacy)

— If indicated, standardized and/or nonstandardized methods to observe and describe the child's or adolescent's writing processes (including planning and organizing, drafting, revising and editing, and creating a final product)

— If indicated, standardized and/or nonstandardized methods to observe and describe the communication and language abilities of a child or adolescent with severe disabilities, who may be using nonconventional means to communicate, including the forms and functions the child or adolescent uses to communicate and the frequency with which individuals in the environment invite, permit, accept, and respond appropriately to such acts

Setting/Equipment Specifications

• Assessment is conducted in a clinical, educational, social, community, or vocational environment conducive to eliciting a representative sample of the child's or adolescent's communication and language abilities in the areas of concern (listening, speaking, reading, writing, cognitive-communication) and in the contexts of concern (e.g., social conversation, following directions, completing math story problems, reading a book).

• Children or adolescents with identified oral and/or written language disorders receive follow-up services to monitor oral and/or written language status and to ensure appropriate treatment. Students using AAC devices and techniques will be assessed in language development and communication use with their devices.

Safety and Health Precautions

• All procedures ensure the safety of the patient/client and clinician and adhere to universal health precautions (e.g., prevention of bodily injury and transmission of infectious disease).

• Decontamination, cleaning, disinfection, and sterilization of multiple-use equipment before reuse are carried out according to facility-specific infection control policies and procedures and according to manufacturer's instructions.

Documentation

- Documentation may include pertinent background information, areas of concern identified by major participants (e.g., child or adolescent, parents, teachers), speech-language assessment results and interpretation, prognosis, and recommendations. Recommendations may include the need for further assessment, follow-up, or referral. When treatment is recommended, information is provided concerning frequency, estimated duration, and type of service (e.g., consultative, classroom based, pullout, clinic based, self-contained program), and home, school, and/or workplace involvement.

- Documentation of hearing status is a critical element.

- Documentation may include a portfolio of the child's or adolescent's communication samples (e.g., audiotaped or videotaped samples of interactions, transcripts of oral conversations or orally read material, descriptions of nonverbal interactions, writing processes, rough drafts, written products).

ASHA Policy and Related References

In addition to the references on p. I-50 [page number refers to original ASHA (1997c) document. Available: http://www.asha.org/library/images/pppslp.pdf.], the following references apply specifically to these procedures:

American Speech-Language-Hearing Association. (1982). Definitions of language. *Asha, 24*(6), 44.

American Speech-Language-Hearing Association. (1990). The role of speech-language pathologists in service delivery for persons with mental retardation and developmental disabilities in community settings. *Asha, 32* (Suppl. 2), 5–6.

American Speech-Language-Hearing Association. (1991). Guidelines for speech-language pathologists serving persons with language, socio-communication, and/or cognitive-communication impairments. *Asha, 33* (Suppl. 5), 21–28.

American Speech-Language-Hearing Association. (1993). Guidelines for caseload size and speech-language service delivery in the schools. *Asha, 35* (Suppl. 10), 33–39.

American Speech-Language-Hearing Association. (1996). Inclusive practices for children and youths with communication disorders. *Asha, 38* (Suppl. 16), 35–44.

National Joint Committee for the Communicative Needs of Persons With Severe Disabilities. (1992). Guidelines for meeting the communicative needs of persons with severe disabilities. *Asha, 34* (Suppl. 7), 1–8.

12.3 Augmentative and Alternative Communication (AAC) Assessment

Procedures to determine the appropriateness of aids, techniques, symbols, and / or strategies to augment or replace speech and enhance communication of patients / clients with expressive and / or receptive communication disorders.

Augmentative and alternative communication (AAC) assessment is conducted according to the Guiding Principles, and the Fundamental Components of Preferred Practice Patterns.

Professionals Who Perform the Procedure(s)

- Speech-language pathologists (often with interdisciplinary or transdisciplinary collaboration)

Expected Outcome(s)

- Individuals with expressive and/or receptive communication disorders are assisted in selecting and obtaining appropriate augmentative and/or alternative communication (AAC) components (aids, techniques, symbols, strategies) to enhance communication.

- Assessment may result in recommendations for AAC strategies, systems, and/or devices, treatment or follow-up, or in referral for other examinations or services.

Clinical Indications

- Individuals of all ages are assessed as needed, requested, or mandated, or when they have impaired communication, or educational, vocational, social, and/or health needs due to their communication status.

- Assessment is prompted by referral or by failure of a speech or language screening (see Procedures 02.0 and 03.0).

Clinical Process

- The parameters of the AAC assessment (e.g., tests, materials) may vary depending on severity, on whether the patient/client is a child or an adult, on whether the expressive or receptive communication disorder is congenital or acquired, and on the individual's communication needs and abilities.

- Assessment includes:

  — Review of auditory, visual, motoric, and cognitive status

  — Examination of specific aspects of voice, speech, language, cognition, and communication systems

  — Observation of posture, gross and fine motor coordination, and any existing adaptive and/or orthotic devices that are currently being used by the patient/client (e.g., wheelchair, neckbraces, communication boards, specialized equipment)

- Selected AAC components are used with the patient/client in various planned communication contexts.

- On completion of the initial AAC assessment, the professional reviews the results of the diagnostic trial with devices, techniques, symbols, and/or strategies, and gives a rationale for the preferred AAC options and system/device characteristics.

- Assessment is conducted periodically as indicated by follow-up protocols.

- Assessment is often an interdisciplinary process.

Setting/Equipment Specifications

- Assessment is conducted in a natural environment (e.g., home or classroom) and/or in a clinical environment that includes a range of AAC aids and components to evaluate the patient's/client's competencies.

- Assessment considers the abilities, needs, and preferences of the patient/client and of those with whom the patient/client will communicate (e.g., family, caregivers, educators, service providers). It also considers the environment in which the AAC component(s) will be routinely used.

Safety and Health Precautions

- All procedures ensure the safety of the patient/client and clinician and adhere to universal health precautions (e.g., prevention of bodily injury and transmission of infectious disease).

- Decontamination, cleaning, disinfection, and sterilization of multiple-use equipment before reuse are carried out according to facility-specific infection control policies and procedures and according to manufacturer's instructions.

Documentation

- Documentation includes pertinent background information, results, interpretation, prognosis, and recommendations. Recommendations may include the need for further assessment, follow-up, or referral. When treatment is recommended, information is provided concerning frequency, estimated duration, and type of service (e.g., individual, group, home program) required.

- All recommendations include a rationale for the preferred AAC options, a description of system/device characteristics, and a description of the AAC intervention program and the patient's/client's response to the recommended system and program.

ASHA Policy and Related References

In addition to the references on p. I-50 [page number refers to original ASHA (1997c) document. Available: http://www.asha.org/library/images/pppslp.pdf.], the following references apply specifically to these procedures:

American Speech-Language-Hearing Association. (1989). Competencies for speech-language pathologists providing services in augmentative communication. *Asha, 31*(3), 107–110.

American Speech-Language-Hearing Association. (1991). Augmentative and alternative communication. *Asha, 33* (Suppl. 5), 8.

American Speech-Language-Hearing Association. (1991). Report: Augmentative and alternative communication. *Asha, 33* (Suppl. 5), 9–12.

12.5 Articulation/Phonology Assessment

Procedures to assess speech articulation / phonology, delineating strengths, deficits, contributing factors, and implications for functional communication.

Articulation/phonology assessment is conducted according to the Guiding Principles and the Fundamental Components of Preferred Practice Patterns.

Professionals Who Perform the Procedure(s)

- Speech-language pathologists.

Expected Outcome(s)

- Assessment is conducted to describe characteristics of speech-sound production and to diagnose a communication disorder.

- Assessment may result in recommendations for treatment or follow-up, or in referral for other examinations or services.

Clinical Indications

- Individuals of all ages are assessed as needed, requested, or mandated, or when they have educational, vocational, social, and health needs caused by impaired communication.

- Assessment is prompted by referral, by the patient's/client's medical status, or by failure of a speech screening (see Procedure 02.0).

Clinical Process

- Assessment includes:

  — Case history

  — Standardized and/or nonstandardized measures to assess developmental and acquired articulation disorders, oral motor skills, segmental and suprasegmental data, phonological processes, and motor speech control

  — Observation of interaction between parent and child or adult and significant other

  — Review of auditory, visual, motoric, and cognitive status

  — Observation or review of voice, fluency, and language

- Patients/clients with identified articulation/phonology disorders receive follow-up services to monitor status and to ensure appropriate treatment.

Setting/Equipment Specifications

- Assessment is conducted in a clinical or natural environment conducive to eliciting a representative sample of the patient's/client's articulation/phonology.

Safety and Health Precautions

- All procedures ensure the safety of the patient/client and clinician and adhere to universal health precautions (e.g., prevention of bodily injury and transmission of infectious disease).

- Decontamination, cleaning, disinfection, and sterilization of multiple-use equipment before reuse are carried out according to facility-specific infection control procedures and manufacturer's instructions.

Documentation

- Documentation includes pertinent background information, results and interpretation, prognosis, and recommendations. Recommendations may include the need for further assessment, follow-up, or referral. When treatment is recommended, information is provided concerning frequency, estimated duration, and type of service (e.g., individual, group, home program) required.

12.6 Fluency Assessment

Procedures to assess aspects of speech fluency, delineating strengths, deficits, contributing and concomitant factors, and implications for functional communication.

Fluency assessment is conducted according to the Guiding Principles and Fundamental Components of Preferred Practice Patterns.

Professionals Who Perform the Procedure(s)

- Speech-language pathologists.

Expected Outcome(s)

- Assessment is conducted to identify disfluent and fluent behaviors and concomitant features and to diagnose the presence of a fluency disorder.

- Assessment may result in recommendations for treatment or follow-up, or in referral for other examinations or services.

Clinical Indications

- Patients/clients of all ages who are at risk for stuttering receive an assessment on the basis of their communication, educational, vocational, social, health, and emotional needs.

- Assessment is prompted by referral (self or other), or by failure of a speech or language screening (see Procedures 02.0 and 03.0).

Clinical Process

- Assessment includes:

  — Elicitation and use of a developmental history through questionnaires and/or interview of patient/ client and/or family members

  — Elicitation of representative speech samples

  — Description of the quantitative and qualitative features of the patient's/client's fluency, including:

- stuttering severity, attitudes toward stuttering and speech, speech naturalness, self-efficacy as a speaker, situational fears, and avoidance behaviors

- categories of disfluency, extent of fluency or nonfluency, and the presence and type of secondary behaviors

- identification and counting of the frequency of primary and secondary stuttering behaviors

- speech rate

- instrumental measurements of oral, laryngeal, and respiratory behavior, if indicated

- other features of communication function, such as muscular tension, emotional reactivity to speech or stuttering behaviors, coping behaviors, nonverbal aspects of communication, or anomalies of social interaction

— Assessment of variables that affect fluency, such as reduced rate; interviewing patient/client or family member about social circumstances, words, listeners, sentence types, speech sounds that present difficulty; modification of interaction style; and/or trial treatment procedures

— Elicitation and use of prognostic information and information that optimizes treatment planning

— Observation or assessment of articulation, language, cognitive, voice, hearing, and vision status

— Communication and interpretation of assessment results and recommendations to relevant professionals, the patient/client, and/or the patient's/client's family and significant others

— Provision of follow-up services to monitor fluency status and to ensure appropriate treatment

Setting/Equipment Specifications

- Assessment is conducted in a clinical or natural environment conducive to eliciting a representative sample of the patient's/client's speech fluency. Instrumental procedures may be used to evaluate the articulatory, laryngeal, and respiratory dynamics that contribute to a patient's/client's fluency.

Safety and Health Precautions

- All procedures ensure the safety of the patient/client and clinician and adhere to universal health precautions (e.g., prevention of bodily injury and transmission of infectious disease).

- Decontamination, cleaning, disinfection, and sterilization of multiple-use equipment before reuse are carried out according to facility-specific infection control policies and procedures and according to manufacturer's instructions.

Documentation

- Documentation addresses the type and severity of the fluency disorder and associated conditions (e.g., medical diagnosis, disability, attitudes toward the fluency disorder).

- Documentation includes pertinent background information, results and interpretation, prognosis, and specific recommendations. Recommendations may include the need for further assessment, follow-up, or referral. When treatment is recommended, information is provided concerning frequency, estimated duration, and type of service (e.g., individual, group, home program) required.

ASHA Policy and Related References *[sic]*

In addition to the references on p. I-50 [page number refers to original ASHA (1997c) document. Available: http://www.asha.org/library/images/pppslp.pdf.], the following references apply specifically to these procedures:

American Speech-Language-Hearing Association. (1995). Guidelines for practice in stuttering treatment, *Asha, 37* (Suppl. 14), 26–35.

12.7 Voice Assessment

Procedures to assess vocal structure and function, identifying strengths, deficits, contributing factors, and implications for functional communication.

Voice assessment is conducted according to the Guiding Principles and Fundamental Components of Preferred Practice Patterns.

Professionals Who Perform the Procedure(s)

- Speech-language pathologists.

Expected Outcome(s)

- Assessment is conducted to diagnose a voice disorder or a laryngeal disorder affecting respiration, describe perceptual phonatory characteristics, measure aspects of vocal function, and examine phonatory behavior.

- Assessment may result in recommendations for treatment or follow-up, or in referral for other examinations or services.

Clinical Indications

- Individuals of all ages are assessed as needed, requested, or mandated; when their vocal function is altered, impaired, or inadequate to meet their communication, educational, emotional, vocational, social, and health needs; or when the impairment has implications beyond vocal status (e.g., neurological dysfunction, inadequate airway, laryngeal dysfunction).

- Assessment is prompted by referral, by the patient's/client's medical status, or by failure of a speech screening (see Procedure 02.0).

Clinical Process

- All patients/clients with voice disorders must be examined by a physician, preferably in a discipline appropriate to the presenting complaint. The physician's examination may occur before or after the voice evaluation by the speech-language pathologist.

- Assessment includes:

  — Case history and vocal use history

  — Perceptual aspects of vocal production/behavior

— Acoustic parameters of vocal production/behavior

— Physiological aspects of phonatory behavior

— Patient's/client's ability to modify vocal behavior

— Emotional/psychological status

— Medical history and associated conditions

— Review of auditory, visual, motoric, and cognitive status

— Observation or review of articulation, fluency, and language

— Functional consequences of the voice disorder

• Assessment includes use of perceptual and/or instrumental measures. Procedures include:

— Perceptual ratings

— Acoustic analysis

— Aerodynamic measures

— Electroglottography

— Imaging techniques such as endoscopy and stroboscopy. (These procedures may be conducted and interpreted in collaboration with other professionals.)

• Patients/clients with identified voice disorders receive follow-up services to monitor voice status and to ensure appropriate treatment.

Setting/Equipment Specifications

• Assessment is conducted in a clinical or natural environment conducive to eliciting a representative sample of the patient's/client's voice production.

Safety and Health Precautions

• All procedures ensure the safety of the patient/client and clinician and adhere to universal health precautions (e.g., prevention of bodily injury and transmission of infectious disease).

• Decontamination, cleaning, disinfection, and sterilization of multiple-use equipment before reuse are carried out according to facility-specific infection control policies and procedures and according to manufacturer's instructions.

Documentation

- Documentation includes pertinent background information, results and interpretation, prognosis, and recommendations. Recommendations may include the need for further assessment, follow-up, or referral. When treatment is recommended, information is provided concerning frequency, estimated duration, and type of service (e.g., individual group, home program) required.

ASHA Policy and Related References

In addition to the references on p. I-50 [page number refers to original ASHA (1997c) document. Available: http://www.asha.org/library/images/pppslp.pdf.], the following references apply specifically to these procedures:

American Speech-Language-Hearing Association. (1992). Position statement and guidelines for evaluation and treatment for tracheoesophageal fistulization/puncture. *Asha, 34* (Suppl. 7), 17–21.

American Speech-Language-Hearing Association. (1992). Position statement and guidelines for vocal tract visualization and imaging. *Asha, 34* (Suppl. 7), 31–40.

American Speech-Language-Hearing Association. (1992). Sedation and topical anesthesia in speech-language pathology and audiology. *Asha, 34* (Suppl. 7), 41–42.

American Speech-Language-Hearing Association. (1993). Position statement and guidelines for oral and oropharyngeal prostheses. *Asha, 35* (Suppl. 10), 14–16.

American Speech-Language-Hearing Association. (1993). Position statement and guidelines on the use of voice prostheses in tracheotomized persons with or without ventilatory dependence. *Asha, 35* (Suppl. 10), 17–20.

ASHA's Preferred Practice Patterns in Intervention

06.0 Consultation—SLP

(as performed by Speech-Language Pathologists)

Procedures to provide professional expertise that may include conferring with other professionals during case staffing and team conferences or in individual communication; providing information to business and industry and public and private agencies; and engaging in program development and evaluation or supervision activities, or providing expert testimony.

Consultation is conducted according to the Guiding Principles and the Fundamental Components of Preferred Practice Patterns.

Professionals Who Perform the Procedure(s)

- Speech-language pathologists

Expected Outcome(s)

- Information is provided about human communication development and processes, communication and related disorders, and assessment and intervention strategies. Goals and expectations of consultation are variable and are negotiated between the consultant and consultee(s).

Clinical Indications

- Consultation services are provided by arrangement or upon request and address:

  — Prevention of communication disorders

  — Identification of persons at risk for communication disorders

  — Assessment and intervention plans and procedures and interpretation of results

  — Environmental assessment and modification

  — Equipment and material needs and/or modifications

  — Program evaluation and management

  — Quality assessment and improvement

  — Education and advocacy

— Second opinion and/or independent educational evaluation

— Expert testimony

Clinical Process

- Consulting activities take many forms. The consultant:

  — Gathers information through observations, interviews, assessments or other direct services, and reviews of records and materials;

  — Assesses the type and extent of assistance required;

  — Makes recommendations or provides information;

  — Provides monitoring and follow-up services. *[sic]*

  — Provides information to federal and state government agencies, business, and industry.

Setting/Equipment Specifications

Consultation services are offered in home, health care, education, business, and industrial settings, for individuals, families, groups, and organizations.

Safety and Health Precautions

- All procedures ensure the safety of the patient/client and clinician and adhere to universal health precautions (e.g., prevention of bodily injury and transmission of infectious disease).

- Decontamination, cleaning, disinfection, and sterilization of multiple-use equipment before reuse are carried out according to facility-specific infection control policies and procedures and according to manufacturer's instructions.

Documentation

The consultant provides written plans or reports to document services rendered as indicated in the agreement made between the parties involved.

ASHA Policy and Related References

In addition to the references on p. I-50 [page number refers to original ASHA (1997c) document. Available: http://www.asha.org/library/images/pppslp.pdf.], the following references apply specifically to these procedures:

American Speech-Language-Hearing Association. (1984). Prevention: A challenge for the profession. *Asha, 26*(8), 35–37.

American Speech-Language-Hearing Association. (1988). Prevention of communication disorders. *Asha, 30*(3), 90.

American Speech-Language-Hearing Association. (1991). A model for collaborative service delivery for students with language-learning disorders in the public schools. *Asha, 33* (Suppl. 5), 44–50.

American Speech-Language-Hearing Association. (1991). The prevention of communication disorders tutorial. *Asha, 33* (Suppl. 6), 15–41.

American Speech-Language-Hearing Association. (1993). Caseload size and guidelines for speech-language pathologists in the schools. *Asha, 35* (Suppl. 10), 33–39.

American Speech-Language-Hearing Association. (1993). Guidelines for audiology services in the schools. *Asha, 35* (Suppl. 10), 24–32.

American Speech-Language-Hearing Association. (1994). Professional liability and risk management for the audiology and speech-language pathology professions. *Asha, 36* (Suppl. 12), 25–38.

American Speech-Language-Hearing Association. (1995). Position statement and guidelines on acoustics in educational settings. *Asha, 37* (Suppl. 14), 15–19.

15.2 Augmentative and Alternative Communication (AAC) System and/or Device Treatment/Orientation

> *Procedures to assist individuals to understand and use their personalized augmentative and alternative communication systems.*
>
> Augmentative and alternative communication (AAC) system and/or device treatment/orientation is conducted according to the Guiding Principles and the Fundamental Components of Preferred Practice Patterns.

Professionals Who Perform the Procedure(s)

- Speech-language pathologists, often with interdisciplinary or transdisciplinary collaboration

Support Personnel Who Perform the Procedure(s)

- Speech-language pathology assistants under the supervision of a certified speech-language pathologist (in accordance with the ASHA Guidelines for the Training, Credentialing, Use, and Supervision of Speech-Language Pathology Assistants).

Expected Outcome(s)

- Augmentative and alternative communication (AAC) system/device treatment/orientation assists individuals to understand and use their individual AAC systems and/or devices and components (e.g., aids, techniques, symbols, and strategies). Treatment/orientation may also assist those persons with whom the patient/client will communicate.

- AAC treatment/orientation results in recommendations for use of the systems and/or devices and components during treatment.

Clinical Indications

- Individuals of all ages receive AAC treatment/orientation services when prior assessment indicates candidacy for a specific system.

Clinical Process

- AAC treatment/orientation considers the abilities, needs, and preferences of the patient/client and of those with whom the patient/client will communicate (e.g., family, caregivers, educators, service providers). It also considers the environment in which the AAC system will be routinely used.

- The AAC treatment/orientation is often part of an interdisciplinary or transdisciplinary approach.

- Treatment should be long enough to accomplish stated objectives/predicted outcomes. The treatment period should not continue when there is no longer any expectation for further benefit. Clinicians should provide to patients/clients and their families/caregivers an estimate of treatment duration.

- Treatment should provide information and guidance to patients/clients, families, and other significant persons about the use of augmentative and alternative communication, and the course of treatment and prognosis for effective communication.

- AAC treatment/orientation includes education in system operation and maintenance for optimum patient/client use, and provision of information about safety and instrument warranty.

- Recommendations for use of the system may address the need for further screening, assessments, treatment, follow-up, or referral.

Setting/Equipment Specifications

- AAC treatment/orientation is conducted in an appropriate planned or natural environment.

Safety and Health Precautions

- All procedures ensure the safety of the patient/client and clinician and adhere to universal health precautions (e.g., prevention of bodily injury and transmission of infectious disease).

- Decontamination, cleaning, disinfection, and sterilization of multiple-use equipment before reuse are carried out according to facility-specific infection control policies and procedures and according to manufacturer's instructions.

Documentation

- Documentation contains information about treatment/orientation provided to patient/client and others.

ASHA Policy and Related References

In addition to the references on p. I-50 [page number refers to original ASHA (1997c) document. Available: http://www.asha.org/library/images/pppslp.pdf.], the following references apply specifically to these procedures:

American Speech-Language-Hearing Association. (1989). Competencies for speech-language pathologists providing services in augmentative communication. *Asha, 31*(3), 107–110.

American Speech-Language-Hearing Association. (1991). Augmentative and alternative communication. *Asha, 33* (Suppl. 5), 8.

American Speech-Language-Hearing Association. (1991). Report: Augmentative and alternative communication. *Asha, 33* (Suppl. 5), 9–12.

15.5 Fluency Treatment

> *Procedures for addressing fluency disorders and concomitant features of fluency disorders.*
>
> Fluency treatment is conducted according to the Guiding Principles, and the Fundamental Components of Preferred Practice Patterns.

Professionals Who Perform the Procedure(s)

- Speech-language pathologists.

Support Personnel Who Perform the Procedure(s)

- Speech-language pathology assistants under the supervision of a certified speech-language pathologist (in accordance with the ASHA Guidelines for the Training, Credentialing, Use, and Supervision of Speech-Language Pathology Assistants).

Expected Outcome(s)

- Treatment is conducted to achieve improved speech behaviors and attitudes.

- Treatment may result in recommendations for reassessment or follow-up, or in referral for other examinations or services.

Clinical Indications

- Individuals of all ages receive treatment when their ability to communicate effectively is impaired and there is reason to believe that treatment will reduce the degree of impairment or disability or lead to improved communication behaviors.

Clinical Process

- Treatment of fluency and related disorders may be intensive or nonintensive in nature.

- Treatment should be long enough to accomplish stated objectives/predicted outcomes. The treatment period should not continue when there is no longer any expectation for further benefit. Clinicians should provide to patients/clients and their families/caregivers an estimate of treatment duration.

- Treatment should provide information and guidance to patients/clients, families, and other significant persons about the nature of stuttering, normal fluency and disfluency, and the course of treatment and prognosis for recovery.

- Treatment should address the complexities of a fluency disorder, including possible reactions, defensive behaviors, and coping strategies of the person who has the fluency disorder and the reactions of significant others in the listening environment.

Depending on assessment results, treatment addresses the following:

- Reduction of the frequency with which stuttering behaviors occur without increasing the use of other behaviors that are not a part of normal speech production.

- Reduction of the severity, duration, and abnormality of stuttering behaviors until they are or resemble normal speech discontinuities.

- Reduction of the use of defensive behaviors (e.g., avoidance behaviors).

- Removal or reduction of processes serving to create, exacerbate, or maintain stuttering behaviors (e.g., parental reactions, listener reactions, client perceptions).

- Assisting the person who stutters make treatment (e.g., adaptive) decisions about how to handle speech and social situations in everyday living.

- Reduction of attitudes, beliefs, and thought processes that interfere with fluent speech production or that hinder the achievement of other treatment goals.

- Reduction of emotional reactions to specific stimuli when they have a negative impact on stuttering behavior or on attempts to modify stuttering behavior.

- Development of plans, including referral, for problems other than stuttering that may accompany the fluency disorder, such as cluttering, learning disability, language/ phonological disorders, voice disorders, psycho-emotional disturbance.

Setting/Equipment Specifications

- Treatment may be conducted in a variety of settings, including residential and nonresidential sites. In any setting, treatment should address the effective transfer of new behaviors to situations in everyday life and should include the provision of monitored practice of newly learned behaviors in natural settings.

- Instrumental procedures may be used to evaluate and monitor the articulatory, laryngeal, and respiratory dynamics addressed in the treatment process.

Safety and Health Precautions

- All procedures ensure the safety of the patient/client and clinician and adhere to universal health precautions (e.g., prevention of bodily injury and transmission of infectious disease).

- Decontamination, cleaning, disinfection, and sterilization of multiple-use equipment before reuse are carried out according to facility-specific infection control policies and procedures and according to manufacturer's instructions.

Documentation

- Documentation includes pertinent background information, treatment goals, results, prognosis, and specific recommendations. Recommendations may include the need for further treatment, follow-up, or referral. When further treatment is recommended, information is provided concerning the frequency, estimated duration, and type of service (e.g., individual, group, home program) required.

- Documentation includes evaluating treatment outcomes and effectiveness.

ASHA Policy and Related References

In addition to the references on p. I-50 [page number refers to original ASHA (1997c) document. Available: http://www.asha.org/library/images/pppslp.pdf.], the following references apply specifically to these procedures:

American Speech-Language-Hearing Association. (1993). Definitions of communication disorders and variations. *Asha, 35* (Suppl. 10), 40–41.

American Speech-Language-Hearing Association. (1995). Guidelines for practice in stuttering treatment, *Asha, 37* (Suppl. 14), 26–35.

15.6 Voice Treatment

Procedures for addressing disorders of voice production, including possible organic, neurologic, behavioral, and psychosocial etiologies, and alaryngeal speech disorders.

Voice treatment is conducted according to the Guiding Principles and the Fundamental Components of Preferred Practice Patterns.

Professionals Who Perform the Procedure(s)

- Speech-language pathologists

Support Personnel Who Perform the Procedure(s)

- Speech-language pathology assistants under the supervision of a certified speech-language pathologist (in accordance with the ASHA Guidelines for the Training, Credentialing, Use, and Supervision of Speech-Language Pathology Assistants).

Expected Outcomes

- Treatment is conducted to achieve improved voice production, coordination of respiration and laryngeal valving, and/or acquisition of alaryngeal speech sufficient to allow for functional oral communication

- Treatment may result in recommendations for reassessment or follow-up, or in referral for other examinations or services.

Clinical Indications

- Individuals of all ages receive treatment when their ability to communicate effectively is impaired and there is reason to believe that treatment will reduce the degree of impairment or disability and lead to improved communication behaviors.

Clinical Process

- Treatment of voice disorders, alaryngeal speech, and/or laryngeal disorders affecting respiration should be long enough for effective change, but should not be continued when there is no longer any further benefit.

- Treatment should provide information and guidance to patients/clients, families, and significant persons about the nature of voice disorders, alaryngeal speech, and/or laryngeal disorders affecting respiration, the goals, procedures, respective responsibilities, and the likely outcome of treatment.

- Treatment plans should address the patient's unique concerns, abilities, or priorities, and be individualized to meet the needs of special populations, including pediatrics, geriatrics, professional voice users, and diverse racial and cultural groups.

- Depending on the assessment results, treatment addresses the following:

  - Appropriate voice care and conservation guidelines, including strategies that promote healthy laryngeal tissues and voice production and reduce laryngeal trauma or strain.

  - Proper use of respiratory, phonatory, and resonatory processes to achieve improved voice production, coordination of respiration and laryngeal valving, with appropriate treatment to enhance these behaviors.

- Patient/client-directed selection of preferred alaryngeal speech communication means, including development of one or more of the following alaryngeal alternatives: esophageal speech, artificial larynx speech, or tracheoesophageal prosthesis speech.

- Assisting the person with a voice disorder, alaryngeal speech, and/or laryngeal disorder that affects respiration to maintain treatment targets in oral communication in occupational and social situations in everyday living.

- Development of plans, including interdisciplinary referrals, for other speech and health problems that may accompany the voice disorder, alaryngeal speech, and/or laryngeal disorder affecting respiration including medical concerns, dysarthria, swallowing difficulty, psycho-emotional disturbance, and other problems.

Setting/Equipment Specifications

- Treatment is conducted in a clinical or natural environment conducive to observing, modifying, and monitoring the patient's/client's voice, alaryngeal speech, and/or laryngeal disorder affecting respiration.

- When available, instrumental measures may be used in treatment to monitor progress and to provide appropriate patient/client feedback of voice production and/or laryngeal function. Instrumental techniques should ensure validity of signal processing, analysis routines, and elimination of task or signal artifacts.

- Laryngeal imaging techniques and selection/placement of tracheoesophageal prostheses must be conducted in settings that have access to emergency medical treatment, if needed.

Safety and Health Precautions

- All procedures ensure the safety of the patient/client and clinician and adhere to universal health precautions (e.g., prevention of bodily injury and transmission of infectious disease).

- Decontamination, cleaning, disinfection, and sterilization of multiple-use equipment before reuse are carried out according to facility-specific infection control policies and procedures and according to manufacturer's instructions.

Documentation

- Documentation includes pertinent background information, treatment goals, results, prognosis, and specific recommendations. Recommendations may include the need for further treatment, follow-up, or interdisciplinary referral. When further treatment is recommended, information is provided concerning the frequency, estimated duration, and type of service (e.g., individual, group, home program) required.

- Documentation includes evaluating treatment outcomes and effectiveness.

ASHA Policy and Related References

In addition to the references on p. I-50 [page number refers to original ASHA (1997c) document. Available: http://www.asha.org/library/images/pppslp.pdf.], the following references apply specifically to these procedures:

American Speech-Language-Hearing Association. (1992). Position statement and guidelines for evaluation and treatment for tracheoesophageal fistulization/puncture. *Asha, 34* (Suppl. 7), 17–21.

American Speech-Language-Hearing Association. (1992). Position statement and guidelines for vocal tract visualization and imaging. *Asha, 34* (Suppl. 7), 31–40.

American Speech-Language-Hearing Association. (1993). Position statement and guidelines for oral and oropharyngeal prostheses. *Asha, 35* (Suppl. 10), 14–16.

American Speech-Language-Hearing Association. (1993). Position statement and guidelines on the use of voice prostheses in tracheotomized persons with or without ventilatory dependence. *Asha, 35* (Suppl. 10), 17–20.

16.0 Speech-Language Instruction

Procedures to teach various communication strategies with the primary goal of providing assistance in academic or vocational areas.

Speech-language instruction is conducted according to the Guiding Principles and the Fundamental Components of Preferred Practice Patterns.

Professionals Who Perform the Procedure(s)

- Speech-language pathologists.

Support Personnel Who Perform the Procedure(s)

- Speech-language pathology assistants under the supervision of a certified speech-language pathologist (in accordance with the ASHA Guidelines for the Training, Credentialing, Use, and Supervision of Speech-Language Pathology Assistants).

Expected Outcome(s)

- Speech-language instruction enhances the interaction between communication and academic or vocational performance.

Clinical Indications

- Individuals of all ages receive speech-language instruction when their academic or vocational performance is adversely affected by their speech or language status.

- Instruction is prompted by referral or by the recommendations of education personnel.

Clinical Process

- Short- and long-term goals and specific objectives are determined from assessment and represent the framework for treatment. They are reviewed periodically to determine appropriateness.

- Instruction should be long enough to accomplish stated objectives/predicted outcomes. Instruction should not continue when there is no longer any expectation for further benefit. Clinicians should provide to patients/clients and their families/caregivers an estimate of instruction duration.

- Instruction addresses effective use of verbal and nonverbal communication in academic, vocational, and social contexts; development of conversational and classroom discourse competence; use of effective listening skills; use of oral language skills for inquiry, identification, description, classification, prediction, and persuasion; use of cognitive/linguistic processes to guide and monitor comprehension of written language; and/or assumption of responsibility for effective communication that is appropriate according to the context and conversational partner.

- Progress is measured by comparing changes in speech-language skills to established performance baselines, including curriculum-based assessments and classroom/workplace observations.

- A communication skills curriculum is one form of instruction.

- Speech-language pathologists serve as members of education teams including special education prereferral teams and problem solving teams (e.g., teacher assistance teams). In addition, speech-language pathologists serve as members of an education team when providing speech-language instruction in the context of the academic program.

Setting/Equipment Specifications

- Instruction is presented in regular or special education classes or in individual/group treatment outside the classroom/workplace setting.

Safety and Health Precautions

- All procedures ensure the safety of the patient/client and clinician and adhere to universal health precautions (e.g., prevention of bodily injury and transmission of infectious disease).

- Decontamination, cleaning, disinfection, and sterilization of multiple-use equipment before reuse are carried out according to facility-specific infection control policies and procedures and according to manufacturer's instructions.

Documentation

- Documentation contains pertinent background information, goals, results of instruction, prognosis, and recommendations. Recommendations may include the need for further treatment, follow-up, or referral. When further treatment is recommended, information is provided concerning the frequency, estimated duration, and type of service (e.g., individual, group, home program) required.

- Documentation may be a part of the patient's/client's individualized education program or class lesson plan.

ASHA Policy and Related References

In addition to the references on p. I-50 [page number refers to original ASHA (1997c) document. Available: http://www.asha.org/library/images/pppslp.pdf.], the following references apply specifically to these procedures:

American Speech-Language-Hearing Association, and Speech Communication Association. (1979). Standards for effective oral communication programs. *Asha, 21*, 1002.

American Speech-Language-Hearing Association. (1991). A model for collaborative service delivery for students with language-learning disorders in the public schools. *Asha, 33* (Suppl. 5), 44–50.

American Speech-Language-Hearing Association. (1993). Caseload size and guidelines for speech-language pathologists in the schools. *Asha, 35* (Suppl. 10), 33–39.

National Joint Committee on Learning Disabilities. (1991). Providing appropriate education for students with learning disabilities in regular education classrooms. *Asha, 33* (Suppl. 5), 15–17.

17.0 Communication Instruction

Procedures designed to improve the communication abilities of an individual who does not exhibit a disorder. Includes instruction in public speaking and modification of dialect.

Communication instruction is conducted according to the Guiding Principles, and the Fundamental Components of Preferred Practice Patterns.

Professionals Who Perform the Procedure(s)

- Speech-language pathologists.

Support Personnel Who Perform the Procedure(s)

- Speech-language pathology assistants under the supervision of a certified speech-language pathologist (in accordance with the ASHA Guidelines for the Training, Credentialing, Use, and Supervision of Speech-Language Pathology Assistants).

Expected Outcome(s)

- Communication instruction is provided to modify and enhance communication abilities in individuals who do not have a communication disorder.

Clinical Indications

- Communication instruction is provided to individuals of all ages as needed or requested, and upon referral. Such referral is made in response to an identified or perceived need for instruction in speaking English as a second language, public speaking, dialect modification, communication effectiveness, interpersonal communication, and other speaking or communication skills.

Clinical Process

- Short- and long-term goals and specific objectives are determined from assessment, including interviews of the individual requesting service, and represent the framework for treatment. They are reviewed periodically to determine appropriateness.

- Instruction covers verbal, nonverbal, cultural, pragmatic, structural, and interpersonal aspects of communication.

- Progress is measured by comparing changes in communication skills to the individual's own performance baselines and evidence of movement toward the client's broader outcome goals.

- Instruction should be long enough to accomplish stated objectives/predicted outcomes. Instruction should not continue when there is no longer any expectation for further benefit. Clinicians should provide to patients/clients and their families/caregivers an estimate of instruction duration.

Setting/Equipment Specifications

- Communication instruction is conducted in a clinical or natural environment conducive to observing, modifying, and monitoring communication behavior.

Safety and Health Precautions

- All procedures ensure the safety of the patient/client and clinician and adhere to universal health precautions (e.g., prevention of bodily injury and transmission of infectious disease).

- Decontamination, cleaning, disinfection, and sterilization of multiple-use equipment before reuse are carried out according to facility-specific infection control policies and procedures and according to manufacturer's instructions.

Documentation

- Documentation contains pertinent background information, treatment goals, results, prognosis, and specific recommendations. Recommendations may include the need for further instruction, follow-up, or referral.

ASHA Policy and Related References

In addition to the references on p. I-50 [page number refers to original ASHA (1997c) document. Available: http://www.asha.org/library/images/pppslp.pdf.], the following references apply specifically to these procedures:

American Speech-Language-Hearing Association and Speech Communication Association. (1979). Standards for effective oral communication programs. *Asha, 21,* 1002.

American Speech-Language-Hearing Association. (1983). Social dialects (and implications). *Asha, 25*(9), 23–27.

American Speech-Language-Hearing Association. (1985). Clinical management of communicatively handicapped minority language populations. *Asha, 27*(6), 29–32.

Communication Profile

Student _____ Date of Birth _____ CA _____

Teacher _____ School _____ Date _____

Examiner/Observer _____ Position _____

Completed for: Eligibility Assessment date _____ date _____ date _____

Annual Review date _____ date _____ date _____

Physiological Considerations: (circle appropriate items)

a. Documented Hearing Loss

b. Visually Impaired

c. Orthopedically Handicapped

d. Specific Syndrome(s)

e. Seizure Disorder

f. Facial Anomaly

g. ADD-ADHD

h. Other

Comments:

Cognitive or Developmental Level Considerations:

Results of Psychological Evaluation: DSM IV

Health Considerations: (circle appropriate items)

a. GI Tube

b. Dysphagia

c. Tracheotomy

d. Medication

e. Compromised Immune System

f. Dietary Restrictions

g. Other

Comments:

Personal Motivation for Communication with Others: (please describe)

Behavioral Considerations: (circle appropriate items)

a. Self stimulation

b. Aggression

c. Self Abuse

d. Perseveration

e. Tantrums

f. Impulsive

g. Distractible

h. Hyperactive

i. Not applicable

Primary Language Considerations: (circle appropriate items)

a. English

b. Spanish

c. Hmong

d. Other

Attendance:

a. Attends Regularly   b. Irregular Attendance   c. Poor Attendance

Comments:

Previous Speech and Language Instruction: (circle appropriate item(s)

a. Consultation/Collaboration   b. Direct Instruction

Circle number of years enrolled:

a. 0 to 2 years   b. 2 to 5 years   c. 5 to 7 years
d. 7 to 9 years   e. 9 to 11 years   f. Not applicable

Comments:

Current System of Communication: (circle appropriate items)

Eye Gaze	Physical Manipulation	Gesture	Vocal
Picture	Written	Signed	Facial Expression
Augmentative Device(s)	Speech	Echolalia (Immediate-Delayed)	

Comments:

Communication Competence; Pragmatics: (circle appropriate items)

With his current system of communication, the student uses his abilities to:

Request	Get Attention	Reject or Refuse
Comment	Give Requested Information	Seek Information
Express Feelings	Social Routines (eg: greetings)	Acknowledge the Speech of Others

Comments:

The Child Demonstrates These Skills of Discourse: (circle appropriate items)

a. Attending to speaker   e. Initiating conversation
b. Turn-taking   f. Maintaining a topic
c. Volunteering/Changing Topic   g. Responding to requests for clarification
d. Questioning   h. Not applicable

Phonemes or Speech Sounds Produced by the Child: (circle appropriate items)

a. Preverbal sounds

b. Speech sounds

c. Babbling-consonant-vowel combinations

d. Jargon

e. Words

f. Not applicable

Comments:

Child Demonstrates Intelligibility at This Level: (circle appropriate items)

a. In known context

b. In unknown context

c. By familiar persons or family

d. By unfamiliar persons

e. Appropriateness of intonation

f. Dysfluencies or stuttering

g. Not applicable

Child Uses These Types of Words: (circle appropriate items)

a. Nouns

b. Verbs

c. Adjectives

d. Adverbs

e. Prepositions

f. Negatives

g. Conjunctions

h. Pronouns

i. Not applicable

Child Expresses These Semantic Relations: (circle appropriate items)

a. Agent (baby)

b. Action (drink)

c. Object (cup)

d. Recurrence (more)

e. Nonexistence (all gone)

f. Cessation (stop)

g. Rejection (no)

h. Location (up)

i. Possession (mine)

j. Agent-Action (baby drink)

k. Action-Object (drink juice)

l. Agent-Action-Object (baby drink juice)

m. Action-Object-Location (throw ball up)

n. Other

o. Not applicable

Child Uses These Morphological Markers: (circle appropriate items)

a. Present progressive (ing)

b. Prepositions (in, on)

c. Regular and irregular past tense (ed, came)

d. Possessives ('s)

e. Not applicable

Child's Mean Length of Utterance from Language Sample:

Applicable   Not applicable

Teacher Sample _____ Therapist Sample _____ Parent Sample _____
             MLU   MLU   MLU

Comments:

Child Demonstrates Language Comprehension By: (circle appropriate items)

a. Demonstrating joint referencing with an adult

b. Responding to common routines or statements
    1. With/Without visual cues

c. Responding to question forms
    1. Yes/No questions
    2. Simple "wh" questions (where, what, who)
    3. Advanced "wh" questions (which, when, why, how)

d. Indicating knowledge of prepositions

e. Other

f. Not applicable

Comments:

If applicable and appropriate, list standardized tests and summarize results:

It is recommended the child receive the following program services: (circle and describe)

Frequency: _____xw   _____xm   Duration: _____minutes

Individual and/or small group instruction

Service Delivery Model: Model I   Model II   Model III   Model IV

Model I

Communicative development will be infused into teacher's daily classroom activities with parents integrating the program at home.

Model II

Pre-language behaviors appear to be at the emergent stage. Communicative development will be infused into teacher's daily classroom activities with parents integrating the program at home.

Model III

Receptive and expressive language skills appear to be lower than cognition. Communicative development will be infused into teacher's daily classroom activities with parents integrating the program at home. Collaborative planning between Speech and Language Specialist and teacher will occur on a regularly scheduled basis.

Model IV

Receptive or expressive communicative skills are less than cognitive skills. Social skills are appropriate for direct service. Communicative development will be infused into teacher's daily classroom activities with parents integrating the program at home. The Speech and Language Specialist will supplement with regularly scheduled services.

❏ Refer to Assistive Technology Specialist

From *Speech and Language Eligibility Criteria* (p. v-8), by C. Hendricks, C. Swenson, and C.L. Huffman, 2000, Merced, CA: Merced County Office of Education. © 1998, 2000 by Merced County Office of Education. Reprinted with permission.

Checklist of Eligibility Guidelines for English Language Learners' Consideration for Special Education or Related Services

Child's name _____ Date _____

School _____ Birthdate _____

Referred by _____

Date of assessment for language disorder _____

Speech-language pathologist _____

Check the appropriate line.

Agree	Disagree	N/A	Indicators
_____	_____	_____	1. A language disorder exists in the student's first language, corroborated by SLP, interpreter, translator, and parent.
_____	_____	_____	2. Student is acquiring English slowly despite ESL support, and school interventions, corroborated by school personnel.
_____	_____	_____	3. Cultural, economic, or experiential differences are not the primary cause of learning problems, verified by interview and evidence.
_____	_____	_____	4. Student is developing at home at a slower rate than siblings as verified by interview and observation.
_____	_____	_____	5. Poor school progress was noted in student's home country if applicable.
_____	_____	_____	6. Student's academic achievements are significantly below verified English proficiency as determined by communication assessment.

Agree	Disagree	N/A	Conclusions based on these indicators
_____	_____	_____	1. Other school resources have been tried and found insufficient to meet student's needs—Chapter 1, ESL, tutoring, etc.
_____	_____	_____	2. Limited English is not the primary cause of the student's communication problems.
_____	_____	_____	3. After this information has been considered, student appears to meet the state's eligibility criteria for a specific communication disability.

SLP decision _____

Team decision _____ Date _____

Eligibility Examples from Five States

These five examples of state criteria for identifying a student with speech or language disabilities demonstrate some of the differences across states. The criteria meet the broad federal definition, while still responding to each state's educational, political, and fiscal views of how children with communication disabilities are selected for services.

North Carolina

(9) Speech-Language Impaired. Children may be identified as needing speech-language evaluations through mass screening efforts and/or referral. Children determined through screening or referral to need evaluations shall be assessed in the areas of articulation, language (form, content, and function), voice and fluency. It is on the basis of such an evaluation that the determination as to the type and intensity of services shall be made.

(a) Articulation/Phonology. For a student to be considered for articulation/phonology intervention, the student's speech should be determined to have a negative impact on academic, social, and/or vocational functioning, and one or both of the following characteristics must exist:

(i) two or more phonemic errors not expected at the student's current age or developmental level are observed during direct testing and/or conversational speech;

(ii) two or more phonological processes not expected at the student's current age or developmental level are observed during direct testing and/or in conversational speech. For a preschool child to be considered for articulation/phonology therapy, the child's speech should be determined to have a negative impact on social-communicative interactions and one or both of the following characteristics must exist:

- Two or more phonemic errors not expected as the child's current age or developmental level are observed during direct testing and/or conversational speech;

- Two or more phonological processes not expected at the child's current age or developmental level are observed during direct testing and/or conversational speech.

(b) Language. A battery of two diagnostic measures is recommended with at least one assessing comprehension and one assessing production of language. Assessment instruments chosen may include normed tests, criterion references tests, and/or a language sample. Scores should be computed in standard scores, language quotients, percentiles, and/or stanines scores when possible. For a student to be considered for intervention, the student's language should be determined to have a negative impact on academic, social, and/or vocational functioning, and one or both of the following characteristics must exist:

(i) norm reference language tests which yield two subtest or total test scores with the following characteristics: 1.5 or more standard deviation below the mean, a language quotient/standard score of 78 (mean of 100), a stanine of two and/or a percentile of eight;

(ii) non-standardized/informal assessment indicates that the student has difficulty understanding and/or expressing ideas and/or concepts to such a degree that it interferes with the student's social/educational progress. For a preschool child to be considered for language intervention, the child's language should be determined to have a negative impact on social-communicative interactions and one or both of the following characteristics must exist:

   a. norm referenced language tests yield two subtest or total test scores with the following characteristics: 1.5 or more standard deviations below the mean, and language quotient/standard score of 78 (mean of 100), a stanine of two and/or a percentile of eight;

   b. non-standardized/informal assessment indicates that the child has difficulty understanding and/or expressing ideas and/or concepts to such a degree that it interferes with the child's social-educational progress.

   Many students, including those with developmental disabilities and, in particular, those classified as mentally disabled, exhibit limitations with expressive and/or receptive communication skills. Not all such students are considered to have a speech-language impairment and in need of therapeutic intervention from the speech-language pathologist. The speech-language pathologist and other members of the IEP team should consider the efficacy of therapeutic intervention for each student and, in determining such, should consider whether or not enrolling a student for speech-language services will significantly change his/her ability to communicate.

(c) Voice. For a student to be considered for placement in a voice therapy program, he/she must demonstrate consistent deviations in vocal production that are inappropriate for chronological/mental age, sex, and ability. Further, the voice disorder should be determined to have a negative impact on academic, social, and/or vocational functioning.

(d) Fluency. For a student to be considered for placement in a fluency therapy program, he/she must demonstrate nonfluent speech behavior characterized by repetitions/prolongations as noted on a regular basis. Further, the fluency disorder should be determined to have a negative impact on academic, social, and/or vocational functioning.

From *Procedures Governing Programs and Services to Students with Disabilities* [Microsoft Word format] (pp. 28–29), by the North Carolina State Board of Education, 2000, Raleigh, NC: Author.

Connecticut

The eligibility statements for speech-language pathology services in Connecticut are spelled out in the state guide in over 22 pages of descriptions of each communication disability and the type of assessment the speech-language pathologist should use.

Eligibility for services is determined by the Pupil Planning Team (PPT), which is held for this purpose and utilizes the report written by the speech-language pathologist. The team reviews results and implications of the speech-language evaluation to decide if the impairment should be addressed as special education, a related service, or a non-special education service. The speech-language pathologist makes suggestions "for developing the child's speech and language intervention plan or participates in determining other service options for children with communication problems who are determined to be ineligible for special education or related services" (Connecticut Department of Education, 1993, p. 39)

Kentucky

Kentucky utilizes the World Health Organization categories (see page 92) combined with a set of severity rating scales for Speech Sound Production (SS), Language (L), Fluency (F), and Voice (V). The severity rating scale is as follows:

0 = Non-disabling condition within normal range

1 = Mild

2 = Moderate

3 = Severe

A score is assigned for each area assessed. These severity rating scores are reported individually and then totaled (T) to arrive at the decision to provide services. Speech-language pathologists include the ratings in their reports in the following form: SS 2, L 3; T 3. Each disability may have an effect, and then the speech-language pathologist determines the total effect on the student's ability to learn. Eligibility is based on documentation that the communication disability is educationally disabling. To be considered by the team, the student's total severity rating must be at least 1 (mild) and the severity rating for adverse effect must be at least 1 (mild) (Kentucky Department of Education, Division of Exceptional Children's Services, 1993).

Ohio

Ohio uses the federal definition and describes each type of communication disability with a schematic that shows how assessment is to be conducted, and the steps the speech-language pathologist and IEP team need to take to arrive at a conclusion that an impairment exists and it has an adverse effect on the student's ability to learn (Ohio Department of Education, 1991). Figure A.1 is their schematic for a language disability.

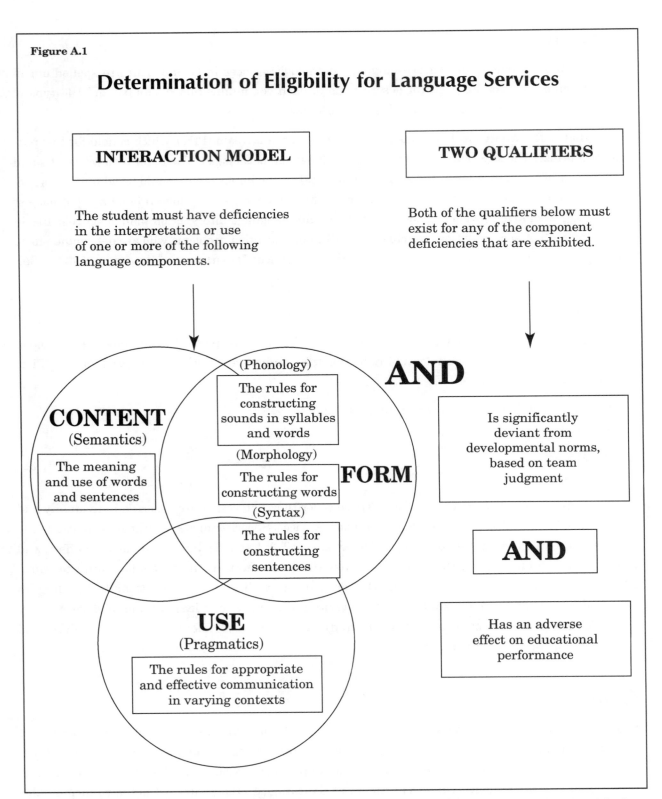

Figure A.1

Determination of Eligibility for Language Services

INTERACTION MODEL

TWO QUALIFIERS

The student must have deficiencies in the interpretation or use of one or more of the following language components.

Both of the qualifiers below must exist for any of the component deficiencies that are exhibited.

AND

CONTENT
(Semantics)

The meaning and use of words and sentences

(Phonology)

The rules for constructing sounds in syllables and words

(Morphology)

The rules for constructing words

FORM

(Syntax)

The rules for constructing sentences

Is significantly deviant from developmental norms, based on team judgment

AND

USE
(Pragmatics)

The rules for appropriate and effective communication in varying contexts

Has an adverse effect on educational performance

From *Ohio Handbook for the Identification, Evaluation, and Placement of Children with Language Problems* (p. 63), by the Ohio Department of Education, 1991, Columbus OH: Author.

Wisconsin

For over 20 years, Wisconsin defined *speech or language impairment* in a brief paragraph that was subject to widely varying interpretations. The need for more uniform guidance resulted in this 2000 revision to the Wisconsin Administrative Code, Chapter PI 11.36 (5).

(5) SPEECH OR LANGUAGE IMPAIRMENT. (a) Speech or language impairment means an impairment of speech or sound production, voice, fluency, or language that significantly affects educational performance or social, emotional or vocational development.

(b) The IEP team may identify a child as having a speech or language impairment if the child meets the definition under par. (a) and meets any of the following criteria:

1. The child's conversational intelligibility is significantly affected and the child displays at least one of the following:

   a. The child performs on a norm-reference test of articulation or phonology at least 1.75 standard deviations below the mean for his or her chronological age.

   b. Demonstrates consistent errors in speech sound production beyond the time when 90% of typically developing children have acquired the sound.

2. One or more of the child's phonological patterns of sound are at least 40% disordered or the child scores in the moderate to profound range of phonological process use in formal testing and the child's conversational intelligibility is significantly affected.

3. The child's voice is impaired in the absence of an acute, respiratory virus or infection and not due to temporary physical factors such as allergies, short-term vocal abuse, or puberty. The child exhibits atypical loudness, pitch, quality or resonance for his or her age and gender.

4. The child exhibits behaviors characteristic of a fluency disorder.

5. The child's oral communication, or for a child who cannot communicate orally, his or her primary mode of communication, is inadequate, as documented by all of the following:

   a. Performance on norm referenced measures that is at least 1.75 standard deviations below the mean for chronological age.

   b. Performance in activities is impaired as documented by informal assessment such as language sampling, observations in structured and unstructured settings, interviews, or checklists.

   c. The child's receptive or expressive language interferes with oral communication or his or her primary mode of communication. When technically adequate norm referenced language measures are not appropriate as determined by the IEP team to provide evidence of a deficit of 1.75 standard deviations below the mean in the area of oral communication, then 2 measurement procedures shall be used to document a significant difference from what would be expected given consideration to chronological age, developmental level, and method of communication such as oral, manual, and augmentative. These procedures may include additional language samples, criterion reference instruments, observations in natural environments and parent reports

(c) The IEP team may not identify a child who exhibits any of the following as having a speech or language impairment:

1. Mild, transitory or developmentally appropriate speech or language difficulties that children experience at various times and to various degrees.

2. Speech or language performance that is consistent with developmental levels as documented by formal and informal assessment data unless the child requires speech or language services in order to benefit from his or her educational programs in school, home, and community environments.

3. Speech or language difficulties resulting from dialectical *[sic]* differences or from learning English as a second language, unless the child has a language impairment in his or her native language.

4. Difficulties with auditory processing without a concomitant documented oral speech or language impairment.

5. A tongue thrust which exists in the absence of a concomitant impairment in speech sound production.

6. Elective or selective mutism or school phobia without a documented oral speech or language impairment

(d) The IEP team shall substantiate a speech or language impairment by considering all of the following:

1. Formal measures using normative data or informal measures using criterion referenced data.

2. Some form of speech or language measures such as developmental checklists, intelligibility ratio, language sample analysis, minimal core competency.

3. Information about the child's oral communication in natural environments.

4. Information about the child's augmentative or assistive communication needs.

(e) An IEP team shall include a department-licensed speech or language pathologist and information from the most recent assessment to document a speech or language impairment and the need for speech or language services.

ASHA's Code of Ethics

(Last Revised January 1, 1994)

Preamble

The preservation of the highest standards of integrity and ethical principles is vital to the responsible discharge of obligations in the professions of speech-language pathology and audiology. This Code of Ethics sets forth the fundamental principles and rules considered essential to this purpose.

Every individual who is (a) a member of the American Speech-Language-Hearing Association, whether certified or not, (b) a nonmember holding the Certificate of Clinical Competence from the Association, (c) an applicant for membership or certification, or (d) a Clinical Fellow seeking to fulfill standards for certification shall abide by this Code of Ethics.

Any action that violates the spirit and purpose of this Code shall be considered unethical. Failure to specify any particular responsibility or practice in this Code of Ethics shall not be construed as denial of the existence of such responsibilities or practices.

The fundamentals of ethical conduct are described by Principles of Ethics and by Rules of Ethics as they relate to responsibility to persons served, to the public, and to the professions of speech-language pathology and audiology.

Principles of Ethics, aspirational and inspirational in nature, form the underlying moral basis for the Code of Ethics. Individuals shall observe these principles as affirmative obligations under all conditions of professional activity.

Rules of Ethics are specific statements of minimally acceptable professional conduct or of prohibitions and are applicable to all individuals.

Principle of Ethics I

Individuals shall honor their responsibility to hold paramount the welfare of persons they serve professionally.

Rules of Ethics

A. Individuals shall provide all services competently.

B. Individuals shall use every resource, including referral when appropriate, to ensure that high-quality service is provided.

C. Individuals shall not discriminate in the delivery of professional services on the basis of race or ethnicity, gender, age, religion, national origin, sexual orientation, or disability.

D. Individuals shall fully inform the persons they serve of the nature and possible effects of services rendered and products dispensed.

E. Individuals shall evaluate the effectiveness of services rendered and of products dispensed and shall provide services or dispense products only when benefit can reasonably be expected.

F. Individuals shall not guarantee the results of any treatment or procedure, directly or by implication; however, they may make a reasonable statement of prognosis.

G. Individuals shall not evaluate or treat speech, language, or hearing disorders solely by correspondence.

H. Individuals shall maintain adequate records of professional services rendered and products dispensed and shall allow access to these records when appropriately authorized.

I. Individuals shall not reveal, without authorization, any professional or personal information about the person served professionally, unless required by law to do so, or unless doing so is necessary to protect the welfare of the person or of the community.

J. Individuals shall not charge for services not rendered, nor shall they misrepresent, in any fashion, services rendered or products dispensed.

K. Individuals shall use persons in research or as subjects of teaching demonstrations only with their informed consent.

L. Individuals whose professional services are adversely affected by substance abuse or other health-related conditions shall seek professional assistance and, where appropriate, withdraw from the affected areas of practice.

For purposes of this Code of Ethics, misrepresentation includes any untrue statements or statements that are likely to mislead. Misrepresentation also includes the failure to state any information that is material and that ought, in fairness, to be considered.

Principle of Ethics II

Individuals shall honor their responsibility to achieve and maintain the highest level of professional competence.

Rules of Ethics

A. Individuals shall engage in the provision of clinical services only when they hold the appropriate Certificate of Clinical Competence or when they are in the certification process and are supervised by an individual who holds the appropriate Certificate of Clinical Competence.

B. Individuals shall engage in only those aspects of the professions that are within the scope of their competence, considering their level of education, training, and experience.

C. Individuals shall continue their professional development throughout their careers.

D. Individuals shall delegate the provision of clinical services only to persons who are certified or to persons in the education or certification process who are appropriately supervised. The provision of support services may be delegated to persons who are neither certified nor in the certification process only when a certificate holder provides appropriate supervision.

E. Individuals shall prohibit any of their professional staff from providing services that exceed the staff member's competence, considering the staff member's level of education, training, and experience.

F. Individuals shall ensure that all equipment used in the provision of services is in proper working order and is properly calibrated.

Principle of Ethics III

Individuals shall honor their responsibility to the public by promoting public understanding of the professions, by supporting the development of services designed to fulfill the unmet needs of the public, and by providing accurate information in all communications involving any aspect of the professions.

Rules of Ethics

A. Individuals shall not misrepresent their credentials, competence, education, training, or experience.

B. Individuals shall not participate in professional activities that constitute a conflict of interest.

C. Individuals shall not misrepresent diagnostic information, services rendered, or products dispensed or engage in any scheme or artifice to defraud in connection with obtaining payment or reimbursement for such services or products.

D. Individuals' statements to the public shall provide accurate information about the nature and management of communication disorders, about the professions, and about professional services.

Competencies Needed by
School-Based Speech-Language Pathologists
Overarching Trend Area: Student Population

Trend	Competency Needed
Student population with increasingly significant needs	Clinical skills and knowledge to provide various treatment approaches (from a researched-based perspective) for children with significant needs, including autistic spectrum disorder, traumatic brain injury, neurologically impaired, and multiple disabilities
	Knowledge of various syndromes, medical advances, implications of genetic research, and associative communication impairments resulting from these
	Knowledge of pharmaceutical intervention and the impact on communication skills
	Ability to determine when speech-language services are indicated: How to make these clinical judgements within the criteria of the code
	Ability to provide services to students who are medically fragile: Knowledge of universal precautions and CPR
	Knowledge and familiarity with augmentative communication, including methods for intervention and devices for use at home and school
Increasingly diverse student population	Knowledge in second language acquisition, differential diagnosis, and the impact of culturally different experiences, and/or lack of school experiences on language acquisition and school success
	Experience working with children from various ethnic/language groups through a trained interpreter
	Ability to conduct least-biased assessment of children who are culturally and linguistically diverse
	Ability to work with bilingual interpreters/translators
	Basic knowledge in a second language

Trend	Competency Needed
Specialized populations	Skills to work with children with cochlear implants
	Skills to work with children with cleft palates
	Diagnostic and intervention decision making for students with attention deficit/hyperactivity disorder (ADHD)
	Expanded skill repertoire for working with students with emotional disabilities and psychiatric conditions
Early Intervention: Infants and toddlers	Clinical experience in assessment and management of infants and toddlers
	Diagnostic and intervention skills with children who are drug-involved, and knowledge of the implication for later learning issues
	Ability to intervene (including counseling) with children and families identified through infant hearing screening procedures
	Ability to work with families addressing family needs which impact the child
Early Intervention: Preschool	Ability to implement programs for children with phonological disorders
	Ability to implement early intervention programs for children with speech-language delays
	Ability to make diagnostic decisions and therapeutic recommendations when services are appropriate

Overarching Trend Area: Intervention

Clinical Expertise (20% of special education identified in the area of speech-language)	Skills and knowledge base required in all areas of speech and language (phonology, language, fluency, voice) for a school-age population
	Clinical skills in oral-motor therapy
	Counseling skills

Trend	Competency Needed
Focus on the general education curriculum	Knowledge of curriculum, performance standards, linking goals and objectives to performance standards
	Knowledge of pedagogy of the general education curriculum, how curriculum is designed, and what skills students need to be successful in the curriculum
	Understanding of brain-based learning theories
	Ability to provide teacher training through demonstration lessons in the classroom
	Ability to incorporate functional therapy activities which can be carried over into the general education curriculum
Prevention/ Intervention services	Ability to assist classroom teachers in the general areas of communication, such as interpersonal communication, listening, and speaking skills
	Ability to demonstrate how interpersonal communication skills can be taught, learned, and reinforced in a meaningful way in natural contexts
Literacy/Reading	Expertise in research related to the developmental process of learning to read
	Skills in early detection and intervention for reading difficulties
	Knowledge of prerequisite reading skills for both decoding and comprehension, including vocabulary and oral language development, as well as phonemic awareness (vs. phonological processing)
	Understanding the role of the speech-language pathologist in prevention and intervention for literacy/reading difficulties
	Skills in working with the continuum of listening/ speaking/reading/writing as it relates to language development and disabilities
	Ability to work as a member of a team at a school site for improvement of literacy skills

Trend	Competency Needed
Changes in service delivery: Classroom-oriented intervention	Ability to support students in the general education program
	Knowledge of various types of alternative service delivery models, how to implement them, and how to decide which type of service delivery is most appropriate for individual students
	Skills and experience providing services to students in small groups, large groups, co-teaching, consultation/collaboration, and other models
	Ability to provide services that focus on curriculum, for example:
	• Reviewing concept vocabulary and syntax expectations for grade-level material
	• Reviewing "test taking vocabulary" and following test directions in preparation for statewide assessment
	Ability to be an ongoing resource to families and support implementation of instructional intervention strategies at home
	Ability to work in an inclusive educational environment, as well as the ability to promote this type of educational philosophy
	Ability to provide services through a consultant/collaborative model (i.e., delivering intervention through the work of others)
	Valuing indirect services provided through consultation/collaboration
	Ability to coordinate services with other service providers
Challenges to eligibility/assessment procedures	Ability to conduct descriptive, prescriptive, performance, and curriculum-based assessments, then describe and evaluate performance based on these models

Trend	Competency Needed
	Ability to make decisions through sound clinical judgements, not solely based on standardized assessments
	Understanding the limitations and drawbacks of standardized assessments
	Ability to relate assessment of student's speech-language functioning to the demands of the classroom
	Ability to describe the student's present levels of performance in terms of a student's needs, strengths, and interests then prescribe adaptations needed for success in the general education curriculum
	Ability to work as a complementary member of the multidisciplinary assessment team, and not in isolation
Use of technology for intervention	Knowledge and expertise in assistive technology for use with students with mild disabilities
	Ability to design application from the Internet for diagnosis, intervention, research, and job management
	Skills and experience with computer assisted intervention programs
Support personnel	Ability to supervise paraprofessionals
	Knowledge of competencies and skills that paraprofessionals can be expected to have and the tasks they are expected to perform
	Understanding of how to coordinate caseloads to allow for time required to provide supervision and direction

Overarching Trend Area: The Educational Reform Environment

Legislative and regulatory changes	Knowledge of the requirements and regulations under IDEA
	Ability to develop IEP goals using benchmarks

Trend	Competency Needed
	Ability to utilize the IEP process in a flexible, functional way allowing for transfer of skills to the classroom
	Ability to write goals and objectives that are attainable by the students
	Understanding of educational organizational structures
	Understanding of obligations under 504
Intensive mastery-based programs	Knowledge of specialized programs (i.e., Fast ForWord, Lindamood-Bell, Lovaas/Discrete Trial) and the ability to address parent requests
	Direct experience with at least one specialized training program
Increased parental participation	Understanding of the parent component of special education
	Understanding of how to involve parents in diagnosis and intervention, and consideration of parent requests for services
	Ability to work with parents: • Encouraging parents to attend therapy and classroom sessions • "Teaching" parents (not just doing direct therapy)
Increasingly litigious environment/ Increase in due process actions	Ability to demonstrate learned competency through maintenance of a professional portfolio
	Knowledge of parent/child due process rights
	Skills in conflict resolution and alternative dispute management
	Skills in avoiding disputes and resolving issues
	Knowledge of legal requirements for their position and the special education system

Trend	Competency Needed

Overarching Trend Area:
Professional Skills and Responsibilities

Educational teaming

Ability to collaborate with other school staff:
- General and special education teachers
- School nurse or health attendant
- Counselors
- Psychologists
- School and district administration (general and special education)
- District or regional services staff
- English Language Learners staff
- Outside agency staff

Ability to effectively communicate with staff and parents

Ability to work as a team member, including knowledge about the contributions of the speech-language pathologist and the contributions of other team members

Understanding of how to become a vital member of a school team

Excellent people skills

Skills for teaming and leadership in the school environment

Ability to design and provide a program that is a critical component of the school that is integral to overall instructional program

Ability to communicate with the school and home to promote generalization of learned skills

Increasing professional responsibilities

Knowledge that being a professional speech-language pathologist means being a lifelong learner who keeps abreast of current trends and changes in the field

Ability to implement new approaches

Networking skills

Understanding of the professional responsibility for professional growth

Trend	Competency Needed
	Knowledge of the resources for seeking new information and ability to utilize this knowledge for challenging issues in areas of diagnostics, intervention, and service delivery
	Understanding of overall issues in special education, including services to children in other disability categories
	Advocacy skills to insure high visibility in order to increase the public's understanding of the complexity of the field and services available
	Knowledge of universal precautions and CPR
Outcomes/Accountability	Experience in how to collect and utilize data to: • Demonstrate effectiveness of intervention • Make decisions about the provision of services • Set intervention goals • Communicate with parents, teachers, students, and staff • Establish exit criteria
Caseloads demands: **Numbers and complexity of cases;** **paperwork requirements**	Expert skills if working with specialized populations Strategies for management Skills in creative scheduling
	Skills for managing paperwork requirements, including report writing
	Understanding of third-party billing and knowledge that such requirements may exist in a school employment setting

Source: Moore-Brown (1999c)

Glossary

If unfamiliar terms are encountered in the following entries, the terms may be found elsewhere in the Glossary. Several sources were used to compile the Glossary and are cited in the entry or listed in the References (American Speech-Language-Hearing Association [ASHA, www.asha.com]; Council for Exceptional Children [www.cec.org]; IDEA [1997, www.ed.gov/office/ OSERS/IDEA]; National Archives and Records Administration [NARA, www.nara.gov]; Nicolosi, Harryman, Kresheck, 1996; Turnbull, 1993; and U.S. Equal Employment Opportunity Commission [EEOC, www.eeoc.gov].

ALTERNATIVE DISPUTE RESOLUTION (ADR): Any of a number of methods (including mediation) for settling disagreements between parents and local educational agencies (LEAs) intended to avoid the need for a due process hearing. ADR methods utilize win-win approaches.

AMERICAN SPEECH-LANGUAGE-HEARING ASSOCIATION (ASHA): The professional, scientific, and credentialing association for more than 99,000 speech-language pathologists; audiologists; and speech, language, and hearing scientists in the United States and around the world. ASHA's mission is to promote the interests of and provide the highest quality services for professionals in audiology, speech-language pathology, and speech and hearing science and to advocate for people with communication disabilities.

AMERICANS WITH DISABILITIES ACT (ADA): Public Law 101-336 passed in 1990 and protected the civil rights of Americans with physical and mental disabilities. The ADA guarantees equal opportunity for individuals with disabilities in public accommodations, employment, transportation, state and local government services, and telecommunications.

ASSESSMENT PLAN: A written plan that indicates assessment procedures and personnel to provide information to an individualized education program (IEP) team.

ASSISTIVE LISTENING DEVICES (ALD): A variety of technology devices used by students to aid them in hearing a teacher and filtering out background noise.

ASSISTIVE TECHNOLOGY (AT): Any item, piece of equipment, or product system acquired commercially off the shelf, modified, or customized to increase, maintain, or improve the functional capabilities of a child with a disability.

AUDITORY PROCESSING: The brain's complex organization of the details of an auditory stimulus to determine meaning, including speech sounds. The details are perceived, discriminated, combined, categorized, and related to recognizable or similar concepts that are stored in memory. The result is an understanding of the auditory stimulus.

Making a Difference
for America's Children

AUGMENTATIVE AND ALTERNATIVE COMMUNICATION (AAC): 1. Any approach designed to support, enhance, or supplement the communication of individuals who are not independent verbal communicators in all situations. **2.** An area of clinical practice that attempts to compensate (either temporarily or permanently) for the impairment and disability patterns of individuals with severe expressive communication disorders. **3.** The use of nonvocal instruments (including picture boards and computer-assisted devices) and approaches by those who cannot communicate vocally.

AUTISM SPECTRUM DISORDER (ASD): Includes any of five diagnoses under the umbrella of Pervasive Developmental Disorders (Autism, Asperger's syndrome, Rett's syndrome, Childhood Disintegrative Disorder, and Pervasive Developmental Disorder-Not Otherwise Specified). Children demonstrate deficits in reciprocal social interactions, verbal and nonverbal communication, and restricted or repetitive behaviors or interests.

AUTISM: A developmental disability, generally evident before age 3, that significantly affects verbal and nonverbal communication and social interaction and that adversely affects a child's educational performance. Other characteristics often associated with autism are engagement in repetitive activities and stereotyped movements, resistance to environmental change or change in daily routines, and unusual responses to sensory experiences.

BENCHMARK: 1. The performance level expected at the end of each grade level. **2.** A major milestone in the curriculum.

BEST PRACTICE: A term commonly used for current, accepted educational methods; the term can be misleading because "best" depends on the individual needs of each child rather than on any particular program or method. (See **GOOD PRACTICE**)

CASE MANAGER: A member of an individualized education program (IEP) team who coordinates the IEP services.

CASELOAD: Students (or the number of students) receiving services from a speech-language pathologist.

CERTIFICATION: Recognition of professional knowledge and skills bestowed by a credentialing body (e.g., the Certificate of Clinical Competence [CCC] in Speech-Language Pathology from the American Speech-Language-Hearing Association [ASHA]).

CHILD FIND: Activities to comply with the Individuals with Disabilities Education Act (IDEA) requirements to annually identify, locate, and evaluate all children with disabilities residing in a local educational agency (LEA) or state educational agency (SEA).

CHRONOLOGICAL AGE (CA): The actual age of an individual derived from date of birth and usually expressed in years, months, and days.

CLASSROOM INSTRUCTION: Teaching and learning interactions that are provided to a class, utilizing a variety of instructional methodologies.

CODE OF FEDERAL REGULATIONS (C.F.R.): A codification of the rules published in the Federal Register by the executive departments and agencies of the federal government.

COLLABORATION: A category of service delivery or a work style in which coequal parties engage voluntarily in shared decision-making toward a common goal of assisting a student to experience school success. The speech-language pathologist may collaborate with another professional in the assessment, intervention, or classroom application of student skills.

COLLABORATIVE CONSULTATION: A form of service delivery in which a student receives intervention that is directed by a speech-language pathologist but may be provided by any trained and supervised person, such as a speech-language pathology assistant (SLPA), a classroom teacher, another special educator, a peer, a parent, or a bus driver, in any relevant setting. The professionals work together using a collaborative style.

COLLABORATIVE INTERVENTION: The delivery of speech-language intervention services by two or more providers, in multiple settings, designed and monitored by the speech-language pathologist.

COMMUNICATION DISORDER: An impairment in one or more of the processes of hearing, speech, or language that results in the inability to comprehend or express thoughts or concepts in oral, manual (e.g., sign language), or written form.

COMMUNICATIVE COMPETENCE: The wide scope of grammatical, cognitive, social, and cultural knowledge that underlies adequate language ability.

COMMUNICATIVE INTENT: The ability to express a range of wants and needs without necessarily using language as a means of communication. Gaze, gesture, and posture are early means of expression for very young children.

CONSULTATION: 1. A category of indirect service delivery models. **2.** A voluntary process in which one professional assists another to address a student's goals using shared participation, effective communication, teamwork, and problem solving.

CONVENTIONAL THERAPY: A category of service delivery models in which intervention is provided directly by a speech-language pathologist in a pullout or in-class setting.

COOPERATIVE LEARNING: A set of instructional methods that include cooperative student to student interaction with subject matter by applying four principles: positive interdependence, individual accountability, equal participation, and simultaneous interaction (Kagan, 1992).

CULTURALLY/LINGUISTICALLY DIVERSE (CLD): A term applied to persons whose experiences vary in their cultural or linguistic contexts. This term does not imply a judgement of competence.

DEAF: 1. When capitalized, a community of individuals sharing a language, which is American Sign Language (ASL), and a culture. **2.** When beginning with a lowercase letter, an audiological condition of an individual whose hearing impairment is so great, even with amplification, that vision becomes the main channel of communication.

DIRECT OUTCOMES: Intended changes in behavior that result from an intervention.

DISCRETE TRIAL TRAINING: A teaching method used with children with autism that uses behavioral therapy; it is often used in intensive all-day programming at home and school.

DUE PROCESS HEARING: The opportunity for a parent, student, or local educational agency (LEA) to present complaints regarding a child's identification, evaluation, placement, or right to free appropriate public education (FAPE). Evidence is presented, and an impartial hearing officer makes a ruling. Also called a fair hearing and an impartial due process hearing.

DYNAMIC ASSESSMENT: A process-oriented approach to assessment that often uses a test-teach-retest format to analyze a child's responses in learning situations, describe the child as a learner, and determine how the child responds to intervention.

EDUCATION FOR ALL HANDICAPPED CHILDREN ACT (EAHCA): Public Law 94-142, passed in 1975, mandated that states provide free appropriate public education (FAPE) in the least restrictive environment (LRE) to meet the needs of children with disabilities from 5 to 21 years of age.

EDUCATION OF THE HANDICAPPED ACT (EHA): Public Law 91-230, passed in 1970, established minimum requirements for states to follow to receive federal assistance for special education.

ELIGIBILITY: A determination based on a child's assessment results as they compare to state or local eligibility criteria for special education. The determination looks at whether the child has a disability and whether that disability requires special education and related services.

EXPULSION: The removal of a student from the educational programs of a school district for a lengthy period of time, generally two semesters or more, imposed by the school board or other governing body. Special education services must continue to be provided to expelled students.

FAMILY EDUCATIONAL RIGHTS AND PRIVACY ACT (FERPA): 20 United States Code (U.S.C.) SS 1232 (g) passed in 1974 and protected the privacy interests of parents and students regarding educational records through standards for record keeping, protocols for parent access to records, and limits to disclosure of records without consent.

FIFTH AMENDMENT: One of two sources of due process protections in the United States Constitution requiring that no person may be deprived of life, liberty, or property, without due process of law.

FOURTEENTH AMENDMENT: One of two sources of due process protections in the United States Constitution requiring that no state may deprive any person of life, liberty, or property, without due process of law.

FREE APPROPRIATE PUBLIC EDUCATION (FAPE): Special education and related services that (a) have been provided at public expense, under public supervision and direction, and without charge; (b) meet the standards of the state educational agency involved; (c) include an appropriate preschool, elementary, or secondary school education in the state involved; and (d) are provided in conformity with the individualized education program (IEP) required under SS 614 (d) of the Individuals with Disabilities Education Act (IDEA).

FRIENDSHIP GROUPS: A method of grouping students for instructional purposes based on students' social relationships.

FUNCTIONAL COMMUNICATION MEASURES (FCMS): A series of seven-point rating scales designed by the American Speech-Language-Hearing Association (ASHA) to describe the different aspects of a patient's or student's abilities over the course of treatment.

FUNCTIONAL OUTCOMES: Measures of a person's actual performance following intervention. Also called performance outcomes.

GOAL: The end result toward which action, muscular or mental, is directed.

GOOD PRACTICE: Current, accepted education or intervention methods that are research-based and effectively address the needs of a student.

HABILITATIVE: Intervention intended to develop skills and abilities that a person has not previously exhibited.

HANDICAPPED CHILDREN'S PROTECTION ACT: Public Law 99-372, passed in 1986, authorized awarding attorneys' fees to families who prevailed in lawsuits under the due process provisions of the Individuals with Disabilities Education Act (IDEA). Also called the Attorneys' Fees Bill.

HEAD START PROGRAM: Established in 1965, a federal program that provides comprehensive services to children from birth to age 5 and their families, targeting those with incomes below the poverty line. Services include education, health, social services, nutrition, and opportunity for parent involvement.

HEALTH MANAGEMENT ORGANIZATION (HMO): A type of managed care organization that provides comprehensive coverage for hospital and health-care practitioner services for a prepaid fixed fee.

HEARING IMPAIRMENT: A generic term that includes all types and degrees of hearing loss, with mild hearing loss being the lowest degree and severe-to-profound hearing impairment being the greatest degree.

INCLUSION MOVEMENT: An educational and social effort to bring students with disabilities into general education classes and environments.

INCLUSION: A philosophy that promotes access for children with disabilities to activities, situations, and environments that are designed for individuals without disabilities by providing the support and accommodations necessary, so the child with disabilities will derive as much benefit from the experience as children without disabilities.

INCLUSIVE PRACTICES: The American Speech-Language-Hearing Association's (ASHA's) position on inclusion that emphasizes serving children and youth in the least restrictive environment (LRE) that meets their needs optimally, taking advantage of the full range of service delivery models and settings.

INDEPENDENT EDUCATIONAL EVALUATION (IEE): An evaluation conducted by a qualified examiner who is not employed by the public agency responsible for a child's education and provided at no expense to parents.

INDIRECT OUTCOMES: Unintended changes in behavior that result from intervention.

INDIVIDUALIZED EDUCATION PROGRAM (IEP): A written statement describing the special education program and placement of each child with a disability that is developed, reviewed, and revised in a meeting in accordance with 34 Code of Federal Regulations (C.F.R.) SS 300.341–300.350.

INDIVIDUALIZED FAMILY SERVICE PLAN (IFSP): A plan developed in place of an individualized education program (IEP) for children 2 years of age and younger. For children 3–5 years of age, the Individuals with Disabilities Education Act (IDEA) permits states to use an IFSP to meet IEP requirements. The IFSP places a family in a central role as recipient, provider, or both of intervention to promote a child's development.

INDIVIDUALIZED TRANSITION PLAN (ITP): 1. A component of the individualized education program (IEP) for each student aged 14 and older. **2.** A statement of a coordinated set of activities designed within an outcome-oriented process to promote movement from school to postschool activities.

INDIVIDUALS WITH DISABILITIES EDUCATION ACT (IDEA): Public Law 105-17, passed in 1990, reauthorized and amended the Education of All Handicapped Children Act (EAHCA).

INDIVIDUALS WITH DISABILITIES EDUCATION ACT (IDEA) AMENDMENTS OF 1997: Revisions to IDEA that placed an emphasis on access to the general curriculum and high expectations for achievement for all students.

INTERDISCIPLINARY TEAM (IDT): A group of special educators from two or more disciplines who address the goals of an individualized education program (IEP). Members work together on the evaluation and treatment team but evaluate and treat a student and family separately. These teams often have formal channels for communication and a functioning case manager (Donahue-Kilburg, 1992).

LANGUAGE DISORDER: A condition characterized by impaired comprehension and/or use of spoken, written, and/or other symbol systems. The disorder may involve the form of language (phonology, morphology, syntax), the content of language (semantics), and/or the function of language in communication (pragmatics).

LEARNING DISABILITIES: A heterogeneous group of disorders that are intrinsic to the individual and presumed to be due to central nervous system dysfunction. These disorders are manifested in significant difficulties in the acquisition and use of listening, speaking, reading, writing, reasoning, or mathematical abilities.

LEAST RESTRICTIVE ENVIRONMENT (LRE): The appropriate educational setting that affords a student the opportunity to learn in an environment that is as close to general education as possible and allows the student as much interaction as possible with nondisabled peers.

LICENSING: The issuance of a legal permit to practice a profession within the jurisdiction of the licensing body.

LITERACY: The condition or quality of being literate, especially the ability to read and write.

LOCAL EDUCATIONAL AGENCY (LEA): A public board of education or other local public authority legally constituted within a state. The board has administrative control or direction of, or performs a service function for, public elementary or secondary schools in a city, county, township, school district, or other political subdivision of a state. The board may also oversee a combination of school districts or counties as are recognized in a state as an administrative agency for its public elementary or secondary schools.

MAINSTREAMING: When students with disabilities are educated with typically developing peers in the same classes, activities, or buildings.

MANIFESTATION DETERMINATION: When an action is contemplated by a local educational agency (LEA) in response to a student's violation of a school's code of conduct, an individualized education program (IEP) team meets to review the child's disability and the behavior subject to disciplinary action. The purpose of this meeting is to make a manifestation determination (i.e., to decide if the behavior was a manifestation of the child's disability). If the behavior was a manifestation of the disability, they must remedy deficiencies found in the student's IEP. If the behavior was not a manifestation of the disability, they must transmit education and discipline records to the disciplinary body.

MEDICARE: A program constituted under the United States Social Security Administration that reimburses hospitals and physicians for health-care services provided to people over 65 years old, those receiving social security payments more than two years, and all citizens who have end-stage renal disease.

MENTAL AGE: An expression of the developmental level of an individual, usually a younger child, that is characteristic of a particular chronological age.

MULTIDISCIPLINARY TEAM (MDT): A group of two or more qualified individuals that performs any needed assessment to provide information to an individualized education program (IEP) team after existing evaluation data are reviewed.

OBJECTIVES: 1. Measurable statements of performance. **2.** Short-term or intermediate steps in reaching an intervention goal.

PERFORMANCE OUTCOMES: Measures of a person's abilities following intervention; also called functional outcomes.

PHONEMIC AWARENESS: The explicit understanding that words are composed of phonemes (i.e., segments of sound smaller than a syllable) plus the knowledge that each of these phonemes has distinctive features (Torgesen, 1999).

PHONICS: Instructional practices that educators use to emphasize how spellings are related to speech sounds in systematic ways (Snow, Burns, and Griffin, 1998).

PHONOLOGICAL AWARENESS: The general ability to attend to the sounds of a language distinct from its meaning, including rhyming, counting syllables, segmenting words, and recognizing onset and rime in words (Snow, Burns, and Griffin, 1998).

PLACEMENT: The description of the program that meets a student's individual educational needs, including the amount, type, frequency, and location of special education and related services.

PREFERRED PRACTICE PATTERNS: Statements developed by the American Speech-Language-Hearing Association (ASHA) that define universally applicable characteristics of activities directed toward individual patients/clients and address structural requisites of the practice, processes to be carried out, and expected outcomes.

PRELITERACY: 1. Skills that are precursors to literacy. **2.** Foundational skills and experiences for reading and writing.

PRESCHOOL AMENDMENTS TO THE EDUCATION OF THE HANDICAPPED ACT: Public Law 99-457, passed in 1986, extended the age of eligibility for special education to include infants and toddlers (birth through 2 years of age) who qualified for services under less-intensive eligibility criteria.

PRESENT LEVELS OF EDUCATIONAL PERFORMANCE: A required component of an individualized education program (IEP), this statement serves as a baseline for functional performance in goal areas and describes how the child's disability affects involvement and progress in the general curriculum.

PRINT FORM: The shape and appearance of written symbols of language.

PRINT MEANING: The meaning represented by written symbols of language.

PROCEDURAL COMPLIANCE: The action of agents of the state correctly following the requirements of due process.

PROCEDURAL DUE PROCESS: 1. The right to challenge an action of the state through an adjudicative procedure before the action may infringe on one's life, liberty, or property. **2.** The procedures followed to protect one's due process rights.

PROSPECTIVE PAYMENT: A Medicare reimbursement system that makes a single payment to cover a defined time period of care for a patient based on a diagnosis and other factors. The payment is intended to cover the costs of all services provided during this time, including therapies.

PULLOUT: In this traditional service delivery model, a student is served directly by a speech-language pathologist individually or in a group of students in a location separate from the classroom.

RANDOM/PURPOSE GROUPS: A method of grouping students for instructional purposes that varies the composition of groups over time based on criteria determined by a speech-language pathologist.

RECIPROCITY: The influence that each person in a relationship has on others in the course of their interactions.

REFERRAL: Written notification sent to a local educational agency (LEA) requesting assessment for a child who is believed to have a disability.

REGULAR EDUCATION INITIATIVE (REI): An educational movement initiated by the document prepared by M. Will for the United States Office of Special Education and Rehabilitation Services (OSERS) in 1986 that outlined reforms in special education, including greater opportunities to include students with disabilities in general education environments.

REHABILITATION ACT: Public Law 93-112, passed in 1973, prohibited discrimination on the basis of disability in programs receiving federal financial assistance, in federal employment, and in the employment practices of federal contractors.

RELATED SERVICE: A service necessary for a student to benefit from special education, including transportation and developmental, corrective, and other supportive services (e.g., speech-language pathology and audiology services; psychological services; physical and occupational therapy; recreation, including therapeutic recreation; social work services; counseling services, including rehabilitation counseling; orientation and mobility services; and medical services, except such medical services that will be for diagnostic and evaluation purposes only) that may be required to assist a child with a disability to benefit from special education. Includes the early identification and assessment of disabling conditions in children.

RESOURCE TEACHERS: Special education or other teachers who provide specialized instruction in the classroom or in a separate location for part of the day.

RESTORATIVE: Intervention intended to restore or recover skills and knowledge lost due to injury or illness.

RESTRUCTURING: All aspects of reform, including instruction, participatory governance, site-based management, the increasing involvement of parents and communities in the development of partnerships and networks, and the redesign of curricula.

SCREENING: An abbreviated procedure to collect information on children's performance and to check for potential developmental or academic concerns that should be further evaluated for possible referral.

SECTION 504: The section of the Rehabilitation Act of 1973 that requires all programs receiving federal funds to be fully accessible to employees and members of the general public who have disabilities.

SEMANTICS: The meaning of words in a language and the relationships between words. Semantics also relates to multiple word meanings, figurative language, and the underlying meanings of words in specific contexts.

SERVICE DELIVERY: The provision of educational or therapeutic services to a target population.

SHARED CAP: As part of the Balanced Budget Act of 1997 (PL105-33), Congress set a limit of $1500 per year on payment for outpatient rehabilitation services provided by skilled nursing facilities, rehabilitation agencies, public health agencies, clinics, and other facilities. The Health Care Financing Administration (HCFA) interpreted the language of this law to mean that speech-language pathology and physical therapy services must share a $1500 payment cap, i.e., total payment for speech-language pathology services, physical therapy services, or a combination of these services could not exceed $1500 per year. In November, 1999, ASHA and other professional organizations won a two-year moratorium on caps for all rehabilitation services.

SHORT-TERM OBJECTIVES: Measurable intermediate steps toward an intervention goal.

SKILL GROUPS: A method of grouping students for instructional purposes based on similar skills or performance levels.

SOUND/SYMBOL CORRESPONDENCE: A phoneme that is mapped onto a graphic symbol, such as a letter or a combination of letters

SPECIAL EDUCATION: Specially designed instruction, provided to identified students at no cost to parents, that meets the unique needs of a child with a disability, including instruction conducted in the classroom, in the home, in hospitals and institutions, and in other settings and instruction in physical education.

SPECIFIC LANGUAGE DEFICIT: A category of language disorder that is usually characterized as a language disorder that cannot be attributed to intellectual or sensory deficits but that substantially affects a child's ability to understand and express verbal and written language. Also called developmental language disorder, specific language impairment, and clinical language disorder.

SPEECH-LANGUAGE PATHOLOGY ASSISTANT (SLPA): Support personnel who provide services in a speech-language program under the supervision of a speech-language pathologist and have a minimum of an associate's degree or equivalent experience.

STANDARDIZED TEST: An assessment measure that provides information concerning the ability of a child in comparison with other children of the same specified group. A standardized test must always be administered in the same manner and under the same conditions to obtain reliability and validity. The standards of interpretation of the student's response behaviors are usually based on the norms of a similar population that has also completed the test.

STATE EDUCATIONAL AGENCY (SEA): The state board of education or other agency or officer primarily responsible for the state supervision of public elementary and secondary schools or, if there is no such officer or agency, an officer or agency designated by the governor or by state law.

STAY PUT: The rule that prohibits a local educational agency (LEA) from changing a child's placement without parental consent while a due process dispute is going on.

STUDENT STUDY TEAM (SST): A group of school staff who meet regularly to problem solve regarding students, recommend in-class modifications, make referrals for specialized services, or refer for special education assessment.

SUBJECT AREA SPECIALIST: An educator who does not have a self-contained classroom of students for the day but sees a class or a small group for part of the day to address a specific subject (e.g., art, music, reading, and biology).

SUPPORT PERSONNEL MODEL: A model of service delivery that uses support personnel (e.g., aides, assistants, or paraprofessionals).

SUSPENSION: The removal of a student from a classroom or school for a limited period of time, generally fewer than or equal to 10 days, as directed by a teacher or principal.

SYNTAX: The part of grammar that regulates the arrangement of words to form meaningful sentences.

TITLE I: A federal program established under the Elementary and Secondary Education Act of 1965 that provided a system of reme-dial education for economically disadvantaged students and provided some entitlements to state-supported or state-operated schools for the "handicapped."

TRANSITION: The movement of a student from one level to another, especially the movement from preschool to elementary school or from high school to postschool.

TRANSDISCIPLINARY TEAM (TDT): A group of special educators from two or more disciplines who share skills, knowledge, and roles as appropriate to address the goals of an individualized education program (IEP). Members divide their work into direct and indirect student services. Not every member works with every student, but all members, including parents and caregivers, consult with each other to carry out the service delivery plans the group designs together (Donahue-Kilburg, 1992).

UNITED STATES CODE (U.S.C.): The written record of the laws of the United States enacted by the legislative branch of the federal government.

UNIVERSAL DESIGN: The design of instructional materials and activities that provides for goals to be achievable by individuals with wide differences in their physical or learning abilities. Alternatives are built into curricular materials and activities to provide students with flexible approaches to meeting instructional objectives.

UNIVERSAL NEWBORN HEARING SCREENING (UNHS) PROGRAM: A system of providing hearing screening for all infants, typically before discharge from the hospital nursery or within 3 months of birth.

References

Adams, M.J. (1999). *Beginning to read: Thinking and learning about print.* Cambridge, MA: MIT Press.

Albanese, B. (2000, January). *Free appropriate public education. What does it mean in the year 2000* [Handout]. Presentation at the Association of California School Administrators Conference, Monterey, CA.

Allington, R.L., and McGill-Franzen, A. (1992). Does high-stakes testing improve school effectiveness? *ERS Spectrum, 10*(2), 3–12.

Allington, R.L., and McGill-Franzen, A. (2000). Looking back, looking forward: A conversation about teaching reading in the 21st century. *Reading Research Quarterly, 35,* 136–153.

American Psychiatric Association (APA). (1995). *Diagnostic and statistical manual of mental disorders* (4th ed.). Washington, DC: Author.

American Psychological Association (APA). (1994). *Publication manual of the American Psychological Association* (4th ed.). Washington, DC: Author.

*American Speech-Language-Hearing Association (ASHA). (1985). Clinical management of communicatively handicapped minority language populations. *Asha, 27,* 29–32.

*American Speech-Language-Hearing Association (ASHA). (1987). Classification of speech-language pathology and audiology procedures and communication disorders. *Asha, 29,* 49–58.

*American Speech-Language-Hearing Association (ASHA). (1989a). Issues in determining eligibility for language intervention. *Asha, 31,* 113–118.

*American Speech-Language-Hearing Association (ASHA). (1989b). *Partnerships in education: Toward a literate America* (No. 17). Rockville, MD: Author.

*American Speech-Language-Hearing Association (ASHA). (1990). Roles of speech-language pathologists in service delivery to infants, toddlers, and their families. *Asha, 32*(Suppl. 2), 4.

*American Speech-Language-Hearing Association (ASHA). (1991a). Augmentative and alternative communication, *Asha, 33*(Suppl. 5), 8.

*American Speech-Language-Hearing Association (ASHA). (1991b). *A building blocks module: Multicultural considerations.* Rockville, MD: Author.

*American Speech-Language-Hearing Association (ASHA). (1994). Code of ethics. *Asha, 40*(Suppl. 18), 43–45.

*American Speech-Language-Hearing Association (ASHA). (1995). *User's guide phase I—group II, National treatment outcome data collection project.* Rockville, MD: Author.

*American Speech-Language-Hearing Association (ASHA). (1996a). Guidelines for training, credentialing, use, and supervision of speech-language pathology assistants. *Asha, 38*(Suppl. 16), 21–34.

*American Speech-Language-Hearing Association (ASHA). (1996b). Inclusive practices for children and youths with communication disorders [Position statement]. *Asha, 38*(Suppl. 16), 35–44.

*ASHA documents are available from American Speech-Language-Hearing Association, 10801 Rockville Pike, Rockville, MD 20852.

*American Speech-Language-Hearing Association (ASHA). (1997a). *Building blocks: Preparing speech-language pathologists to serve infants, toddlers, and their families.* Rockville, MD: Author.

*American Speech-Language-Hearing Association (ASHA). (1997b). *Omnibus survey results.* Rockville, MD: Author.

*American Speech-Language-Hearing Association (ASHA). (1997c). *Preferred practice patterns for the profession of speech-language pathology.* Rockville, MD: Author.

*American Speech-Language-Hearing Association (ASHA). (1997d). Trends and issues in school reform and their effects on speech-language pathologists, audiologists, and students with communication disorders. *ASHA Desk Reference* (Vol. 4, pp. 310–310i). Rockville, MD: Author.

*American Speech-Language-Hearing Association (ASHA). (1998a, September 8). Medicare: How the new payment system will affect you. *ASHA Leader Extra,* pp. 11–14.

*American Speech-Language-Hearing Association (ASHA). (1998b). *Speech-language pathology assistants* [Information series]. Rockville, MD: Author.

*American Speech-Language-Hearing Association (ASHA). (1998c). Students and professionals who speak English with accents and nonstandard dialects: Issues and recommendations. *Asha, 40*(Suppl. 18), 28–31.

*American Speech-Language-Hearing Association (ASHA). (1998d). *Survey of speech-language pathology services in school-based settings* [Final report]. Rockville, MD: Author.

*American Speech-Language-Hearing Association (ASHA). (1998e). *User's guide: National treatment outcome data collection project.* Rockville, MD: Author.

*American Speech-Language-Hearing Association (ASHA). (1999a, December). *American Speech-Language-Hearing Association priority issues and outcomes: 2000.* Retrieved May 21, 2000, from the World Wide Web: http://www.asha.org /association/workplan1.htm

*American Speech-Language-Hearing Association (ASHA). (1999b, October). *Detailed analysis of the final IDEA Part B regulations available to members.* Retrieved January 29, 2001, from the World Wide Web: http://www.asha.org/idea/idea _final_analysis.htm

*American Speech-Language-Hearing Association (ASHA). (1999c). *Guidelines for the roles and responsibilities of the school-based speech-language pathologist.* Rockville, MD: Author.

*American Speech-Language-Hearing Association. (ASHA). (1999d). *1999 ASHA workforce study.* Rockville, MD: Author.

*American Speech-Language-Hearing Association (ASHA). (1999e). *Proposed criteria for approval of technical training programs for speech-language pathology assistants.* Rockville, MD: Author.

*American Speech-Language-Hearing Association. (ASHA). (1999f). *Proposed criteria for registration of speech-language pathology assistants.* Rockville, MD: Author.

*American Speech-Language-Hearing Association (ASHA). (2000a). *Frequently asked questions about speech-language pathology assistants.* Retrieved February 19, 2001, from the World

*ASHA documents are available from American Speech-Language-Hearing Association, 10801 Rockville Pike, Rockville, MD 20852.

420

Wide Web: http://www.asha.org/information/faq _slpasst.htm

*American Speech-Language-Hearing Association (ASHA). (2000b). *IDEA and your caseload: A template for eligibility and dismissal criteria for students ages 3–21.* Rockville, MD: Author.

*American Speech-Language-Hearing Association (ASHA). (2000c, January). *Responding to the changing needs of speech-language pathology and audiology students in the 21st century: A briefing paper for academicians, practitioners, employers, and students.* Retrieved January 30, 2001, from the World Wide Web: http://www.asha .org/students/changing.htm

*American Speech-Language-Hearing Association (ASHA). (2000d). *Roles and responsibilities of speech-language pathologists with respect to reading and writing in children and adolescents.* Rockville, MD: Author.

*American Speech-Language-Hearing Association (ASHA). (2000e, February). *Why be certified by ASHA?* Retrieved January 29, 2001, from the World Wide Web: http://www.asha.org/member

*American Speech-Language-Hearing Association (ASHA). (2000f). *Working for change: A guide for speech-language pathologists and audiologists in schools.* Rockville, MD: Author.

Americans with Disabilities Act (ADA), 42 U.S.C. § 12101 *et seq.* (1990).

Amiot, A. (1998). Policy, politics, and the power of information: The critical need for outcomes and clinical trials data in policy-making in the schools. *Language, Speech, and Hearing Services in Schools, 29,* 245.

Anderson, R.J. (1992). Educational reform: Does it all add up? *Teaching Exceptional Children, 24*(2), 4.

Angelo, D.H., and Lowe, R.J. (1993). An overview of the profession of speech-language pathology in the schools. In R.J. Lowe (Ed.), *Speech-language pathology and related professions in the schools* (pp. 1–20). Boston: Allyn and Bacon.

Apel, K. (1993, November). *Index of state's definition of language impairment and qualification for service* [Handout]. Presentation at the annual convention of the American Speech-Language-Hearing Association, Anaheim, CA.

Apel, K. (1999). An introduction to assessment and intervention with older students with language-learning impairments: Bridges from research to clinical practice. *Language, Speech, and Hearing Services in Schools, 30,* 228–230.

Apel, K., and Swank, L. (1999). Second chances: Improving decoding skills in the older student. *Language, Speech, and Hearing Services in Schools, 30,* 231–242.

Arvedson, J.C. (2000). Evaluation of children with feeding and swallowing problems. *Language, Speech, and Hearing Services in Schools, 31,* 28–41.

Audette, B., and Algozzine, B. (1992). Free and appropriate education for all students: Total quality and the transformation of American public education. *Remedial and Special Education, 13*(6), 8.

Audette, B., and Algozzine, B. (1997). Re-inventing government? Let's re-invent special education. *Journal of Learning Disabilities, 30,* 378–383.

Autism Society of America. (1996, July-August). Definition of autism. *Advocate, 3,* 1.

*ASHA documents are available from American Speech-Language-Hearing Association, 10801 Rockville Pike, Rockville, MD 20852.

Bain, B.A., and Dollaghan, C.A. (1991). The notion of clinically significant change. *Language, Speech, and Hearing Services in Schools, 22,* 264–270.

Bateman, B.D., and Linden, M.A. (1998). *Better IEPs: How to develop legally correct and educationally useful programs* (3rd ed.). Longmont, CO: Sopris West.

Battle, D.E. (1998). *Communication disorders in multicultural populations.* Boston: Butterworth-Heineman.

Baum, H.M. (1998). Overview, definitions, and goals for ASHA's treatment outcomes and clinical trials activities (What difference do outcome data make to you?). *Language, Speech, and Hearing Services in Schools, 29,* 246–249.

Bettleheim, B., and Zelan, K. (1982). *On learning to read: The child's fascination with meaning.* New York: Vintage.

Biemiller, A. (1999). *Language and reading success.* Cambridge, MA: Brookline.

Biklin, D. (1992). *Schooling without labels: Parents, educators and inclusive education.* New York: Teachers College Press.

Biklin, D., and Cardinal, D.N. (Eds.). (1997). *Contested words, contested science: Unraveling the facilitated communication controversy.* New York: Teachers College Press.

Blackstone, S.W. (Ed.). (2000). AAC approaches for infants and toddlers. *Augmentative Communication News, 12*(6), 1–8.

Blackstone, S., and Pressman, H. (1996, August). *Treatment outcomes in AAC.* Presentation at the biennial convention of the International Society for Augmentative and Alternative Communication, Vancouver, British Columbia, Canada.

Bland, L.E. (1998, May). School speech and language services. *Language Learning and Education, 5,* 33–35.

Bland, L.E. (1999, October). Interview with Diane L. Eger on the implications of IDEA '97 and accountability. *Language Learning and Education, 6,* 8–10.

Blosser, J.L., and Kratcoski, A. (1997). PACs: A framework for determining appropriate service delivery options. *Language, Speech, and Hearing Services in Schools, 28,* 99–107.

Board of Education v. Rowley, 458 U.S. 176 (1982).

Bondy, A.S., and Frost, L.A. (1994). The picture exchange communication system. *Focus on Autistic Behavior, 9,* 1–19.

Boudreau, D.M., and Hedberg, N.L. (1999). A comparison of early literacy skills in children with specific language impairment and their typically developing peers. *American Journal of Speech Language Pathology, 8,* 249–260.

Brannen, S.J., Cooper, E.B., Dellegrotto, J.T., Disney, S.T., Eger, D.L., Ehren, B.J., Ganley, K.A., Isakson, C.W., Montgomery, J.K., Ralabate, P.K., Secord, W.A., and Whitmire, K.A. (2000). *Developing educationally relevant IEPs: A technical assistance document for speech-language pathologists.* Rockville, MD: American Speech-Language-Hearing Association.

Break down barriers between general and special education. (2000). *Inclusive Education Programs, 7*(1), 1, 9.

Brekken, L., Carr, A., and Cranor, L. (1988). *Team assessment in early childhood special education: A trainer's resource guide* (2nd ed.). Sacramento, CA: Resources in Special Education.

Brice, A. (1993). *Understanding the Cuban refugee.* San Diego, CA: Los Amigos Research Associates.

Brice, A.E. (2000). Which language for bilingual speakers? Factors to consider. *Communication Disorders and Sciences in Culturally Linguistically Diverse Populations, 6,* 1–7.

Brown v. Board of Education, 347 U.S. 483 (1954).

Bucaro, F.C. (2000). Professionalism and ethics: How do you spell success? *The Communication Connection, 14*(2), 1–2, 4.

Buekelman, D.R., and Miranda, P. (1998). *Augmentative and alternative communication: Management of severe communication disorders in children and adults.* (2nd ed.). Baltimore: Brookes.

Butler, K.G. (1997). Using dynamic approaches to support assessment and intervention: New approaches. In N.W. Nelson and B. Hoskins (Eds.), *Strategies for supporting classroom success: Focus on communication* [Cassette recording, audio-workshop] (Cassette No. 7, pp. 1–8). San Diego, CA: Singular.

Butler, K.G. (Ed.). (1999). Many voices, many tongues: Accents, dialects and variations. *Topics in Language Disorders, 19*(4), iv–v.

Calculator, S.N. (1999). Look who's pointing now: Cautions related to the clinical use of facilitated communication. *Language, Speech, and Hearing Services in Schools, 30,* 408–414.

California Department of Education. (1997). *Guidelines for language, academic, and special education services required for limited-English-proficient students in California public schools, K–12.* Sacramento, CA: Author.

California Department of Education. (1998). *English-language arts content standards for California public schools: Kindergarten through grade twelve.* Sacramento, CA: Author. .

California Department of Education. (1999a). *Best practices for designing and delivering effective programs for individuals with autism spectrum disorders.* Sacramento, CA: Author

California Department of Education. (1999b). *The California reading initiative and special education in California: Critical ideas to focus meaningful reform.* Sacramento, CA: Author.

California Department of Education. (1999c). *California special education programs: A composite of laws.* Sacramento, CA: Author.

California Department of Education. (1999d). *Reading / Language arts framework for California public schools: Kindergarten through grade twelve.* Sacramento, CA: Author.

California Department of Education. (1999e). *Special education rights of parents and children.* Sacramento, CA: Author.

California education code: 2000 desktop edition. (2000). Eagan, MN: West Group.

California Speech-Language-Hearing Association (CSHA). (1996). *Technical report on the utilization of speech aides in the public schools.* Sacramento, CA: Author.

Camarata, S.M. (1996). On the importance of integrating naturalistic language, social intervention, and speech-intelligibility training. In L.K. Koegel, R.L. Koegel, and G. Dunlop, *Positive behavioral support* (pp. 31–49). Baltimore: Brookes.

Campbell, D. (1999a). Focus on function in the schools. *Advance, 9*(51), 7–8.

Campbell, D. (1999b). Improving student outcomes. *Advance, 9*(35), 10–11.

Catts, H.W., and Kamhi, A.G. (1999). *Language and reading disabilities*. Boston: Allyn and Bacon.

Center for the Improvement of Early Reading Achievement (CIERA). (2001, January). *CIERA homepage*. Retrieved January 29, 2001, from the World Wide Web: http://www.ciera.org/ciera/publications/report-series/inquiry-2/2-002 ann.pdf

Center for Special Education Finance (CSEF). (1999a, September). *Frequently asked questions*. Retrieved January 29, 2001, from the World Wide Web: http://csef.air.org/faq1-3.html

Center for Special Education Finance (CSEF). (1999b, September). *Frequently asked questions*. Retrieved January 29, 2001, from the World Wide Web: http://csef.air.org/faq2-1.html

Centers for Disease Control (CDC). (1999). *Training manual for volunteer screening program of Special Olympics games*. Atlanta, GA: Author.

Cernosia, A. (1999, March). *Individuals with Disabilities Education Act–1997 reauthorization* [Handout]. Presentation at the Special Education Division, California Department of Education, Sacramento, CA.

Cetron, M.J., and Gayle, M.E. (1990, September-October). Educational renaissance: 43 trends for the U.S. schools. *The Futurist,* 33–40.

Chard, D.J. (1999). Case in point: Including students with disabilities in large-scale testing. *Journal of Special Education Leadership, 12*(2), 39–42.

Charlotte-Mecklenburg Schools, Exceptional Children Department. (2000). *Handbook for speech-language pathologists*. Charlotte, NC: Author.

Cheng, L-R.L. (1999a). Many voices, many tongues: Accents, dialects, and variations [Foreword]. *Topics in Language Disorders, 19*(4), vi–vii.

Cheng, L-R.L. (1999b). Moving beyond accent: Social and cultural realities of living with many tongues. *Topics in Language Disorders, 19*(4), 1–10.

Church, G., and Glennen, S. (1992). *The handbook of assistive technology*. San Diego, CA: Singular.

Cirrin, F.M. (1996, April). Discrepancy models: Implications for service in public schools. *Language Learning and Education, 3,*(1), 9–10.

Cirrin, F.M., and Penner, S.G. (1995). Classroom-based consultative service delivery models for language intervention. In. M.E. Fey, J. Windsor, and S.F. Warren (Eds.), Language intervention: Preschool through the elementary years (pp. 333–362). Baltimore: Brookes.

Code of Federal Regulations (C.F.R.). Assistance to states for the education of children with disabilities and the early intervention program for infants and toddlers with disabilities; Final regulations, C.F.R., Title 34, § 300, 301, and 303 (1999).

Cole, K.N., Dale, P.S., and Thal, D.J. (Eds.). (1998). *Assessment of communication and language.* Baltimore: Brookes.

Cole, L. (1983). Implications of the position on social dialects. *Asha, 25*(9), 25–27.

Collins, M., and Dowell, M.L. (1998). Discipline and due process. *Thrust for Educational Leadership, 28*(2), 34–36.

Connecticut Department of Education. (1993). *Guidelines for speech and language programs.* Hartford, CT: Author.

Contra Costa Special Education Local Plan Area (SELPA). (1998, November). *Outcome Measures* [Handout]. Presentation to state SELPA directors, Sacramento, CA.

Cook, L., Weintraub, F., and Morse, W. (1995). Ethical dilemmas in the restructuring of special education. In J.L. Paul, H. Rosselli, and D. Evans (Eds.), *Integrating school restructuring and special education reform* (pp. 119–139). Fort Worth, TX: Harcourt Brace.

Cooley, E. (1995). Special education: At the crossroads. *Policy Update, 4,* 1–2.

Cooper, K.J. (1999, December 3). '89 education summit's goals still unmet. *The Washington Post,* p. A2.

Council of Administrators of Special Education (CASE). (1999a). Guidelines for using benchmarks in the IEP process. *In CASE, 41*(2), 8–9.

Council of Administrators of Special Education (CASE). (1999b). *Section 504 and the ADA: Promoting student access.* (2nd ed.). Albuquerque, NM: Author.

Council for Exceptional Children (CEC). (1997a, September). CEC policy manual. Retrieved January 29, 2001, from the World Wide Web: http://www.cec.sped.org/pp/policies/ch3.htm

Council for Exceptional Children (CEC). (1997b). A history of special education. *Teaching Exceptional Children, 29*(5), 5–50.

Council for Exceptional Children (CEC). (1999). Special educators share their thoughts on special education teaching conditions. *CEC Today, 5*(9), 1–5.

Council of Language, Speech, and Hearing Consultants in State Education Agencies (CLSHCSEA). (1998). *Council of Language, Speech, and Hearing Consultants in State Education Agencies regular (active) members* [Membership list]. Charleston, WV: Author.

Council of Language, Speech, and Hearing Consultants in State Education Agencies (CLSHCSEA). (1999). *CLSHCSEA* [Brochure]. Charleston, WV: Author.

Crais, E.R. (2000). Ecologically valid communication assessment of infants and toddlers. In L.R. Watson, E. Crais, and T.L. Layton (Eds.), *Handbook of early language impairment in children: Assessment and treatment* (pp. 1–37). Albany, NY: Delmar.

Crawford, H. (1998). Applying outcomes. *Advance, 8*(35), 6–9.

Creaghead, N.A. (1992). *Classroom language intervention: Developing schema for school success.* Columbus, OH: Educom.

Creaghead, N.A. (1999). Evaluating language intervention approaches: Contrasting perspectives. *Language, Speech, and Hearing Services in Schools, 30,* 335–338.

Damico, J.S., Secord, W.A., and Wiig, E.H. (1992). Descriptive language assessment at school: Characteristics and design. *Best Practices in School Speech-Language Pathology, 2,* 1–8.

Danforth, S., Rhodes, W., and Smith, T. (1995). Inventing the future: Postmodern challenges in educational reform. In J.L. Paul, H. Rosselli, and D. Evans (Eds.), *Integrating school restructuring and special education reform* (pp. 214–236). Fort Worth, TX: Harcourt Brace.

Daniel R.R. v. State Board of Education, 874 F. 2d 1036 (5th Cir. 1989).

Deno, E. (1970). The cascade of special education services. *Exceptional Children, 39,* 495.

Deveres, L., and Pitasky, V. (1999a). *Student behavior: Intervention and prevention strategies that work.* Horsham, PA: LRP Publications.

Deveres, L., and Pitasky, V. (1999b). *Understanding student behavior: A guide to functional behavioral assessments.* Horsham, PA: LRP Publications.

Donahue, M.L., Syzmanski, C.M., and Flores, C.W. (1999). When Emily Dickinson met Steven Spielberg: Assessing social information processing in literacy contexts. *Language, Speech, and Hearing Services in Schools, 30,* 274–284.

Donahue-Kilburg, G. (1992). *Family-centered early intervention for communication disorders.* Gaithersburg, MD: Aspen.

Duchan, J.F. (1999). Views of facilitated communication: What's the point? *Language, Speech, and Hearing Services in Schools, 30,* 401–407.

Education for All Handicapped Children Act (EAHCA), 20 U.S.C. § 14000 *et seq.* (1975).

Education Amendments of 1974, 20 U.S.C. § 1703 (1974).

Education of the Handicapped Act (EHA), 20 U.S.C. § 1471 (1970).

Education of the Mentally Retarded Children Act, Pub. L. No. 85-926, § 2, 72 Stat. 1777 (1958).

Ehren, B.J. (2000). Maintaining a therapeutic focus and sharing responsibility for student success: Keys to in-classroom speech-language services. *Language, Speech, and Hearing Services in Schools, 31,* 219–229.

Elementary and Secondary Education Act (ESEA), 20 U.S.C. § 2701 *et seq.* (1965).

Enderby, P., and Emerson, J. (1995). *Does speech and language therapy work?* London: Whurr.

Erickson, K., and Koppenhaver, D. (1995). Developing a literacy program for children with severe disabilities. *Reading Teacher, 48,* 676–684.

Evans, D., and Panacek-Howell, L. (1995). Restructuring education: National reform in regular education. In J.L. Paul, H. Rosselli, and D. Evans (Eds.), *Integrating school restructuring and special education reform* (pp. 30–42). Fort Worth, TX: Harcourt Brace.

Family Educational Rights and Privacy Act (FERPA), 20 U.S.C. § 1232g (1974).

Federal Interagency Forum on Child and Family Statistics. (1999). *America's children: Key national indicators of well-being.* Washington, DC: U.S. Government Printing Office.

Ferguson, M.L. (1991). Collaborative consultative service delivery: An introduction. *Language, Speech, and Hearing Services in Schools, 22,* 147.

Ferguson, M.L. (1992). The transition to collaborative teaching. *Language, Speech, and Hearing Services in Schools, 23,* 371–372.

Ferguson, M.L. (1994–1995). Surviving the changing schools: A call for treatment efficacy research. *Tejas, XX*(2), 7–9.

Fey, M.E. (1996, April). Cognitive referencing in the study of children with language impairments. *Language Learning and Education, 3,* 7–8.

Fey, M. (1999, Winter). Speech-language pathology and the early identification and prevention of reading disabilities. *Perspectives,* 13–17.

Fisher, R., Ury, W., and Patton, B. (1991). *Getting to yes: Negotiating agreement without giving in* (2nd ed.). New York: Penguin.

Florida Department of Education, Bureau of Instructional Support and Community Services. (1995). *A training resource manual for the implementation of state eligibility criteria for the speech and language impaired.* Tallahassee, FL: Author.

Florida Department of Education, Bureau of Instructional Support and Community Services. (1997). *A training and resource manual for the implementation of state eligibility criteria for the speech and language impaired* [Addendum]. Tallahassee, FL: Author.

Folkins, J. (1999, November). *The language used to describe individuals with disabilities.* Rockville, MD: American Speech-Language-Hearing Association. Retrieved February 3, 2001, from the World Wide Web: http://www.asha.org/publications/folkins.htm

Fullan, M. (1995). *Change forces.* Bristol, PA: Falmer Press.

Fung, F., and Roseberry-McKibbon, C. (1999). Service delivery considerations in working with clients from Cantonese speaking backgrounds. *American Journal of Speech-Language Pathology, 8,* 309–318.

Gajewski, N., Hirn, P., and Mayo, P. (1998). *Social skill strategies.* Eau Claire, WI: Thinking Publications.

Garcia, S.B., and Ortiz, A.A. (1988). *Preventing inappropriate referrals of language minority students to special education* (New Focus Series No. 5). Wheaton, MD: National Clearinghouse for Bilingual Education.

Gartner, A., and Lipsky, D.K. (1987). Beyond special education: Toward a quality system for all students. *Harvard Educational Review, 57,* 367–395.

German, D. (1992). Word-finding intervention for children and adolescents. *Topics in Language Disorders, 13*(1), 33–50.

Gillam, R.B. (1999a). Computer-assisted language intervention using Fast ForWord: Theoretical and empirical considerations for clinical decision-making. *Language, Speech, and Hearing Services in Schools, 30,* 363–370.

Gillam, R.B. (1999b, May). Phonological awareness after the primary grades. *Language Learning and Education, 6*(1), 20–21.

Gillon, G.T. (2000). The efficacy of phonological awareness intervention for children with spoken language impairment. *Language, Speech, and Hearing Services in Schools, 31,* 126–141.

Gilyard, K. (1999, March). *Student suspension and expulsion.* Presentation of the law firm of Atkinson, Andleson, Loya, Ruud, and Romo, Ontario, CA.

Glennen, S. (2000, January). AAC: An historical perspective. Presentation at the ASHA Division 12 Leadership in AAC institute, Sea Island, GA.

Goals 2000: Educate America Act, H.R. 1804, 103d Cong., 2d Sess. (1994).

Goldberg, B. (1996). Imagining tomorrow: What's ahead for our professions. *Asha, 38,* 22–28.

Goldsworthy, C.L. (1996). *Developmental reading disabilities: A language-based treatment approach.* San Diego, CA: Singular.

Goldsworthy, C.L. (1998). *Sourcebook of phonological awareness activities.* San Diego, CA: Singular.

Goodlad, J.I. (1984). *A place called school.* New York: McGraw-Hill.

Gorn, S. (1997a). *The answer book on individualized education programs.* Horsham, PA: LRP Publications.

Gorn, S. (1997b). *The answer book on special education law* (2nd ed.). Horsham, PA: LRP Publications.

Goss v. Lopez, 419 U.S. 565 (1975).

Graham, S., and Harris, S.R. (1999). Assessment and intervention in overcoming writing difficulties: An illustration from the self regulated strategy development model. *Language, Speech, and Hearing Services in Schools, 30,* 255–264.

Greenspan, S.I. (1992). *Infancy and early childhood: The practice of clinical assessment and intervention with emotional and developmental challenges.* Madison, CT: International Universities Press.

Greenspan, S.I., and Wieder, S. (1999). A functional developmental approach to autism spectrum disorders. *Journal of the Association for Persons with Severe Handicaps, 24,* 147–161.

Griffer, M.R. (1999). Is sensory integration effective for children with language-learning disorders?: A critical review of the evidence. *Language, Speech, and Hearing Services in Schools, 30,* 393–400.

Grimes, A.M. (1997). Audiology treatment outcomes. *CSHA Magazine, 26*(2), 10–11.

Guarneri, G., Carr, A., and Brekken, L. (1988). *Team assessment in early childhood and special education* (2nd ed.). Sacramento, CA: California Department of Education.

Gutierrez-Clellen, V.F. (1999). Language choice in intervention with bilingual children. *American Journal of Speech-Language Pathology, 8,* 291–302.

Hall, G.E., and Hord, S.M. (1987). *Change in schools: Facilitating the process.* Albany, NY: State University of New York Press.

Handicapped Children's Protection Act/Attorneys' Fees Bill, 20 U.S.C. § 1400 (1986).

Hanson, M. (1984). *Atypical infant development.* Baltimore: University Park Press.

Hardman, M.L., Drew, C.J., and Egan, M.W. (1999). *Human exceptionality: Society, school, and family* (6th ed.). Boston: Allyn and Bacon.

Harris, D.M., and Evans, D.W. (1994). Integrating school restructuring and special education reform. *Case in Point, 8*(12), 7–19.

Hart, B., and Risley, T.R. (1995). *Meaningful differences in the everyday experience of young American children.* Baltimore: Brookes.

Haywood, H.C., Brown, A.L., and Wingenfeld, S. (1990). Dynamic approaches to psycho-educational assessment. *School Psychology Review, 19,* 411–422.

Hehir, T.F. (1999). The changing roles of special education leadership in the next millennium: Thoughts and reflections. *Journal of Special Education Leadership, 12*(1), 3–8.

Helfand, D. (2000, July 2). Boldly going beyond the printed page. *Los Angeles Times,* p. B6.

Hendricks, C., Swenson, C., and Huffman, C.L. (2000). *Speech and language eligibility criteria.* Merced, CA: Merced County Office of Education.

Herer, G.R. (1989). Communication: The key to education. In American Speech-Language-Hearing Association (ASHA), *Partnerships in education: Toward a literate America* (No. 17, pp. 1–3) [ASHA Reports]. Rockville MD: ASHA.

Herer, G.R., and Glattke, T.J. (2000, November 16). Making newborn hearing screening a reality. Presentation at the annual convention of the American Speech-Language-Hearing Association, Washington, DC.

Hocutt, A., and McKinney, D. (1995). Moving beyond the regular education initiative: National reform in special education. In J.L. Paul, H. Rosselli, and D. Evans (Eds.), *Integrating school restructuring and special education reform* (pp. 43–62). Fort Worth, TX: Harcourt Brace.

Homer, E.M. (2000a). Dysphagia. In E. Pritchard Dodge (Ed.), *The survival guide for school-based speech-language pathologists* (pp. 399–421). San Diego, CA: Singular.

Homer, E.M. (2000b). Scheduling and collaborative planning. In E. Pritchard Dodge (Ed.), *The survival guide for school-based speech-language pathologists* (pp. 1–56). San Diego, CA: Singular.

Homer, E.M., Bickerton, C., Hill, S., Parham, L., and Taylor, D. (2000). Development of an interdisciplinary dysphagia team in the public schools. *Language, Speech, and Hearing Services in Schools, 31,* 62–75.

Honig v. Doe, 484 U.S., 305 (1988).

Hoskins, B. (1990). Collaborative consultation: Designing the role of the speech-language pathologist in a new educational context. *Best Practices in School Speech-Language Pathology, 1,* 29–36.

Hoskins, B. (1995). *Developing inclusive schools.* Bloomington, IN: Indiana University, Smith Research Center.

Hoskins, B. (1997). *Conversations.* Eau Claire, WI: Thinking Publications.

How to address the shortage of speech and language pathologists. (1999). *The Special Educator, 14*(3), 1–10.

Idol-Maestas, L., Paolucci-Whitcomb, P., and Levin, A. (1986). *Collaborative consultation.* Austin, TX: Pro-Ed.

Illinois State Board of Education, Blackhawk Area Special Education District. (1993). *Speech language impairment: A technical assistance manual.* Springfield, IL: Author.

Indiana Speech-Language-Hearing Association (ISHA). (1997). *Indiana's overview of good practice in schools.* Noblesville, IN: Author.

Individuals with Disabilities Education Act (IDEA), 20 U.S.C. § 1400 *et seq.* (1990).

429

Individuals with Disabilities Education Act (IDEA) Amendments, 20 U.S.C. § 1400 *et seq.* (1997).

Interdisciplinary Council on Developmental and Learning Disorders (ICDL). (2000). *ICDL Clinical practice guidelines: Redefining the standards of care for infants, children, and families with special needs.* Bethesda, MD: ICDL Press.

Issakson, C. (2000). Working through the complexities of cognitive referencing: Connecticut's eligibility criteria. *Language Learning and Education, 7*(1), 21–25.

Johnson, D.W., and Johnson, R.T. (1989). *Cooperation and competition: Theory and research.* Edina, MN: Interaction Books.

Johnson, W., Brown, S.F., Curtis, J.F., Edney, C.W., and Keaster, J. (1956). *Speech handicapped school children.* New York: Harper and Row.

Kagan, S. (1994). *Cooperative learning.* San Clemente, CA: Kagan.

Kamhi, A. (1991). Treatment efficacy: An introduction. *Language, Speech, and Hearing Services in Schools, 22,* 254.

Kari H. v. Franklin Special School District, 23 IDELR 538 (6th Cir. 1995).

Kauffman, J.M., and Hallahan, D.P. (Eds.). (1995). *The illusion of full inclusion: A comprehensive critique of a current special education bandwagon.* Austin, TX: Pro-Ed.

Kavale, K., and Reese, B., (1992). The characteristics of learning disabilities: An Iowa profile. *Learning Disabilities Quarterly, 15*(2), 74–94.

Kendall, J.S., and Marzano, R.J. (1996). *Content knowledge: A compendium of standards and benchmarks for K–12 education.* Aurora, CO: Mid-Continent Regional Educational Laboratory.

Kentucky Department of Education, Division of Exceptional Children's Services. (1993). *Kentucky eligibility guidelines for communication disabilities.* Frankfort, KY: Author.

Kist, W. (2000). Beginning to create the new literacy classroom: What does the new literacy look like? *Journal of Adolescent and Adult Literacy, 43,* 710–718.

Kliewer, C., and Landis, D. (1999). Individualizing literacy instruction for young children with moderate to severe disabilities. *Exceptional Children, 66*(1), 85–100.

Koegel, R.L., Schreibman, L., Good, A., Cerniglia, L., Murphy, C., and Koegel, L. (1989). How to teach pivotal behaviors to children with autism: A training manual. Santa Barbara, CA: University of California.

Koppenhaver, D.A., and Yoder, D.E. (1993). Classroom literacy instruction for children with severe speech and physical impairments (SSPI): What is and what might be. *Topics in Language Disorders, 13*(2), 1–15.

Krassowski, E., and Plante, E. (1997). IQ variability in children with SLI: Implications for use of cognitive referencing in determining SLI. *Journal of Communication Disorders, 30*(1), 1–9.

Kubicek, F.C. (1994). Special education reform in light of select state and federal court decisions. *The Journal of Special Education, 28*(1), 27–42.

Kurjan, R.M. (2000). The role of the school-based speech-language pathologist serving preschool children with dysphagia: A personal perspective.

Language, Speech, and Hearing Services in Schools, 31(1), 42–49.

Langdon, H. (1999). Collaborating with oral language interpreters and translators. *CSHA Magazine, 28*(2), 10–11.

Langdon, H.W. (2000). Diversity. In E. Pritchard Dodge (Ed.), *The survival guide for school-based speech-language pathologists* (pp. 367–397). San Diego, CA: Singular.

Langdon, H.W., and Cheng, L. (in press). *Working successfully with interpreters and translators in speech-language pathology and audiology.* Eau Claire, WI: Thinking Publications.

Langdon, H.W., and Saenz, T.I. (1996). *Language assessment and intervention with multicultural students: A guide for speech-language-hearing professionals.* Oceanside, CA: Academic Communication Associates.

Larson, V. Lord, and McKinley, N.L. (1987). *Communication assessment and intervention: Strategies for adolescents.* Eau Claire, WI: Thinking Publications.

Larson, V. Lord, and McKinley, N.L. (1995a). Characteristics of adolescents' conversations: A longitudinal study. *Clinical Linguistics and Phonetics, 12*, 183–203.

Larson, V. Lord, and McKinley, N. (1995b). *Language disorders in older students: Preadolescents and adolescents.* Eau Claire, WI: Thinking Publications.

Larson, V.L., McKinley, N.L., and Boley, D. (1993). Service delivery models for adolescents with language disorders. *Language, Speech, and Hearing Services in Schools, 24*, 36–42.

Learning Disabilities Association of America (LDA). (1993). Inclusion: Position paper of the Learning Disabilities Association of America. Retrieved January 30, 2001, from the World Wide Web: http://www.ldanatl.org/positions/inclusion.shtml

Lewis, M. (1984). Developmental principles and their implications for at-risk and handicapped infants. In M. Hanson (Ed.), *Atypical infant development* (pp. 143–158). Baltimore: University Park Press.

Lidz, C.S. (1991). *Practitioner's guide to dynamic assessment.* New York: Guilford Press.

Lieberman, G. (1995/96, Fall/Winter). Accountability for all students: A report of the NASDSE Accountability Focus Group. *Case in Point, 9*(2), 46–50.

Lipsky, D.K., and Gartner, A. (1996). Inclusion, school restructuring, and the remaking of American society. *Harvard Educational Review, 66*, 762–796.

Lombardi, T.P., and Ludlow, B.L. (1996). *Trends shaping the future of special education.* Bloomington, IN: Phi Delta Kappa Educational Foundation.

Lord, C., Bristol, M.M., and Scholper, E. (1993). Early interaction for children with autism and related developmental disabilities. In E. Schopler, M. Van Bourgondien, and M. Bristol (Eds.), *Preschool issues in autism* (pp. 111–129). New York: Plenum Press.

Lovaas, O.J. (1996). The UCLA young autism model of service delivery. In C. Maurice, G. Green, and S. Luce (Eds.), *Behavioral intervention for young children with autism* (pp. 241–348). Austin, TX: Pro-Ed.

Lowe, R.J. (Ed.). (1993). *Speech-language pathology and related professions in the schools*. Boston: Allyn and Bacon.

Luke, A., and Elkins, J. (2000a). Redefining adolescent literacies. *Journal of Adolescent and Adult Literacy, 43*, 212–215.

Luke, A., and Elkins, J. (2000b). Re/mediating adolescent literacies [Special themed issue]. *Journal of Adolescent and Adult Literacy, 43*, 396–398.

Lyon, G.R. (1998). *Overview of reading and literacy initiatives*. Testimony provided to the Committee on Labor and Human Resources, United States Senate. Bethesda, MD: National Institute of Child Health and Human Development.

Madell, J.R. (1999). Auditory integration training: One clinician's view. *Language, Speech, and Hearing Services in Schools, 30*, 371–377.

Maloney, M.H. (1997). *The seven deadly sins: Common mistakes that lead to due process hearings* [Video]. Horsham, PA: LRP Publications.

Maloney, M.H., and Pitasky, V.M. (1996). *The special educator 1996 desk book*. Horsham, PA: LRP Publications.

Martin, E.W., Martin, R., and Terman, D.L. (1996). The legislative and litigation history of special education. *The Future of Children: Special Education for Students with Disabilities, 6*(1), 25–39.

Martin, R., and Weatherly, C. (1996, November). *The 1996 fall regional institutes on special education law*. Presentation of LRP Publications, San Francisco, CA.

Marvin, C. (1994). Home literacy experiences of preschool children with single and multiple disabilities. *Topics in Early Childhood Special Education, 14*, 436–454.

Marzano, R.J. (2000). 20th century advances in instruction. In R.S. Brandt (Ed.), *Education in a new era* (pp. 67–95). Alexandria, VA: Association for Supervision and Curriculum Development.

Mastropieri, M.A., and Scruggs, T.E. (2000). *The inclusive classroom*. Upper Saddle River, NJ: Merrill.

Mauer, D.M. (1999). Issues and applications of sensory integration theory and treatment with children with language disorders. *Language, Speech, and Hearing Services in Schools, 30*, 383–392.

Maugh, T.H. (2000, May 4). Test identifies newborns likely to develop autism. *Los Angeles Times*, p. 4.

McDonnell, L.M., McLaughlin, M.J., and Morison, P. (Eds.). (1997). *Educating one and all: Students with disabilities and standards-based reform*. Washington, DC: National Academy Press.

McEllistrem, S., Roth, J.A., and Cox, G. (1998). *Students with disabilities and special education*. Rosemount, MN: Data Research.

McGill-Franzen, A., and Allington, R.L. (1993). Flunk 'em or get them classified: The contamination of primary grade accountability data. *Educational Researcher, 22*(1), 19–22.

McGregor, G., and Vogelsberg, R.T. (1998). *Inclusive schooling practices: Pedagogical and research foundations*. Baltimore: Brookes.

McGrew, K.S., Thurlow, M.L., Shriner, J.G., and Spiegel, A.N. (1992). *Inclusion of students with disabilities in national and state data collection programs* (Technical Report No. 2). Minneapolis, MN: National Center on Educational Outcomes.

McLaughlin, M.J. (1999). Access to the general education curriculum: Paperwork and procedure or redefining "special education." *Journal of Special Education Leadership, 12*(1), 9–14.

McLaughlin, M.J., Nolet, V., Morando Rhim, L., and Henderson, K. (1999). Integrating standards: Including all students. *Teaching Exceptional Children, 31*(3), 66–71.

McWhirt by McWhirt v. Williamson County School, 23 IDELR 509 (6th Cir. 1994).

Menyuk, P. (1999). *Reading and linguistic development.* Cambridge, MA: Brookline Books.

Merced County Office of Education. (1998). *Speech and language eligibility criteria.* Merced, CA: Author.

Merritt, D.D., and Culatta, B. (1998). *Language intervention in the classroom.* San Diego, CA: Singular.

Miller, L. (1989). Classroom based language intervention. *Language, Speech, and Hearing Services in Schools, 20,* 153–169.

Miller, L. (1999). *What we call smart: A new narrative for intelligence and learning.* San Diego, CA: Singular.

Mills v. D.C. Board of Education, 348 F. Supp. 866 (D.D.C. 1972).

Moje, E.B., Young, J.P., Readence, J.E., and Moore, D.W. (2000). Reinventing adolescent literacy for new times: Perennial and millennial issues. *Journal of Adolescent and Adult Literacy, 43,* 400–409.

Montgomery, J.K. (1990). Building administrative support for collaboration. *Best Practices in School Speech-Language Pathology, 1,* 1, 75–79.

Montgomery, J.K. (1992). Clinical forum: Implementing collaborative consultation: Perspectives from the field. *Language, Speech, and Hearing Services in Schools, 23,* 363–364.

Montgomery, J.K. (1993a). The law and the school professional. In R.J. Lowe (Ed.), *Speech-language pathology and related professions in the schools* (pp. 67–85). Boston: Allyn and Bacon.

Montgomery, J.K. (1993b). Writing shared goals for special education services. *Curriculum and Instruction Update, Fountain Valley School District, 2*(1), 22–24.

Montgomery, J.K. (1994a). Federal legislation affecting school settings. In R. Lubinski and C. Frattali (Eds.), *Professional issues in speech-language pathology and audiology* (pp. 201–217). San Diego, CA: Singular.

Montgomery, J.K. (1994b). Service delivery issues for schools. In R. Lubinski and C. Frattali (Eds.), *Professional issues in speech-language pathology and audiology* (pp. 218–231). San Diego, CA: Singular.

Montgomery, J.K. (1995, November). *President's address: Plenary session.* Presentation at the American Speech-Language-Hearing Association Annual Convention, Orlando, FL.

Montgomery, J.K. (1997a). Inclusion in the secondary school. In L. Power-de-Fur and F.P. Orelove (Eds.), *Inclusive education* (pp. 181–192). Gaithersburg, MD: Aspen Publications.

Montgomery, J.K. (1997b). Using functional outcomes in the schools. *CSHA Magazine, 26*(2), 7–8.

Montgomery, J.K. (1998). Reading and the SLP: Using discourse, narratives and expository text. *CSHA Magazine, 27*(3), 8–9.

Montgomery, J.K. (1999a). Accents and dialects: Creating a national professional statement. *Topics in Language Disorders, 19,* 78–89.

Montgomery, J.K. (1999b). Treatment outcomes and reimbursement: Aren't they related? *Communication Connection, Wisconsin Speech-Language-Hearing Association, 13*(1), 1–3.

Montgomery, J.K. (2000a, June). The Golden SLPA Project: *Training culturally competent speech-language pathology assistants in a community college* [Handout]. Presentation at 5th Biannual Head Start Research Conference, Washington, DC.

Montgomery, J.K. (2000b, April). *Inclusive practices in the middle school.* Presentation at Hewes Middle School, Tustin Unified School District, Tustin, CA.

Montgomery, J.K., and Bonderman, I.R. (1989). Serving preschool children with severe phonological disorders. *Language, Speech, and Hearing Services in Schools, 20,* 76–84.

Montgomery, J.K., and Herer, G.R. (1994). Future watch: Our schools in the 21st century. *Language, Speech, and Hearing Services in Schools, 25,* 130–135.

Moore-Brown, B. (1992). Writing meaningful IEPs. *Clinically Speaking, 9*(2), 1–2.

Moore-Brown, B. (1998). *Individualized education programs and standards.* Unpublished doctoral dissertation, University of Southern California, Los Angeles.

Moore-Brown, B. (1999a, April). *Multicultural issues for the professions.* Presentation at the Fourth Annual Communication Disorders Multicultural Conference of the National Student Speech-Language-Hearing Association, Fullerton, CA.

Moore-Brown, B. (1999b, April). *President's address: Plenary session.* Presentation at the California Speech-Language-Hearing Association Annual State Conference, Pasadena, CA.

Moore-Brown, B. (1999c, July). *Skills and competencies needed by the school-based speech-language pathologist in the 21st century: Implications of educational trends.* Presentation at the American Speech-Language-Hearing Association Council on Professional Standards in Speech-Language Pathology and Audiology, Rockville, MD.

Moore-Brown, B. (2000, March). *Skills and competencies needed by the school-based speech-language pathologist in the 21st century: Implications of educational trends.* Presentation at the Speech-Language Pathologists of Area Education Agency 6, Marshalltown, IA.

Moore-Brown, B., Cooper, C., and Ferguson, M. (1998). When supervisor and supervisee disagree. *Asha 40*(2), 56, 42.

Moore-Brown, B., and Montgomery, J. (1999). [Survey of Council of State Association Presidents]. Unpublished raw data.

Moore-Brown, B., Montgomery, J., Biehl, L., Karr, S., and Stein, M. (1998, November). *Accountability, outcomes and functional goals: Part II.* Presentation at the American Speech-Language-Hearing Association Annual Convention, San Antonio, TX.

Moore-Brown, B., Robinson, T.L., Williams, R., Claussen, R., and Martinez, S. (1998). *Using speech-language pathology assistants in the schools: What's going on?* Presentation at the ASHA Teleseminar, Rockville, MD.

Mulkerne, S.M. (1992). Emerging at-risk populations: Implication for special education reform. *Preventing School Failure, 36*(4), 20–23.

Mullen, R. (2000). Data report available for K–6 schools component of NOMS. *ASHA Special Interest Division 16* [Newsletter], *1*(3), 18.

Myers, R., and Sobehart, H. (1995). Creating a unified system—The road less traveled. *Case in Point, 9*(1), 1–9.

National Association of State Boards of Education (NASBE). (1999). *NASBE state profiles.* Retrieved January 30, 2001, from the World Wide Web: http://www.nasbe.org/edprofiles.html

National Association of Year Round Education (NAYRE). (2001). Retrieved February 8, 2001, from the World Wide Web: http://www.nayre.org/about.html

National Center for Learning Disabilities (NCLD). (1994). *Statement on inclusion.* New York: Author.

National Commission on Excellence in Education. (1983). *A nation at risk: The imperative for educational reform.* Washington, DC: U.S. Government Printing Office.

National Council on Disability (NCD). (1993). *Serving the nation's students with disabilities: Progress and prospects* [Report]. Washington, DC: Author.

National Education Goals Panel (NEGP). (1999). *Complete information for all goals.* Retrieved January 30, 2001, from the World Wide Web: http://www.negp.gov/page3-1.htm

National Joint Committee on Learning Disabilities (NJCLD). (2001). A reaction to full inclusion: A reaffirmation of the right of students with learning disabilities to a continuum of services. In NJCLD, *Collective perspectives on issues affecting learning disabilities: Position papers and statements* (pp. 123–125). Austin, TX: Pro-Ed.

National Literacy Act of 1991, 20 U.S.C. § 1203 *et seq.* (1991).

Neidecker, E.A. (1987). *School programs in speech-language: Organization and management* (2nd ed.). Englewood Cliffs, NJ: Prentice Hall.

Neidecker, E., and Blosser, J. (1993). *School programs in speech-language: Organization and management.* Needham, MA: Allyn and Bacon.

Nelson, N.W. (1990). Only relevant practices can be best. *Best Practices in School Speech-Language Pathology, 1,* 15–28.

Nelson, N.W. (1992). Targets of curriculum-based language assessment. In W. Secord and J. Damico (Eds.), *Best practices in school speech-language pathology: Descriptive nonstandardized language assessment* (pp. 73–85). San Antonio, TX: Psychological Corporation.

Nelson, N. (1996, April). Discrepancy models and the discrepancy between policy and evidence: Are we asking the wrong questions? *Language Learning and Education, 3,* 3–5.

Nelson, N. (1999, February). *Building language and making connections: Opportunities of a computer supported writing lab.* Presentation at the 8th Annual Symposium on Disabilities and Literacy, Chapel Hill, NC.

Nelson, N., Cheng, L., Shulman, B., and Westby, C. (1994, November). Factors influencing speech language eligibility and service. *Language Learning and Education, 1,* 8–13.

Nelson, N.W., and Hoskins, B. (1997). *Strategies for supporting classroom success* [Audiotape set]. San Diego, CA: Singular.

Neubert, D.A. (1997). Time to grow. *Teaching Exceptional Children, 29*(5), 5–17.

Neuman, S.B., Smagorinsky, P., Enciso, P.E., Baldwin, R.S., and Hartman, D.K. (2000). Snippets: What will be the influences on literacy in the next millennium? *Reading Research Quarterly, 35,* 276–282.

New Jersey Department of Education. (1999). *Parental rights in special education.* Retrieved January 30, 2001, from the World Wide Web: http://www.state .nj.us/njded/parights/prise_b_w.pdf

North Carolina Department of Public Instruction, Division of Exceptional Children. (1985). North Carolina public school guidelines for speech-language programs. Raleigh, NC: Author.

North Carolina State Board of Education (2000) Procedures governing programs and services for children with disabilities [Microsoft Word format]. Raleigh, NC: Author. Retrieved January 29, 2001, from the World Wide Web: http://www.dpi.state.nc .us/ec/procedures.htm

Nye, C., and Montgomery, J.K. (1989). Identification criteria for language disordered children: A national survey. *Hearsay, 4,* 26–33.

Oberti v. Board of Education of Borough of Clementon School District, 995 F. 2d 1204 (3d Cir. 1993).

O'Connell, P.F. (1997). *Speech, language, and hearing programs in schools: A guide for students and practitioners.* Gaithersburg, MD: Aspen Publications.

O'Donnell, D.G. (1999). *A guide for understanding and developing IEPs.* Madison, WI: Wisconsin Department of Public Instruction.

Office for Civil Rights (OCR). (1999). *Section 504 and education.* Retrieved January 30, 2001, from the World Wide Web: http://www.ed.gov/offices/OCR /regs/34cfr104.html

Office of Special Education and Rehabilitative Services (OSERS). (1999, March). *IDEA '97.* Retrieved January 30, 2001, from the World Wide Web: http://www.ed.gov/offices/OSERS/IDEA/IDEA.pdf

Ohanian, S. (2000). Goals 2000: What's in a name? *Phi Delta Kappan, 81,* 344–355.

Ohio Department of Education. (1991). *Ohio handbook for identification, evaluation, and placement of children with language problems.* Columbus, OH: Author.

Orkwis, R., and McLane, K. (1998). *A curriculum every student can use: Design principles for student access* (ERIC/OSEP Topical Brief). Reston, VA: Council for Exceptional Children.

Ortiz, A.A., Garcia, S.B., 1988). A prereferral process for preventing inappropriate referrals of Hispanic students to special education. In A. Ortiz and B.A. Ramirez (Eds.), *Schools and the culturally diverse exceptional student: Promising practices and future directions* (pp. 27–31). Reston, VA: Council for Exceptional Children.

Osborne, A.G., Jr. (1988). *Complete legal guide to special education services: A handbook for administrators, counselors, and supervisors.* West Nyack, NY: Parker.

Osborne, A.G., Jr. (1992). Legal standards for an appropriate education in the post-Rowley era. *Exceptional Children, 54,* 488–493.

Osborne, A.G., Jr., and DiMattia, P. (1995). IDEA's LRE mandate: Another look. *Exceptional Children, 61,* 582–584.

O'Shea, D., and O'Shea, L.J. (1997). Collaboration and school reform: A twenty-first-century perspective. *Journal of Learning Disabilities, 30,* 449–462.

O'Toole, T.J. (2000). Legal, ethical, and financial aspects of providing services to children with swallowing disorders in the public schools. *Language, Speech, and Hearing Services in Schools, 31,* 56–61.

Palacio, M. (2000). Distinct, not deficient: Structured teaching for children with autism. *Advance, 10*(1), 8–9.

Parent Advocacy Coalition for Educational Rights (PACER) Center. (1989). *It's the "person first"— Then the disability.* (Document PHP-c31). Minneapolis, MN: Author.

Parrish, T.B., and Chambers, J.G. (1996). Financing special education: The future of children. *Special Education for Students with Disabilities, 6,* 121–138.

Paul, J.L., and Evans, D. (1995). The national context of reform in general and special education: Reshaping the agenda [Introduction: Part I]. In J.L. Paul, H. Rosselli, and D. Evans (Eds.), *Integrating school restructuring and special education reform* (pp. 1–8). Fort Worth, TX: Harcourt Brace.

Paul, J.L., and Rosselli, H. (1995). Integrating the parallel reforms in general and special education. In J.L. Paul, H. Rosselli, and D. Evans (Eds.), *Integrating school restructuring and special education reform* (pp. 188–213). Fort Worth, TX: Harcourt Brace.

Paul, J.L., Yang, A., Adiegbola, M., and Morse, W. (1995). Rethinking the mission and methods: Philosophies for educating children and the teachers who teach them. In J.L. Paul, H. Rossellini, and D. Evans (Eds.), *Integrating school restructuring and special education reform* (pp. 9–29). Forth Worth, TX: Harcourt Brace.

Paul-Brown, D., and Caperton, C.J. (in press). Treatment settings and service delivery models for children with communication disorders in the context of early childhood inclusion. In M.J. Guralnick (Ed.), *Early childhood inclusion: Focus on change.* Baltimore: Brookes.

Pena, E. (1996). Dynamic assessment: The model and its language applications. In K.N. Cole, P.S. Dale, and D.J. Thal (Eds.), *Assessment of communication and language* (pp. 281–307). Baltimore: Brookes.

Pena, E. (2000). Measurement of modifiability in children from culturally linguistically diverse backgrounds. *Communication Disorders Quarterly, 21*(3) 87–97.

Pena, E., and Gillam, R. (in press). Dynamic assessment of children referred for speech and language evaluations. In C.S. Lidz (Ed.), *Dynamic assessment: Prevailing models and applications.* New York: JAI.

Pena, E., Miller, L., and Gillam, R. (1999). Dynamic assessment of narrative ability. *CSHA Magazine, 28*(2), 12–18.

Pena, E., Quinn, R., and Iglesias, A. (1992). The application of dynamic methods to language assessment: A nonbiased procedure. *The Journal of Special Education, 26,* 269–280.

437

Pennsylvania Association for Retarded Citizens (PARC) v. Commonwealth of Pennsylvania, 334 F. Supp. 1257, 343 F. Supp. 279 (E.D.Pa. 1971).

Pennsylvania Department of Education (1999). EISC—Interpreting the educational imperative [Online]. Available: http://www.pde.psu.edu /bbpages_reference /40005/40005100.html

Peters-Johnson, C. (1998). Action: School services, survey of speech-language pathology services in school-based settings national study final report. *Language, Speech, and Hearing Services in Schools, 29,* 120–126.

Pickett, J.P. (2000). Due process. In *The American Heritage Dictionary* (4th ed., p. 553). Boston: Houghton Mifflin.

Picus, L.O., and Wattenbarger, J.L. (1996). *Where does the money go? Resource allocation in elementary and secondary schools.* Thousand Oaks, CA: Corwin Press.

Polmanteer, K., and Turbiville, V. (2000). Family responsive individualized family service plans for speech-language pathologists. *Language, Speech, and Hearing Services in Schools, 31(1),* 4–14.

Poolaw v. Bishop, 67 F. 3d 830 (9th Cir. 1995).

Power-deFur, L., and Orelove, F.P. (Eds.). (1997). *Inclusive education: Practical implementation of the least restrictive environment.* Gaithersburg, MD: Aspen.

Prelock, P.A. (2000). Multiple perspectives for determining the roles of speech-language pathologists in inclusionary classrooms. *Language, Speech, and Hearing Services in Schools, 31,* 213–218.

Preschool Amendments to the Education of the Handicapped Act 20 U.S.C. § 1471 *et seq.* (1986).

Price, B.J., Mayfield, P.K., McFadden, A.C., and Marsh, G.E. (2000). *Collaborative teaching: Special education for inclusive classrooms.* Retrieved January 30, 2001, from the World Wide Web: http://www/parrotpublishing.com

Pritchard Dodge, E. (1994). *Communication lab.* East Moline, IL: LinguiSystems.

Pritchard Dodge, E. (Ed.). (2000). *The survival guide for school-based speech-language pathologists.* San Diego, CA: Singular.

Putnam, J.W., Spiegel, A.N., and Bruininks, R.H. (1995). Future directions in education and inclusion of students with disabilities: A Delphi investigation. *Exceptional Children, 61,* 553–577.

Quinn, R., Goldstein, B., and Pena, E.D. (1996). Cultural linguistic variation in the United States and its implications for assessment and intervention in speech-language pathology: An introduction. *Language, Speech, and Hearing Services in Schools, 27,* 345–346.

Raber, S., Roach, V., and Fraser, K. (Eds.). (1998). *The push and pull of standards-based reform.* Alexandria, VA: Center for Policy Research on the Impact of General and Special Education Reform.

Raskind, M. (2000). Assistive technology for children with learning difficulties [Booklet]. San Mateo, CA: Schwab Foundation for Learning.

Rehabilitation Act Amendments of 1992, Pub. L. No. 102-569, § 508, 106 Stat. 4430 (1992).

Retherford, K.S. (1996). Normal communication acquisition: An animated database of behaviors [Computer software]. Eau Claire, WI: Thinking Publications.

Ripich, D.N., and Creaghead, N.A. (1994). *School discourse problems* (2nd ed.). San Diego, CA: Singular.

Romski, M.A., and Sevcik, R.A. (1996). Breaking the speech barrier: Language development through augmented means. Baltimore: Brookes.

Rooney-Moreau, M.R., and Fidrych H. (1998). *ThemeMaker*. Easthampton, MA: Discourse Skills Productions.

Rooney-Moreau, M.R., and Fidrych-Puzzo, H. (1994). *The story grammar marker*. Easthampton, MA: Discourse Skills Productions.

Roseberry-McKibbon, C. (1999). Service delivery to Asian-American families: Principles and practices. *CSHA Magazine, 28*(2), 17–18.

Roseberry-McKibbon, C., and Eicholtz, G.E. (1994). Serving children with limited English proficiency in the schools: A national survey. *Language, Speech, and Hearing Services in Schools, 25,* 156–164.

Rosenbek, J.C. (1984). Treating the dysarthric talker. *Seminars in Speech and Language, 5*(4), 359–384.

Rosetti, L.M. (1993). Enhancing early intervention services to infants and toddlers and their families. *Journal of Childhood Communication Disorders, 15*(2), 1–6.

Sacramento City Unified School District v. Rachel H., 14 F. 3d 1398 (9th Cir. 1994).

Sailor, W. (1991). Special education in the restructured school. *Remedial and Special Education, 12*(6), 8–22.

Sailor, W., and Skrtic, T. (1995). Modern and postmodern agendas in special education: Implications for teacher education, research, and

policy development. In J.L. Paul, H. Rosselli, and D. Evans (Eds.), *Integrating school restructuring and special education reform* (pp. 418–432). Fort Worth, TX: Harcourt Brace.

Sanders, M. (2001). *Understanding dyslexia and the reading process: A guide for educators and parents.* Boston: Allyn and Bacon.

Sanger, D., and Moore-Brown, B. (2000, November). *Advancing the discussion on communication and violence.* Presentation at the annual convention of the American Speech-Language-Hearing Association, Washington, DC.

Sanger, D., Moore-Brown, B., and Alt, E. (2000). Advancing the discussion on communication and violence. *Communication Disorders Quarterly, 22*(1), 43–48.

Schnaiberg, L. (1996, January 17). *Oberti and the law.* Retrieved January 30, 2001, from the World Wide Web: http://www.edweek.org/ew/1996/17law.h15

Schraeder, T., Quinn, M., Stockman, I.J., and Miller, J. (1999). Authentic assessment as an approach to preschool speech language screening. *American Journal of Speech-Language Pathology, 8,* 195–200.

Schreibman, L., Koegel, R.L., Charlop, M.H., and Egel, A.L. (1990). Infantile autism. In A.S. Bellack, M. Hersen, and A.E. Kaxdin (Eds.), *International handbook of behavior modification and therapy* (pp. 763–789). New York: Plenum Press.

Scott, J., Clark, C., and Brady, M. (2000). *Students with autism.* San Diego, CA: Singular.

Seal, B.C. (1997). Educating students who are deaf and hard of hearing. In L.A. Power-deFur and F.P. Orelove (Eds.), *Inclusive Education:*

Practical implementation of the least restrictive environment (pp. 259–271). Gaithersburg, MD: Aspen.

Secord, W.A. (1998, Summer). *Assessment materials.* Presentation at the summer schools conferences on "Achieving Successful Outcomes in Schools" of the American Speech-Language-Hearing Association, Washington, DC.

Secord, W.A. (1999). *School consultation: Concepts, models, and procedures.* Flagstaff, AZ: Northern Arizona University.

Secord, W.A., and Damico, J.S. (1998, Summer). *Let's get practical: 49 ways to work with teachers in the classroom.* Presentation at the summer schools conferences on "Achieving Successful Outcomes in Schools" of the American Speech-Language-Hearing Association, Washington, DC.

Section 504 of the Rehabilitation Act of 1973, 29 U.S.C. § 794. (1973).

Seymour, H.N., Bland-Stewart, L., and Green, L. (1998). Difference versus deficit in child African-American English. *Language, Speech, and Hearing Services in Schools, 29,* 96–108.

Shriner, J.G., Kim, D., Thurlow, M.L., and Ysseldyke, J.E. (1993). *IEPs and standards: What they say for students with disabilities* (Technical Report No. 5). Minneapolis, MN: National Center on Educational Outcomes.

Siegel, L.M. (1999). *The complete IEP guide: How to advocate for your special ed child.* Berkeley, CA: Nolo.com.

Simmons, D.C., and Kame'enui, E.J. (1998). *What reading research tells us about children with diverse learning needs: Bases and basics.* Mahwah, NJ: Lawrence Erlbaum Association.

Singer, B.D., and Bashir, A.S. (1999). What are executive functions and self-regulation and what do they have to do with language learning disorders? *Language, Speech, and Hearing Services in Schools, 30,* 265–273.

Slavin, R.E. (1990). *Cooperative learning: Theory, research, and practice.* Englewood Cliffs, NJ: Prentice Hall.

Smith Lang, J. (2000, May/June). Newborn infant hearing screening: A shift to prevention in dealing with hearing loss in children. *CSHA Magazine, 28*(7), 8–10.

Snow, C.E., Burns, M.S., and Griffin, P. (Eds.). (1998). *Preventing reading difficulties in young children.* Washington, DC: National Academy Press.

Spahr, J.C. (1996, August). Outcome data prove value of SLP services. *ASHA Leader, 1,* 1–2.

Sparks, S.N., Clark, M.J., Erickson, R.L., and Oas, D.B. (1990). *The professional's role in the home or center: Infants at risk for communication disorders.* Tucson, AZ: Communication Skill Builders.

Stainback, W., and Stainback, S. (Eds.). (1996). *Controversial issues confronting special education: Divergent perspectives* (2nd ed.). Boston: Allyn and Bacon.

Stewart, S., Gonzalez, L.S., and Page, J.L. (1997). Incidental learning of sight words during articulation training. *Language, Speech, and Hearing Services in Schools, 28,* 115–126.

Strong, C.J., and Hoggan North, K. (1996). *The magic of stories.* Eau Claire, WI: Thinking Publications.

Technology counts '99: Building the digital curriculum. (1999). *Education Week, XIX,* 19.

Tharpe, A.M. (1999). Auditory integration training: The magical mystery cure. *Language, Speech, and Hearing Services in Schools, 30,* 378–382.

The Association for Severe Handicaps (TASH) (2000, March). *TASH resolution on inclusive education.* Retrieved January 30, 2001, from the World Wide Web: http://www.tash.org/resolutions /R33INCED.html

Threats, T. (2000, September). The World Health Organization's revised classification: What does it mean for speech-language pathology? *Journal of Medical Speech Language Pathology, 8*(3), xiii–xviii.

Throneburg, R.N., Calvert, L.K., Sturm, J.J., Paramboukas, A.A., and Paul, P.J. (2000). A comparison of service delivery models: Effects on curricular vocabulary skills in the school setting. *American Journal of Speech-Language Pathology, 9*(1), 10–20.

Thurlow, M.L., and Thompson, S.J. (1999). District and state standards and assessments: Building an inclusive accountability system. *Journal of Special Education Leadership, 12*(2), 3–10.

Tierney, R.J., Johnston, P., Moore, D.W., and Valencia, S.W. (2000). Snippets: How will literacy be assessed in the next millennium? *Reading Research Quarterly, 35,* 244–250.

Torgeson, J.K. (1998). Catch them before they fall: Identification and assessment to prevent reading failure in young children. *American Educator, 22*(1–2), 32–39.

Turnbull, H.R., III. (1993). *Free appropriate public education: The law and children with disabilities* (4th ed.). Denver, CO: Love.

Ukrainetz, T.A., Harpell, S., Walsh, C., and Coyle, C. (2000). A preliminary investigation of dynamic assessment with Native American kindergartners. *Language, Speech, and Hearing Services in Schools, 31,* 142–154.

Unger, H.G. (1996). Year-round school. In *Encyclopedia of American Education* (Vol. III, p. 1095). New York: Facts on File.

U.S. courts affirm the need for a full continuum of services. (1996). *CEC Today, 3*(1), 4–5.

U.S. Department of Commerce. (1993). *We the American children.* Washington, DC: U.S. Government Printing Office.

U.S. Department of Education. (1998). *Twentieth annual report to Congress on the implementation of the Individuals with Disabilities Education Act.* Washington, DC: Author.

U.S. Department of Education. (1999). *Twenty-first annual report to Congress on the implementation of the Individuals with Disabilities Education Act.* Washington, DC: Author.

U.S. Department of Education (2000a, August). *The challenge of overcrowded schools is here to stay: Growing pains.* Retrieved January 30, 2001, from the World Wide Web: http://www.ed.gov/pubs/bbecho00/part2.html

U.S. Department of Education. (2000b). *Twenty-second annual report to Congress on the implementation of the Individuals with Disabilities Education Act.* Washington D.C.: Author.

U.S. Department of Justice. (1999). *Americans with Disabilities Act home page.* Retrieved November 26, 1999, from the World Wide Web: http://www.usdoj.gov/crt/ada/adahom1.htm

Valdez, F.M., and Montgomery, J.K. (1997). Outcomes from two treatment approaches for children with communication disorders in Head Start. *Journal of Children's Communication Development, 18*(2), 65–71.

van Kleeck, A. (1998). Preliteracy domains and stages: Laying the foundations for beginning reading. *Journal of Children's Communication Development, 20*(1), 33–51.

Veale, T.K. (1999). Targeting temporal processing deficits through Fast ForWord: Language therapy with a new twist. *Language, Speech, and Hearing Services in Schools, 30,* 353–363.

Vygotsky, L.S. (1978). *Mind in society: The development of higher mental processes.* Cambridge, MA: Harvard University Press.

Wallach, G.P., and Butler, K.G. (Eds.). (1994). *Language-learning disabilities in school age children and adolescents.* New York: Merrill.

Webb, D.L., Greer, J.T., Montello, P.A., and Norton, S.M. (1987). *Personnel administration in education: New issues and new needs in human resource management.* Columbus, OH: Merrill.

Wetherby, A. (1998, July). *Improving early identification of communication disorders: Engaging parents in the process.* Presentation at the Fourth Biannual Head Start Research Conference, Washington, DC.

Wetherby, A. (2000, July). Understanding and enhancing communication and language. Two Day Institute at Northern Arizona University, Flagstaff, AZ.

Wetherby, A., and Prizant, B. (1992). Profiling young children's communicative competence. In S. Warren and J. Reichle (Eds.), *Causes and effects in communication and language intervention* (pp. 217–253). Baltimore: Brookes.

Wetherby, A., and Prizant, B. (1998). *Communication and symbolic behavior scales development profile* [Research edition]. Chicago: Applied Symbolix.

Whaley, C.E., and Whaley, H.F. (1986). *Future images: Future studies for grades 4 to 12.* New York: Trillian Press.

The White House. (2000). *The Clinton-Gore administration: From digital divide to digital opportunity* [Online]. Available: http://www.whitehouse.gov /WH/New/digitaldivide

Whitmire, K. (1999). Action: School services. *Language, Speech, and Hearing Services in Schools, 30,* 427–434.

Whitmire, K. (2000a). Action: School services: ASHA's 1999 priority issue I: Resources for school-based members. *Language, Speech, and Hearing Services in Schools, 31,* 194–199.

Whitmire, K. (2000b). Action: School services: Dysphagia services in schools. *Language, Speech, and Hearing Services in Schools, 31,* 99–103.

Whitmire, K., Karr, S., and Mullen, R. (2000). Action: School services. *Language, Speech, and Hearing Services in Schools, 31,* 402–406.

Wilcox, M.J. (1997). Considerations in promoting language-based learning readiness for children in Head Start. In J. Heller (Ed.), *Head Start university partnerships: Issues in child development research and practice* (pp. 61–79). Washington, DC: Administration for Children and Families.

Will, M. (1986). *Educating students with learning problems: A shared responsibility.* Washington, DC: U.S. Department of Education.

Williams, D. (2000). AAC interventions for children with autism. In J. Scott, C. Clark, and M. Brady (Eds.), *Students with autism* (pp. 214–215). San Diego, CA: Singular.

Williams, J.M. (2000, June 21). Bush: "The ADA is a good law." *Business Week Online.* Retrieved January 25, 2001, from the World Wide Web: http://www.businessweek.com/bwdaily/dnflash/june/2000/nf00621d.htm

Winget, P., Boyle, S., and Reynolds, V. (1994, September/October). Courts, congress, associations debate LRE. *The Special Edge, 7,* 1:14.

Wisconsin Administrative Code. (2000). Chapter PI 11.36 (5).

Wisconsin Department of Public Instruction. (June, 2000). *Revised sample special education forms* [Microsoft Word format]. Retrieved January 30, 2001, from the World Wide Web: http://www.dpi.state.wi.us/dpi/dlsea/een/form_int.html

Wisconsin Special Education Mediation System. (2001). Retrieved February 3, 2001, from the World Wide Web: http://www.cesa7.k12.wi.us/sped/wsems/index.htm

Wolf, K.E. (1997). Outcomes data: Quantifying accountability for the professions. *CSHA Magazine, 26*(2), 4–5.

Wolf, K.E., and Calderon, J.L. (1999). Cultural competence: The underpinning of quality health care and education services. *CSHA Magazine, 28*(2), 4–6.

Wolfberg, P.J., and Schuler, A.L. (1993). Integrated play groups: A model for promoting the social and cognitive dimensions of play in children with autism. *Journal of Autism and Developmental Disorders, 23,* 467–489.

Wolfram, W. (1991). *Dialects and American English.* Englewood Cliffs, NJ: Prentice Hall.

Wolfram, W., and Fasold, R.W. (1974). *Study of social dialects in American English.* Englewood Cliffs, NJ: Prentice Hall.

World Health Organization (WHO). (1980). *WHO: International classification of impairments, disabilities and handicaps.* Geneva, Switzerland: Author.

Wyatt, T. (1999). Current clinical perspectives in the delivery of speech and language services to African-American children. *CSHA Magazine, 28*(2), 14–16.

Yell, M.L., Katsiyannis, A., Bradley, R., and Rozalski, M.E. (2000). Ensuring compliance with the discipline provisions of IDEA '97: Challenges and opportunities. *Journal of Special Education Leadership, 13,* 3–18.

Yoder, D.E., and Koppenhaver, D.A. (1993). In D.E. Yoder and D.A. Koppenhaver (Eds.), Literacy Learning and Persons with Severe Speech Impairments [Foreword]. *Topics in Language Disorders, 13*(2), vi–vii.

Yopp, H.K. (1995). A test for assessing phonemic awareness in young children. *Reading Teacher, 49*(1), 20–29.

Ysseldyke, J.E., Thurlow, M.L., McGrew, K.S., and Shriner, J.G. (1994). *Recommendations for making decisions about the participation of students with disabilities in statewide assessment programs* (Synthesis Report 15). Minneapolis, MN: National Center on Educational Outcomes.

Zirkel, P. (2000, May). *Section 504 and ADA.* Presentation of LRP Publications, Irvine, CA.

Indexes

Author Index

Subject Index

Page references in *italics* refer to information contained in illustrations or charts.

accents, 210–11

access issues, 264–65

accountability, in special education, 41, 142–43, 335

activities

    children and, 15

adolescents

    characteristics, 198, *199–200*

    goals, 198–201

    strategies for, 202, *203,* 204

    transition process, 198, 201

African American families, 13, 211

aides, 166–67, 290–91

alternative dispute resolution (ADR), 247

American Federation of Teachers (AFT), 129, 130

American Psychological Association (APA)

    People First language guidelines, 29

American Speech-Language-Hearing Association (ASHA), 4

    activities of, 299–300

    Certificate of Clinical Competence (CCC), 271, 272, *273,* 315, 316

    Code of Ethics, 296, 395–97

    continuing education, 315–16

    functional status measures, *145–46*

    inclusion position statement, 130, 131

    Legislative Council issues, 159

    literacy position statements, 181, 330–31

    Multi-Cultural Affairs Division, 85

    preferred practice patterns in assessment, 341–65

    preferred practice patterns in intervention, 366–82

    reading/literacy guidelines, 184–86

    scope of practice statements, 312, 336

    service delivery options guidelines, 157

    special interest divisions, 300

    speech-language pathology assistants (SLPAs), 290–92

    students in, 300, 312

    web site contents, 312

Americans with Disabilities Act (ADA) (P.L. 101-336), 27, 264–65

annual review, of IEP, 113–14

applications, job, 274–75

applied behavior analysis, 220

articulation therapy

    assessment, 358–59

    exit criteria, 116–17

ASHA. *See* American Speech-Language-Hearing Association (ASHA)

assessment

    articulation, 358–59

    ASHA preferred practice patterns, 341–65

    assessment plan, 245

    assessment report, 76–77

    for assistive technology, 229–30

    augmentative and alternative communication (AAC), 71

    common elements of, *75*

    consent, 245

    dynamic testing, 73–74

    fluency, 360–62

    functional communication measures (FCMs), 152–54, *153*

    independent educational evaluations, 77–78, 243